# Chinese Medicine in East Africa

**Series:** Epistemologies of Healing
**General Editors:** David Parkin and Elisabeth Hsu, University of Oxford

This series publishes monographs and edited volumes on so-called traditional medical treatment, alternative and complementary medicine, and ethnobiological studies that relate to health and illness. The emphasis of the series is on different forms of healing, knowing and doing, in comparison with other practices, and in recognition of the fluidity between them.

*Recent volumes:*

**Volume 20**
*Chinese Medicine in East Africa: An Intimacy with Strangers*
Elisabeth Hsu

**Volume 19**
*Configuring Contagion: Ethnographies of Biosocial Epidemics*
Edited by Lotte Meinert and Jens Seeberg

**Volume 18**
*Fierce Medicines, Fragile Socialities: Grounding Global HIV Treatment in Tanzania*
Dominik Mattes

**Volume 17**
*Capturing Quicksilver: The Position, Power, and Plasticity of Chinese Medicine in Singapore*
Arielle A. Smith

**Volume 16**
*Ritual Retellings: Luangan Healing Performances through Practice*
Isabell Herrmans

**Volume 15**
*Healing Roots: Anthropology in Life and Medicine*
Julie Laplante

**Volume 14**
*Asymmetrical Conversations: Contestations, Circumventions, and the Blurring of Therapeutic Boundaries*
Edited by Harish Naraindas, Johannes Quack and William S. Sax

**Volume 13**
*The Body in Balance: Humoral Medicines in Practice*
Edited by Peregrine Horden and Elisabeth Hsu

**Volume 12**
*Manufacturing Tibetan Medicine: The Creation of an Industry and the Moral Economy of Tibetanness*
Martin Saxer

**Volume 11**
*Fortune and the Cursed: The Sliding Scale of Time in Mongolian Divination*
Katherine Swancutt

*For a full volume listing, please see the series page on our website:*
*https://www.berghahnbooks.com/series/epistemologies-of-healing*

# Chinese Medicine in East Africa
## An Intimacy with Strangers

Elisabeth Hsu

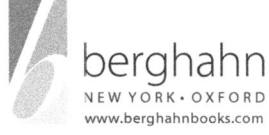

berghahn
NEW YORK · OXFORD
www.berghahnbooks.com

First published in 2022 by
Berghahn Books
www.berghahnbooks.com

© 2022, 2025 Elisabeth Hsu
First paperback edition published in 2025

All rights reserved. Except for the quotation of short passages
for the purposes of criticism and review, no part of this book
may be reproduced in any form or by any means, electronic or
mechanical, including photocopying, recording, or any information
storage and retrieval system now known or to be invented,
without written permission of the publisher.

Library of Congress Cataloging-in-Publication Data
Names: Hsu, Elisabeth, author.
Title: Chinese medicine in East Africa : an intimacy with strangers / Elisabeth Hsu.
Other titles: Epistemologies of healing ; v. 20.
Description: New York : Berghahn Books, 2022. | Series: Epistemologies of healing; volume 20 | Includes bibliographical references and index.
Identifiers: LCCN 2022004880 (print) | LCCN 2022004881 (ebook) | ISBN 9781800735569 (hardback) | ISBN 9781800735576 (ebook)
Subjects: LCSH: Medicine, Chinese—Africa, East—History—21st century. | Medicine, Chinese—Practice—Africa, East—History—21st century. | Traditional medicine—Africa, East—History—21st century.
Classification: LCC R651.A353 H78 2022 (print) | LCC R651.A353 (ebook) | DDC 610.96—dc23/eng/20220201
LC record available at https://lccn.loc.gov/2022004880
LC ebook record available at https://lccn.loc.gov/2022004881

British Library Cataloguing in Publication Data
A catalogue record for this book is available from the British Library

EU GPSR Authorized Representative
LOGOS EUROPE, 9 rue Nicolas Poussin, 17000, LA ROCHELLE, France
Email: Contact@logoseurope.eu

ISBN 978-1-80073-556-9 hardback
ISBN 978-1-83695-084-4 paperback
ISBN 978-1-83695-219-0 epub
ISBN 978-1-80073-557-6 web pdf

https://doi.org/10.3167/9781800735569

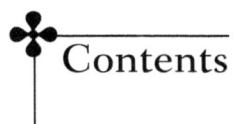
# Contents

| | |
|---|---|
| List of Illustrations | vii |
| Acknowledgements | viii |
| A Note on Transcription | ix |
| Introduction | 1 |

### Part I. Moving through the Practico-Sensory Realm of Space

| | | |
|---|---|---|
| 1. | Spatial Textures of the Clinical Encounter | 45 |
| 2. | Misunderstandings, and the Spaces They Create | 82 |

### Part II. Emplacement, Emplotment, 'Empotment'

| | | |
|---|---|---|
| 3. | Patients, Practitioners and Their *Pots* | 119 |
| 4. | The Patients | 145 |
| 5. | The Practitioners | 190 |
| 6. | The *Pots*: Orientations | 238 |

### Part III. Pots, 'Pots' and *Pots*

| | | |
|---|---|---|
| 7. | What Is in a 'Pot'? Industrially Produced Chinese Formula Medicines | 263 |

## Contents

8. What Makes a *Pot* Efficacious? Social Distance, and the Potencies of *Pots* — 303
9. 'The Chinese Antimalarial' as 'Pot' and *Pot* — 343

**Conclusion.** Kaleidoscopic Refractions — 367

**References** — 374

**Index** — 413

# Illustrations

**Figures**

**1.1.** A figure–ground image.     47

**1.2 a–b.** A figure–ground image affected by and affecting different textures.     48

**1.3 a–b.** The in-between space as pot in a medical encounter.     49

**1.4.** Chinese medical practice in Kariakoo, Dar es Salaam, 2002.     62

**1.5.** Spatial textures of a traditional African healer's practice in Bagamoyo, 2002.     66

**Maps**

**0.1.** East Africa and its Chinese medical teams.     21

**0.2.** The People's Republic of China and the Chinese practitioners' provenance.     23

**Tables**

**1.1.** Co-opting local expertise: laboratory technicians and their services.     63

**2.1.** Grice's four maxims for the principle of cooperation (*and their flouting*).     106

# Acknowledgements

## Funding

This research was funded by the Swiss National Foundation, stipend no.1115-05574, in 2001; the British Academy, small grant, SG-33849 and a Wellcome travel award, in 2002; the British Institute of Eastern Africa (BIEA), large grant, in 2003; the Chiang Ching-kuo Foundation for International Scholarly Research, personal allowance for international expert on the project *shentigan*/bodily-felt sensory attentiveness, in 2004–5; the British Academy Commonwealth conference grant in 2007/08, apart from yearly research allowances of the Institute of Social and Cultural Anthropology and Queen Elizabeth House, both at the University of Oxford.

## Research and Ethics Approval

The research was approved by COSTECH (Commission for Science and Technology), no. 2001-349-NA-2001-122 'Patients' perceptions of Chinese and Tanzanian traditional medicines'. Research was carried out following the ethical guidelines of the ASA (Association of Social Anthropologists). I was assigned as host and mentor the medical anthropologist Dr Edmund Kayombo at the Traditional Medicine Unit, Muhimbili hospital, Dar es Salaam, whom I thank warmly for his continued support.

Overall, the author wishes to express her indebtedness to the research participants in the field, to her colleagues, friends and family in Africa, China and Europe, as well as to the publisher and their most supportive staff. The research, its writing up and its publication benefitted from the unfailing encouragement by David Parkin.

# A Note on Transcription

Chinese words in *putonghua* 普通话 are transcribed into *pinyin* 拼音. Chinese characters are given in simplified script, unless pre-1900 texts are quoted. Swahili and other non-English words are given in italics. In modern standard Chinese phrases and sentences are made up of polysyllabic words, while in classical Chinese each character is transcribed as a separate syllable.

# Introduction

Do you enjoy your time here?
*It's all the same.*
So, why did you come here?
*To do business.*
Medicine as business?
*I first tried growing vegetables . . .*
Growing vegetables as business?
*All you need is a garage, plastic tubs, water, beans and lots of working hands [to grow bean sprouts or make tofu] . . .*
. . . And, I guess, a taste for your produce to have a clientele?
*There are too few Chinese restaurants here, that's why I changed to doing medicine . . .*

—Excerpt of a conversation with a
Chinese medicine practitioner, 2001

The early twenty-first century has seen an acceleration of movement across national and transnational landscapes. Social scientists speak of hubs and whirls, diversity, superdiversity, mobility, hybridity and assemblages. These 'theoretical minima' refer to the processes of globalisation, glocalisation, creolisation, worlding and entangled histories, which in anthropology and the history of science, technology and medicine used to be discussed in terms of 'cultural exchange' or 'technology transfer' less than half a century ago. Textures of transformation and the social relatedness relevant to the study of medicoscapes, medical diversity, medicine and mobility, alongside the multiple dynamics instigated by body techniques, sensory and other articulations, everyday tactics, and sexual and life history transitions are the focus of this book.

When, between 2001 and 2008, I conducted ethnographic fieldwork on the introduction of 'Chinese medicine' (defined in more detail below) into East Africa, that is, Tanzania, Kenya and Uganda, I soon realised that this research was not addressing a pressing problem for public health.[1] This was primarily for reasons of quantity. There were too few private Chinese medical practitioners, numbering only about twenty per country, in countries with about 35–42 million people (in Tanzania), 31–37 million (in Kenya) and 25–32 million (in Uganda) at the time. Yet however insignificant they were in number, these private practitioners who styled themselves 'Traditional Chinese Medicine' doctors were culturally visible. The first Chinese medical practices opened as private enterprises in Kenya in the late 1980s, in Uganda in 1995 and in Tanzania in 1996.[2] They catered to a primarily regional, local and transnational East African clientele, men, women, infants and children, and, as this research will show, benefitted from the sterling work of the earlier socialist Chinese medical delegations (for the latter, see e.g. Li 2011, Langwick 2011).

It soon became clear that the phenomenon I focused on was part of a larger social landscape that was not left unaffected by the diplomatic and other relations between China and Africa (e.g. Alden et al. 2008, Bräutigam 2009). As specialised as the topic of 'Chinese medicine in East Africa' would appear, it evidently confronted me with questions fundamental to living beings' entanglement and basic to anthropology as a discipline. Where the media reinforced the view of an unsurmountable 'culture clash' between 'The Africans' and 'The Chinese',[3] this ethnography – with its focus on healing – has drawn inspiration from a principle of intimate co-existence that the evolutionary theoretician and microbiologist Lynn Margulis (1991) emphasised, also known as 'the intimacy of strangers'. The great achievements in evolution, Margulis argued, arose from cooperation and collaboration (further explained in Chapter 6).

Committed to 'slow research' (Adams et al. 2014),[4] I continued post-fieldwork research, not least through e-communication, conference participation, letters of correspondence, brief in-person visits, and exchanges of goods and ideas with African and Africanist anthropologists over more than a decade,[5] such that I felt compelled – as a medical anthropologist – to think about concepts as fundamental to anthropology as that of 'culture'. Specifically, I started to ask: in cases where treatment was successful and led to a recovery of the patient, what instigated this process of healing between mostly

Introduction

African patients and Chinese practitioners? Is there another way of thinking about these encounters than in terms of a 'culture clash'?

## The Core Concern: *Uzima*, Wholeness and Health

'Healing' is linguistically cognate with 'wholeness'. In Swahili, *uzima*, which means wholeness, is the word for health (Iliffe 1998: 11), and for well-being in a broad sense (Obrist 2003: 281).[6] Yet Chinese medicine patients rarely spoke of 'holism'. Meanwhile, their doings were suggestive of a sense of 'incompleteness' (Nyamnjoh 2021).[7] Very evidently, they were searching, open to 'trying out' opportunities on offer.[8] Some were in search of '*words* of wholeness and well-being', what Dilger (2007: 65) calls the neo-Pentecostal 'Gospel of Prosperity (*neno la uzima*) and, intricately related to it, the concepts of "awakening" (*uamsho*) and "salvation" (*uokovu*)'. Others were seeking *dawa*, medicines: 'natural', 'herbal' or 'natural herbal' treatment, paradoxically in modern and 'advanced' Chinese medical clinics in urban East Africa. As we will see later, when they spoke of 'natural herbs', they alluded to a configuration – or according to Norbert Elias (1978) a 'figuration' – of a wholeness that connected the patient to the plant and the plant to the place of their ancestors (Chapters 3 and 8). In a similar vein, 'good health' (*afya mzuri*) was related to place, such as the 'conditions of living' (*hali ya maisha*, cf. Obrist 2003). *Uzima* was also linked to the political anthropologically identified concern with autochthony (Fayers-Kerr 2018),[9] which extended much beyond the idea of a healthy body-enveloped-by-skin, even if it involved becoming entangled with strangers, momentarily, in commercialised and commodified transactions.

The English word *whole* has been etymologically traced to the Middle English *hool*, 'healthy', 'unhurt', 'entire', and mentioned alongside *hale*, 'fresh' and *holy*, 'sacred', 'consecrated'; it comes from Old English *hal*, akin to Old High German *heil*, 'healthy', 'unhurt', and Old Norse *heill* (Oxford English Dictionary, 2nd Edition, 1989). However, neither religious piety, as implied by *Heilung*, *Heiland* and *Heil*, nor a New Age appropriation of this etymology in terms of 'holism' shall provide the framing of this book.

Keeping *the body in balance* (Horden and Hsu 2013) is central not only to European but also to Islamic and South and East Asian medicines,[10] and has been identified as a concern throughout the vast expanses of Bantu-speaking Africa as well (Parkin 2013; see also Janzen 1992). Although people did not speak much about it, in daily life they did show concern with the regulation of the flow of bodily fluids and other nourishing things. Conversations on the Swahili-speaking East African coastline with the respective medical experts (during fieldwork 2001–5) furthermore brought to the fore Ayurvedic and Arabic medical manuscripts or printed texts, featuring notions of balancing and bolstering, countering and countervailing, and the openings and closings that regulate the flows within the body, as well as into and out of it.

## Openings and Closings, Flows and Blockages

Anthropologists of Africa have long noted that 'openings' and 'closings' are a matter of concern, not only for the individual body, but also for the social body and the body politic. This seems to be so particularly in times of rapid changes and exchanges, and also when it comes to questions of fecundity and fertility (which involve an exchange of fluids). Devisch (1993) has vividly demonstrated this in regard to fertility rites among the Yaka of Central Africa, and likewise Boddy (1989) in regard to genital cutting and stitching in Hofriyat in northern Sudan. The closure that keeps the waters in the womb, like in a watermelon, ensures fecund moisture. Bodily regulated openness and closure has been shown to be directly related to enhancing flows of life.

Taylor (1988, 1992) took this preoccupation with openings and closings a step further, and highlighted that body-technological efforts of dancing and cutting would affect the flow of fluids: the flow of water, milk, blood, saliva, urine and sexual fluids. His ethnography went beyond a focus on the body-enveloped-by-skin and highlighted that the transaction of cattle for marriage or the mixing of fluids in sexual intercourse were motivated by a concern with ensuring and instigating flows, as those were considered generative of the matter that perpetuates life. Taylor's fieldwork was in Rwanda, and his concern was not to argue that the healers he worked with were just as concerned with balance and regulation, as Asian medical practitioners are. Rather, he emphasised that the treatment rationale concerned with regulatory efforts towards a harmonious balancing of different components competed with several others.

*Introduction*

In a similar vein, Parkin has long lamented the fact that African thought tends to be excluded from the discussion of scholarly medical learning preoccupied with regulatory balancing, when in fact it is also much preoccupied with it. In a paper with subtitle 'The View from the Office, and the Voice from the Field', Parkin (1990) argues that sensory aspects of evidentiality may have caused this bias in anthropological theory, with visually perceived written information being privileged over orally – and aurally – transmitted knowledge. Arguing against taking the 'lack' of a literate tradition as evidence for a 'lack' of complex social stratification and scholarly medico-moral systems that value balance, Parkin (2013) made a case for a 'relational balance' in the cosmologies of Bantu-speaking Africans. His argument presents convincing linguistic evidence for postulating overlapping orally transmitted transregional semantic fields. Yet his focus is on only one sort of social and sexual transgression, called *chira*, and its bodily retribution through wasting; hence considered a case of keeping the body in balance.[11] Indeed, the medico-moral nexus of Asian medical learning advocates avoidance of excessive consumption and immoral conduct too, but mostly through a 'regulatory balancing' of ethnophysiological flows of blood or *qi* (breath, wind or air).

Notwithstanding, the 'difference' between African and Chinese medical cultures has tended to loom large in peoples' perceptions, as well as in the imagination of social and bioscientific researchers, whether 'African', 'Chinese' or 'Other'. Political and economic asymmetries have heightened this difference. However, the difference may not be as pronounced as generally assumed, as hinted at with the above discussion pertaining to openings and closings, flows and blockages, and relational as well as regulatory balancing.

## *The Spatial Production of Wholeness*

This book starts with the usual questions regarding multiple efficacies in general, and in Chinese medical treatment in particular, by asking what sorts of wholeness medical treatment supposedly effects. If an individual in crisis affects and is affected by the surrounding social spaces, is the healing of individual bodies in any discernible way linked to the production of wholeness in social space? And how might a medical encounter's making of wholeness become reflected in a visible and tangible 'production of space' (Lefebvre

1974, [1974] 1991)? Is it possible, by attending to a concerted healing effort to which people from different provenances contribute, that we can start thinking about 'culture' differently? Rather than identifying traits of sameness in provenance to define culture,[12] might such a joint effort towards 'making whole', as represented by healing efforts, be regarded as an intrinsically culture-making process?

Even though 'culture' has become a 'do-not-use-it' taboo word in anthropology, it is in constant use in public life – on the radio, in the newspaper and on TV. Sometimes, it is referred to in ways that cry out for its reappropriation by anthropology, and social anthropology in particular. Here our discipline has created a term central to both its theorising and its method of generating evidence through fieldwork, but we have disengaged ourselves from the term without being able to distance ourselves entirely from the implications for anthropological theory that this entails. As a result, anthropologists today find themselves in the passive position of seeing the concept of 'culture' put centre stage in the public arena but imbued with essentialising meanings that even the inventors of the term had meant to overcome (e.g. Boas 1911: 14). This essentialising tendency comes to the fore particularly when commentators speak of cultural 'difference' and 'other' cultures.[13]

By contrast, already Marcel Mauss suggested that a research focus on technique and technology ([1906] 1979a, [1935] 1979b, [1913–1953] 2006b, [1967] 2007) had the potential to do away with 'sameness' as the defining feature of culture.[14] Admittedly, the remarkable twelve texts, chronologically assembled and thoughtfully edited by Nathan Schlanger (Mauss 2006b), do not form a highly structured argumentative piece. Nevertheless, the messages they contain, alongside insights gleaned from his *Manual of Ethnography* (2007) and a careful reading of his *Seasonal Variations* (1979a) combined with his famous essay on 'Les techniques du corps' ([1936], 1950, [1935] 1973, [1935] 1979b, [1935] 2006a), open up to-date insufficiently explored ways of approaching 'skilled activity' – an apt category for thinking through any medical intervention.[15]

Mauss argued that techniques and skills are partially learned and transferred, adopted piecemeal and transformed. Some can easily be imitated, while others are used in ways that involve skilful finetuning. Importantly, such kaleidoscopically assembled techniques, rearranged in consideration of possible complementarity to each other, can lead to an emerging and mutually negotiated sort of 'wholeness', fundamentally different from the 'wholeness through sameness' that the term 'culture' usually invokes.

This shifting of focus towards an ethnography of hands-on techniques and bodily skills that are always oriented towards being situation-specifically effective takes us away from abstractions like language and religion. Mauss insisted on studying 'social morphology' and material 'objects' in their relation to each other, and rejected the idea that a cartography of the distribution of objects would lead to an identification of 'culture', as any such undertaking was grounded in circular reasoning.[16] The distribution of 'cultural' objects on their own provided no evidence for the expanse of a 'culture'. Rather, it was the responsive interdependency between humans and the materials they engaged with that, as Mauss argued, make culture (inclusive of what some call 'more-than-humans', or what we will refer to below as living *pots*).

Mauss thereby critiqued the homogenising concept of culture that his uncle had formulated. Mauss's focus on technique allowed for a concept of society and culture that was less interested in boundaries and boundary reinforcement, separation and the exclusion of non-members on the grounds of abstract ideas – the well-known 'collective representations', which, thanks to the 'science' of anthropology, would become a scientifically described and lived reality. Rather than studying 'culture', Mauss's attention was on studying specific 'cultural efforts', say, the cultivation and perfection of the craftsman's skills and technologies. This process, he emphasised, involved the 'borrowing' of whatever from whoever. Cultural effort was thus likened to craftsmanship intent on advancing itself, through the making of crafts. It required an attitude of curiosity and openness towards the other and the unknown, we might say, motivated by a sense of what Nyamnjoh (2021) calls 'incompleteness', which in the context of craftsmanship makes probing and 'trying out' into a virtue.

Today we can take the discussion a step further. The Maussian study of concrete 'joint efforts', which involves a focus on both an individual's skills and the material object simultaneously, diverts the researcher's gaze away from the individual. Rather than focusing on the individual body, their gaze actively explores the textures of the spaces that the individual creates and partakes in (Lefebvre 1991), and these bodily skills and techniques, in turn, can be interpreted as working towards an individual's place-making, emplacement and 'empotment', a process that involves the negotiation of materialities.

## *China in Africa, Africa in China (CA/AC)*

The Chinese government's current 'One Belt – One Road' (Belt and Road Initiative, BRI) project has tended to style the distance between China and Africa as merely geographic, and twenty-first-century Chinese socialism-cum-capitalism was to shrink this geographical distance.[17] Although the rhetoric of South–South win-win commerce committed to technology and engineering that was strangely reminiscent of the nineteenth and twentieth centuries' projects of capitalism and of the North–South colonialism that it claimed to overcome, I saw it proliferate throughout East Africa in the early twenty-first century. The promise of Deng Xiaoping (1904–97) accompanying the endorsement from 1978 onwards of his vision of economic reforms in the People's Republic of China (PRC), which was that they would bring economic prosperity to everyone, and wealth would eventually percolate down from the super-rich, seemed to be embraced by promoters of late liberalism as well. Admittedly, in the early 2000s, the idea of 'development' no longer had the same traction that it had shortly after independence in many African states in the 1950s and 1960s. Nevertheless, the hubs and whirls in the cityscape were able to spur a belief in a better future.

Shortly after I returned from this project's final field trip to East Africa, one of the first edited volumes on China in Africa and Africa in China (CA/AC) relations was to be published (Alden et al. 2008), and would be foundational to a field in area studies that had grown rapidly.[18] Research on CA/AC relations does not generally foreground cultural issues. Rather, education (e.g. student grants for Africans to study in China), finance, health care, technical assistance (e.g. agriculture; see 'growing vegetables' above), material aid and infrastructure figure prominently.[19] Bräutigam (2011: 19) addresses the big questions that loom in everyone's mind: 'Does China's non-interference policy provide cover for pariah regimes in Sudan and Zimbabwe? Has China's growing presence in Africa worsened efforts to build good governance, improve human rights and reduce corruption? Are the Chinese leading a 'race to the bottom' in social and environmental issues? Does their active support for Chinese business present unfair competition?'

Analysts have differentiated between private and official finance, where the latter comprises two parts: (a) the equivalent to 'official development assistance' (ODA) that China has offered Africa, which consists of grants, zero-interest loans, debt relief and concessional loans; and (b) 'other official flows' (OOF) of specified credits and loans. In contrast to OECD countries, China's OOF finances have generally been larger than the official development assistance (Bräutigam 2011). 'In 2008, China probably disbursed about US$1.2 billion in ODA in Africa, compared with the World Bank (US$4.1 billion), the United States (US$7.2 billion) and France (US$3.4 billion)' (ibid.: 211). These figures referred, however, only to official development assistance spending in that year. Meanwhile, as case studies of large infrastructure projects (dams, railways) have demonstrated, the Chinese investment projects could be financed through different channels. This made it possible to provide ethically questionable levels of debt finance (ibid.). Evidently, China's financial involvement in African nation states was and is complex.

So, how was China's current wave of aid and other economic collaborations to affect African 'development', and how would it affect the 'industrialization challenge'? 'Will China catalyze or crush African manufacturing?' (Bräutigam 2011: 211). Political scientists were and are interested in large-scale aid programmes, public and private, and in public-private investments that overlap in multiple ways. Bräutigam called for a balanced view: 'Why does China give aid?' she asked. 'The conventional answer is: to get access at resources. Yet . . . this is *at best* a partial and misleading answer. Fundamentally, foreign aid is a tool of foreign policy' (Bräutigam 2009: 17). No doubt, China's foreign aid would affect China's health care diplomacy.

The expert on health care diplomacy and Chinese medicine provision in Africa is Li Anshan whose studies on the topic are foundational for anyone entering the field (Li 2006, 2009, 2011, 2021). However, these publications unfortunately did not yet exist at the time of my fieldwork. Studies from the 1970s by Bruce Larkin (1971), Alan Hutchison (1975), Philip Snow (1988) and many others prepared me for the field.

## Review of Some Key Texts: From 'Asian Medical Systems' to Their Globalisation

This book traces its genealogy to work that was foundational to medical anthropology as a subdiscipline of social anthropology. Charles Leslie's *Asian Medical Systems* (1976) combined ethnographic and historical research on the 'great traditions', emphasising 'culture' for understanding 'medicine'. It discussed the history, politics and social movements that led to the institutionalisation in modern health care of learned medicine in the Middle East and South and East Asia. These modernist movements reflected an era, after independence, when growing economies inspired confidence.

A second volume, *Paths to Asian Medical Knowledge* (Leslie and Young 1992), on these literate traditions that had been rendered up-to-date and legitimised by scholar-physicians through interpretive and exegetical work, also focused on epistemological questions. Published fifteen years later, this volume contained vintage pieces by the first generation of medical anthropologists who had done long-term fieldwork on the practices of Asian medical 'traditions', spoke the language and had the reading skills to engage with the technical aspects of these traditions' texts.

Another decade later, two further edited volumes on Asian medicines and their globalisation were published: *Countervailing Creativity: Patient Agency in the Globalisation of Asian Medicines* by Elisabeth Hsu and Erling Høg (2002) and *Asian Medicine and Globalisation* by Joseph S. Alter (2005a). Neither volume became as well known as the previous two, but both are relevant for this monograph, as they both engaged with the social dynamics of globalisation. This was when so-called 'international health' care, as moderated by the WHO, had started to be superseded by so-called 'global health' (Brown et al. 2006; Cueto et al. 2019), and when the World Bank was taking increasingly important financial-cum-medical decisions in increasingly commercialised and commodified health markets. The 2002 volume *Countervailing Creativity* discussed countervailing currents to those of the 'Coca-Cola and blue jeans' globalisation that went 'from the West to the rest' of the world, in that these currents – in the editors' framing – consisted of an East-to-South flow (rather than being subsumed into the South–South relations currently discussed in CA/AC circles). *Countervailing Creativity* comprised six

*Introduction*

original articles on: Ayurveda in Germany, Tibetan medicine in the USA, Shiatsu practices in the UK and Japan, Korean medicine in Kazakhstan, Chinese medicine in Tanzania and acupuncture in post-socialist Russia, all of which provided ethnographies of 'patient agency'. With its focus on globalisation and patients as actively involved in the shaping of Asian medical practice, *Countervailing Creativity* aimed to complement the earlier two volumes' focus on Asian medical knowledge and doctors in Asia.

The other edited volume, *Asian Medicine and Globalisation*, published a couple of years later, has an introduction by Joseph S. Alter (2005b) that is relevant for us here, as he, like us, was apprehensive of globalised forms of 'Asian medicine' being reduced to TM/CAM.[20] For one thing, as declared in his introduction's first sentence, Alter was interested in how 'coherence' is produced, and how it related to 'health, broadly defined'. Incidentally, Alter's questions resonate directly with our own observations regarding the Swahili word for health and wholeness, *uzima*, which opened this book. Alter's writing must have affected my gaze, as I read it long ago in the field. As stated on the first page, Alter's ultimate concern was with 'culture'. However, although Alter problematised the two themes of 'health and wholeness' and 'medicine and culture' very succinctly in his introductory chapter, these important questions were barely addressed in the book's later chapters.

Alter suggested not to think of 'Asian medicine' as an 'Asian form of medicine' but 'as being various experimental techniques, concerned with embodied life and longevity' (Alter 2005b: 18). As Alter had it, these 'experimental techniques' cannot be studied on their own in a decontextualised way. Rather, they are enacted in fields where they must be legitimised as a 'form of an "Asian medicine"'. The medical fields, as defined by East Africa's governments, insisted on Chinese practitioners being categorised as 'traditional medicine' practitioners selling 'natural herbs'. Meanwhile, the 'worlding' of Chinese medicine through transnational frames (Zhan 2009), regardless of whether it is in Dar es Salaam, Singapore or San Francisco, has meant that the emerging styles of medical practice have transmuted from one into another. They were ever elusive, like quicksilver (Smith 2018). Zhan's and Smith's ethnographies endorse Alter's understanding of Asian medical cultures, beyond the clearly bounded medicalised forms of Asian medical TM/CAM.

These volumes of 1976, 1992 and 2002/2005 form a set because their authors are medical anthropologists and historians, and they reference each other. The first volume focused on social aspects of reformist movements, the second on medical knowledge and epistemologies and the third two volumes on their globalisation. All authors were, broadly speaking, concerned with what Alter called the 'nationalistic politics of culture', the 'when, why and how' of their extension beyond 'bounded frameworks of legitimation' and the 'modernisation' of 'traditional' medical knowledge. This was the state of the art in the medical anthropology of Asian medicines over twenty years ago, when I embarked on my first field trip for this project.

## Asian Pharmaceuticals, Acupuncture and the RCT (Randomised Controlled Trial)

Meanwhile, another cluster of medical anthropological literatures would emerge on Asian medical pharmaceuticals with more health-scientific or science studies orientations (or both), starting with Adams (2002), who took issue with the double-blind randomised controlled trials (RCTs) to which Tibetan pharmaceuticals were and still are subject. Alongside several co-authored articles (e.g. Adams et al. 2005), other publications followed suit on Tibetan pharmaceuticals, in particular studies undertaken by social and medical anthropologists (e.g. Craig and Glover 2009; Craig 2012; Gerke 2013, 2021; Saxer 2013; Blaikie et al. 2015; Schrempf and Springer 2015; Van der Valk 2017; Kloos 2010, 2017).

In the field of Chinese medicine, studies on RCTs have been concerned mostly with acupuncture. They no doubt impacted acupuncture practice overseas in important ways, as assessed in the doctoral theses by Iven Tao (2008, 2009) on acupuncture in Germany, Lucia Candelise (2008, 2011) on acupuncture in France and Italy, and Gry Sagli (2003, 2010) on acupuncture in Norway. In line with this trend, Scheid and McPherson (2011) assembled complementary and alternative health research that included articles critiquing treatment evaluation by means of RCTs.

The Chinese medical formulas (*fangji* 方剂), which consist of decoctions (*tangye* 汤液) constituted by carefully selected Chinese *materia medica* (*zhong yao* 中药) and are applied in a personalised way specific to each individual patient's distemper, are still in use today. However, by definition, no legitimation industry has been put in motion in defence of their efficacy. Conceptualised by some as material culture remnants of bygone times, they have been superseded by industrially produced proprietary medicines, which in this monograph will be referred to as 'Chinese formula medicines' (*zhongchengyao* 中成药; see, in particular, Part III).

Anthropological and historical research on medicine and related practices in South Asia[21] has in recent years led to an outpouring of publications on industrially produced Ayurvedic and other South Asian pharmaceuticals.[22] The most relevant for our purposes will be Pordié and Gaudillière (2014; see Chapter 7).

How a Vietnamese family's medical formula became implicated in industrial production is compellingly documented by Wahlberg (2006, 2008a, 2008b, 2012), and the legendary so-called pharmacy debate in South Korea is discussed in an eight hundred-page thesis by Ma Eunjeong (2008). Wahlberg and Ma have in common that they discuss Vietnamese and Korean medicine as what in Joseph S. Alter's understanding features as a 'medicalised' form of Asian medicine. Theirs are substantial ethnographic studies that masterfully address issues raised in science studies. By contrast, this monograph will emphasise sensory anthropological aspects of Chinese formula medicines and how they have become part of East Africa's urban spatial practices.

In addition to the dyad of patient and practitioner (Chapters 4–5), this research is concerned with the materiality of the medicines (Chapters 6–9). How did patients perceive and handle them, and what made them constitutive of spatial practices in urban East Africa? Rather than providing biographies of each medicine, and investigating their social lives and changing values (Whyte et al. 2003), this research investigates ontological questions regarding body techniques of daily life, more so than hospital technology (Mol 2002), as well as the medicines' sensed materialities and how those made them constitutive of their 'playing fields'. To find answers, we have to become attuned to textured spatialities (Chapters 1–3).

## *A Not-Untrivial Note on Terminology*

In this context, more thought needs to be given to the term 'Chinese medicine'. It provides a literal translation of the Chinese word *zhongyi* 中医. Since *zhongyi* refers to a wide range of different Chinese medical routines, medical anthropologists and historians nowadays use the term 'Chinese medicine' to refer to *zhongyi* in this broad sense, past and present (as proposed by Farquhar 1994: 1–2; Hsu 1999: 7; Scheid 2002; Zhang 2007: 1). However, the term *zhongyi* came into being only in the nineteenth century (Croizier 1968, 1976), in contradistinction to the newly imported *xiyi*, so-called 'Western medicine' (which was subject to multiple and major paradigm shifts at the time). So, in Republican times (1911–49), the term *Zhonghua yixue* referred to 'Western medicine' as practised and theorised in China (as, for instance, in 中華醫學雜誌, the *National Medical Journal of China*, lit. China's medicine journal). However, after the socialist revolution in 1949, the term *zhongyi* eventually became used to refer to the Chinese medicine that the communist state promoted from the mid-1950s onwards in educational institutions,[23] and publications in Chinese started rendering the term *zhongyi* in English translation as TCM, 'Traditional Chinese Medicine' (Sivin 1987: 429; Hsu 1999: 7, 2022; Taylor 2001, 2005). So, in order to give themselves the prestige of practising a legitimate form of 'Chinese medicine', many Chinese medicine practitioners in Africa said that they were TCM doctors.

## *Medicine and Migration: A Matter of Creolisation, Hybridity or Superdiversity?*

In the public arena, the idea of cultivating an 'accommodating' and 'tolerant' culture towards foreign labourers, refugees, migrants and mobile sojourners tends to be seen as progressive. The phrase certainly expresses a well-meant attitude to the 'other'. However, it also implies a paternalising generosity that is ultimately interested in maintaining asymmetries between 'us' and 'them'. Such 'generosity' helps perpetuate an utterly patronising stance towards the 'other', as it inadvertently endorses the idea that cultural harmony would in an ideal world be ensured by cultural 'sameness' and the cultural 'assimilation' (in the 1950s) of otherness. Although 'hybridisation' (in the 1990s) attends to heterogeneity, the subtext is similar: we live in a world that is messy and not ideal, and hence we should be 'tolerant' of others' otherness.

Such a condescending attitude towards 'the other' not only distorts the potential of a fruitful encounter between self and other. It also perpetuates those aspects of the idea of 'culture' that the discipline of anthropology has so loudly critiqued. A focus on identifying what stabilises a cultural given will inevitably tacitly 'essentialise' cultural difference.[24]

In globalisation and migration studies a number of analytical terms have been coined with a view to foregrounding cultural diversity and heterogeneity between and within cultures. However, even if we acknowledge that cultures are diverse, this does not do away with the idea of culture defined by sameness, that is, participants sharing the same collective representations.[25]

Terms like 'creolisation' have a several-centuries-old history of celebrating otherness and the mixtures that the engaged self produces in a creative encounter with the other, not only in eroticised colonial settings. 'The creole' often has an intriguing ring, particularly in French literature, being associated with a straddling of boundaries, and their transgression. The word tends to allude to the aesthetic, and can connote striking beauty and unusual novelty in taste. However, when it was introduced into anthropology, the sensuous allusions to aesthetics were kept to a minimum (Hannerz 1987; see also Harré and Rampton 2002).

'Hybridity' is another term that aims to capture the social mixing that mobility and migration entails. The term itself was developed in the context of the natural sciences, in biology. Social scientists will be particularly familiar with its use in Mendelian genetics, where 'hybrids' are mixtures of 'pure races' or varieties. However, there is valuable sociological research on the 'hybridisation' of Chinese medical practices (e.g. Frank and Stollberg 2004). This sociological understanding of hybridisation is vehemently opposed to the idea of any initially pure culture. Pieterse (1994: 80) in particular advanced 'the hybridization of hybrid cultures' and explores creative, playful processes of recombining what is at hand (see also Pieterse 1995). Nevertheless, even if the sociological research undertaken with this terminology is non-essentialising and compelling, the term remains infelicitous due to its Mendelian connotations.

More recently, another term has gained a notable following: 'superdiversity'. Steven Vertovec, who coined the term, notes that he was influenced by the ideas developed around

> cultural complexity as considered by Fredrik Barth . . . and Ulf Hannerz . . . , particularly their thinking about modes of cultural confluence, the coexistence of multiple historical streams and the ways individuals in

complex settings relate to each other from different vantage points. (Vertovec 2005: 1026)

It was not that the 'new immigrants' were increasing in number. Rather, Vertovec identified various qualitative changes at a time when transnational migration and mobility had become increasingly normative: empirical studies in London showed that while migrants would settle in clusters, they now spread over several boroughs, effecting a high ethnic mix. Furthermore, their degree of staying connected to their homelands was unprecedented, evidenced for instance by the volume of international telephone calls, which facilitated, for example, participation in the development of the homeland or in intermarriages. Vertovec did not identify recurrent patterns of conflict, but acknowledged challenges for policy.

> Compared to the large-scale immigration of the 1950s–early 1970s, the 1990s–early 2000s have seen more migrants from more places entailing more socio-cultural differences going through more migration channels leading to more, as well as more significantly stratified, legal categories (which themselves have acted to internally diversify various groups), and who maintain more intensely an array of links with places of origin and diasporas elsewhere. Super-diversity is now all around the UK, and particularly in London. (Ibid.: 1043)

Superdiversity ranges from culinary adventures, fashion and clothing to multilingualism and experimental architecture. It makes transcultural encounters look exciting, comes across as hype and has a buzz to it. After all, the term was coined when London as the 'world in one city' bid for and got to host the Olympics in 2012. This was in the historically interesting period after the Berlin Wall had fallen in 1989. It was also after the Tian'anmen incident earlier in the same year, 1989, which would lead to the opening up of the PRC to the world, and this, as we will see below in respect to East African health fields, would leave the global economy of late liberalism not unaffected. The encounters between perceived culturally 'other' African patients and Chinese physicians can indeed be studied as an aspect of 'superdiversity'.

Superdiversity, as used in migration and mobility studies, has importantly also inspired linguistic anthropological research (e.g. Blommaert 2013: 44–48, summarised in Parkin 2016). For instance, adverts for accommodation in urban neighbourhoods written in both

*Introduction*

simplified and traditional Chinese characters (*jiantizi* 简体字 and *fantizi* 繁體字) would aim to attract 'Chinese' customers from both the PRC and Taiwan. Superdiversity has evidently been accounted for through other inter- and transdisciplinary research as well, not least as it aims to cultivate a speedy critical responsiveness to the ever-changing immigration policies and population movements. However, as fluid, carnivalesque and postmodern as the phenomena that superdiversity studies are, its concept of 'diversity' hinges on its implicit contrast to 'sameness', the sameness implied by the bounded culture concept that we aim to overcome.

Alongside Vertovec's research into superdiversity, medical anthropologists at the Max Planck Institute in Goettingen started pursuing research into 'medical diversity' (Parkin, Krause and Alex 2013; Krause, Parkin and Alex 2014). This happened in an effort to 'update' medical pluralism. The latter is a term coined in the 1970s (Leslie 1980; Nichter and Lock 2002), at a time when information technology and the mobility of labour were not yet as developed as they are today, when overlapping 'medicoscapes' on a global scale are common (Wolf and Hörbst 2003). Whereas the study of 'medicoscapes' was to align itself with science and technology studies on so-called 'boundary objects' (Star and Griesemer 1989) as the locus where different cultures intersected, a sensitivity to 'medical landscapes' (Hsu 2008a) requires medical anthropologists to relinquish the objectifying bird's-eyes view and attend to the moving body's ever-changing horizons in both foreground and background.

The emphasis on fluidity – this rhetoric that cultural processes are always in flow – supersedes the earlier, and in anthropology now historical, concept of 'culture as an enduring unit'. Indeed, in the current, fast-moving, interconnected world, everything is experienced as being in constant flux, looping, braided, transforming and transmuting into other things. Without denying this speed, multiple mixing and complicating of complexity, it nevertheless is worth asking oneself whether there are any limitations to this fluidity.

## *Re-arranging Kaleidoscopic Refractions*

The term 'kaleidoscopic refractions' alludes to solid but fractured pieces. As the kaleidoscope is turned, the pieces will reconfigure. Fractures are more likely along certain lines than along others. As the viewer turns the kaleidoscope, the fractured is reassembled. In a kaleidoscope this happens in self-symmetrical fashion. The colourful parts that make up the whole are each different, yet each is chunky and solid, and some of these chunky pieces are remarkably long-lived. The chunky fragments do not dissolve entirely into a hydrodynamic whirl of change, nor are they part of a heterogeneous assemblage, a term that despite being ill defined from the start (Phillips 2006) for the lack of a better choice still enjoys great currency (e.g. Kloos 2017).

The notion of kaleidoscopic refractions resonates to a certain degree with recent discussions in medical anthropology on so-called 'transfigurations', which aim to bring Norbert Elias's concept of 'figuration' into conversation with Marilyn Strathern's notion of 'sociality' (for details, see Mattes et al. 2020).[26] Elias (1969) aimed to overcome the impasse within which studies found themselves if they plotted the individual against society. With a study on the nobility in Europe (France, in particular) from the Middle Ages to the early modern period, he laid the foundations for a 'historical sociology' of how people's 'psychological household' changed over time. He found that the psychological household of the individuals studied showed continuities with the sociological milieu in which they lived. The analytic concept of 'figurations' that he thereupon formulated accounted for the melding of sociological milieu and psychological disposition.

In a kaleidoscope, there is a continuity between the chunky glass pieces that remain internally intact and remarkably unaltered when they are reassembled in entirely new reconfigurations: the refractions are self-symmetrical. The becoming they enable would accordingly be that certain chunky pieces are picked up and rearranged in a self-symmetrical manner, much like the bird's nest is built – in a self-symmetrical manner – to the proportions of the bird's body.

Tim Ingold already noted that becoming involves self-symmetrical realignments, although that was not his most central concern in the following quote:

> Imagine a bird's nest, for example. The bird collects twigs and other materials from here and there. In no sense are these materials parts of the nest until they are assembled there. That is to say, they *become* parts in the course of the work, and only as they settle – and as they adjust themselves and progressively hold each other in place. (Ingold 2013: 69)

## Introduction

Although the nest may subsequently be redone, that work of mutual adjustment can never be recovered. For the coherence of the nest – that *wholeness* which renders its constituents as parts – is no more prefigured in the constituents themselves than is the pattern of a knitted garment prefigured in a hank of wool. . . . Through the bird's own activity, and not through the imposition of any plan or blueprint, the nest is shaped *to the proportions* of its body. (Ingold 2014: 5; italics added)

We see that through the bird's activity the assembled materials became parts of a whole, without themselves having been predestined to occupy the position into which they adjust themselves. Ingold's claim that a cultural constellation is created (or might we say, following Elias, a figuration), shaped to the proportions of the bird's own body, implicitly takes the body as the starting point whence culture is generated and hints at growth along 'automorphic symmetries'.

Herrmann Weyl (1952) long ago suggested that there was a tendency for all living organisms to reassemble themselves according to an 'automorphic symmetry' (regardless of whether they had a radial symmetry like a starfish or a seahorse's bilateral symmetry), and he posited that this re-assemblance applied, regardless of scale and size, even to atmospheric particles. Independently, Benoit Mandelbrot (1983) advanced the concept of 'self-similarity', after identifying an algorithm for how parts relate to wholes with respect to any phenomena in nature, irrespective of scale. Lynn Margulis (1997) became a widely known spokesperson of 'autopoiesis' and spontaneous recalibration; this was in the swinging sixties, and after she joined forces with James Lovelock to advance the Gaia Hypothesis (cf. Onori and Visconti 2012). More recently, Donna Haraway (2016) introduced Margulis's thinking into science and technology studies. However, in the course of doing so, Haraway also added her own ethically guided thinking when she suggested to speak of a process of 'sympoiesis' rather than 'autopoiesis' among higher-order organisms. Meanwhile, it would appear that such a hierarchical differentiation between lower- and higher-order organisms that the concept of sympoiesis draws on is precisely what the research by Weyl, Mandelbrot and Margulis was aiming to overcome.

The above thinkers have in common that they all underlined that there is no hand that turns the kaleidoscope and no creator at the steering wheel. Two were particularly daring, as they suggested that biological organisms, and many if not all phenomena in nature, are marked by 'automorphic symmetry' (Weyl) or by 'self-similarity' (Mandelbrot). Although, as we will see, some of the transformations discussed in this book showed traits of self-similarity between the given parts and emergent wholes studied, these ethnographic findings are too fragmented to construct a stringent argument, even if some can be interpreted to point in the direction of an automorphic symmetrical texturing of the emergent socialities and spatialities. Yet as feminist scholarship tells us, such 'situated knowledges', even if fragmented, are valuable and legitimate in themselves (Haraway 1988).

## The Fieldwork: Why East Africa?

John Iliffe's *East African Doctors* (1998) was published precisely in the period of preparation for this research. Its superb scholarship, communicated in succinct prose, was one of the main reasons that I started to be drawn to East Africa rather than South or West Africa for my fieldwork. Iliffe states clearly on the first page that his book is not a sociology of the East African medical profession but a 'collective biography' of East African doctors, with a focus on Black Africans, 'covering many aspects of their experience since ... the 1870s'. This made his study foundational to this medical anthropological project. Iliffe's intricate knowledge of the region and its history, and the questions he brought to it, provided an ideal entry point into the new field site for the novice that I was and still am, and structured my research accordingly.

At the time I had already researched twentieth-century Chinese medicine for over a decade, in regard to 'Westernisation' and 'modernisation',[27] not without contesting those terms (e.g. by replacing discussion of 'modernisation' with that of 'standardisation' as a project that strong government had periodically endorsed in China's history of scholarly medicine). Interested in general epistemic issues, I compared different modes of knowledge transmission.[28] So, the initial question I had for this project was: How would Chinese medical learning affect and be affected by the medical landscapes in East Africa?

'It will be argued', writes Iliffe (1998: 5), 'that modern doctors in East Africa have not been seriously threatened by competition from indigenous medicine, largely because in East Africa, unlike India or

*Introduction*

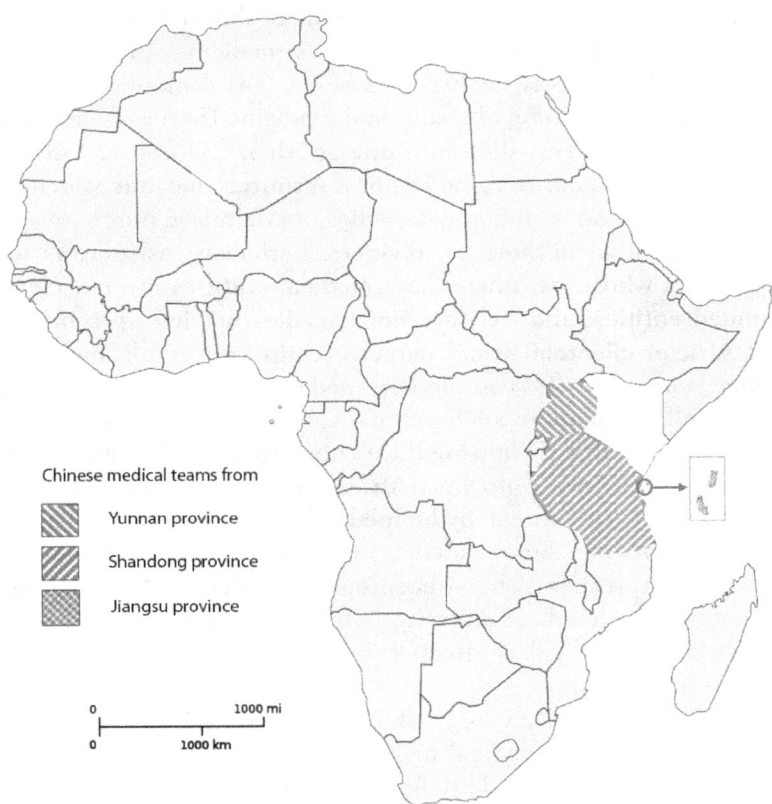

**Map 0.1.** East Africa and its Chinese medical teams. East Africa comprises the nation states Uganda, Kenya and Tanzania (inclusive of Zanzibar, which includes the two islands Unguja and Pemba). Socialist China despatched and continues to despatch Chinese medical teams from Shandong province to Tanzania, from Jiangsu province to Zanzibar, and from Yunnan province to Uganda. Kenya was a stronghold of the Allied Forces during the Second World War and received no Chinese medical teams (information gathered in fieldwork, 2001–8). Source: Wikimedia Commons, modified by the author, September 2021. https://commons.wikimedia.org/wiki/File:Blank_Map-Africa.svg.

China, that medicine lacked a literate tradition to provide a basis for its modernisation.' Instead, he suggested: 'The real threat to professional medicine, has come from the illicit sale of modern drugs for self-medication, an outgrowth of the dominant position which chemo-therapy has gained within modern medicine.'

Iliffe worked with a concept of 'medical pluralism' that allowed him to differentiate between 'indigenous medicine' and 'self medication'.[29] However, as fieldworkers know, it is sometimes difficult to disentangle the doing of traditional medicine from self-care practices because the two slide into one another.[30] Different forms of indigenous medicine were no doubt a resource that was widely relied upon, starting with home remedies, marketplace purchases and visits to spiritual authorities, diviners, herbalists, astrologers and neighbours who were 'uncles'. Yet medical cultures are not clearly bounded entities, and they are not like tiles making up a mosaic. East African clientele would perceive Chinese formula medicines (*zhongchengyao* 中成药) as 'modern medicines', and their consumption as self-medication; such practices would thus fall into the domain of 'illicit sales'. Following Iliffe's observations, the introduction of Chinese medicine into East Africa would likely accordingly be perceived as a 'real threat' by biomedical professionals. This monograph will provide some evidence in support of this, although the concept of 'threat' will be conceptualised differently, in line with recent work on 'medical diversity' (which adds the spatial to social analysis) and 'medical landscapes' (which comprehends the social through the spatial).

When I started fieldwork in Dar es Salaam in 2001, the 'mushrooming' of Chinese medical practices was a matter of contention among local journalists. This fieldwork finding suggests that they were perceived as a 'threat'. I was also informed by a foreign expert about the killing of a Chinese medical doctor on the doorstep of his home as he was returning from the celebrations of an auspicious event for his business with Tanzanian officials. On my last visit to Dar es Salaam in 2007, I learned that one of the firms that had set up a chain of Chinese medical practices all over the country no longer existed. Its directors were criminals. They had been put on trial the year before, and sent to jail. I am not an investigative journalist. Under the circumstances, I decided not to research whether, and if so to what extent, the sort of private Chinese medical practices that were seen to be 'mushrooming', particularly in Dar es Salaam at the turn of the millennium, posed an enduring threat.

As already stated, this book responds to the general perception of 'culture' as impeding 'transcultural' communication and interaction.

*Introduction*

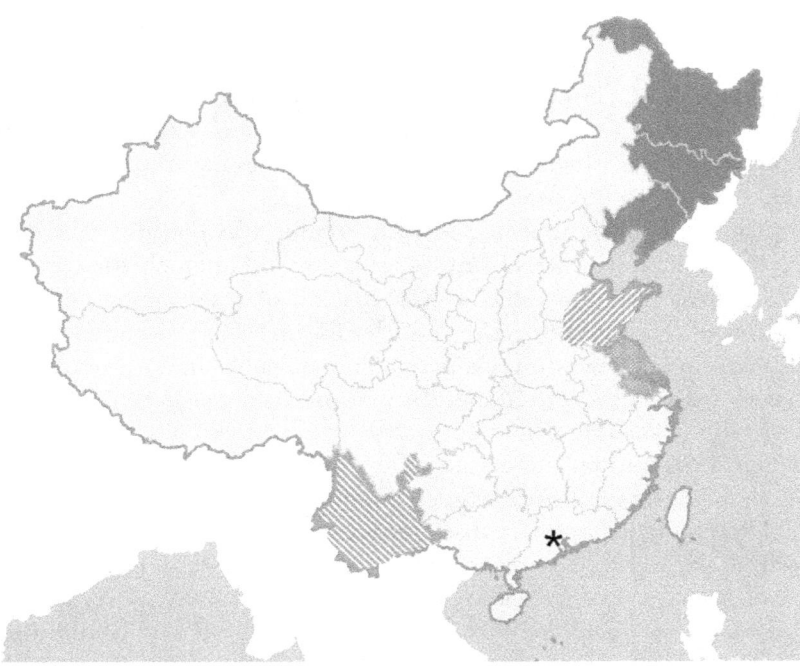

**Map 0.2.** The People's Republic of China and the Chinese practitioners' provenance. Socialist China despatched and continues to despatch Chinese medical teams from Shandong province to Tanzania, from Jiangsu province to Zanzibar (including Unguja and Pemba islands) and from Yunnan province to Uganda. Kenya was a stronghold of the Allied Forces and received no Chinese medical teams. Enterprising people from Southeast China settled, scattered throughout East Africa, during the interwar years and after the Second World War (e.g. Shunde, * in map). Northeast China became the main sending region of entrepreneurial Chinese medical practitioners about ten years after Chairman Mao's death in 1976, when Deng Xiaoping's reforms started to be implemented more vigorously (information gathered in fieldwork, 2001–8). https://commons.wikimedia.org/wiki/File:Map_of_PRC.svg. Source: Wikimedia Commons, modified by the author, September 2021.

Therefore, I chose to focus particularly on those clinical encounters that were successful insofar as they were perceived to lead to the patient's recovery. I ask which Chinese medical procedures were deemed successful in East African health fields and to what extent these procedures involved an effort to cultivate sorts of 'wholeness'. For some people, there are more interesting and pressing issues regarding CA/AC, but I chose to design this study so as to better understand what the necessary preconditions are to enable healing to happen, and to what extent healing means making whole, whatever that involves in the concrete situation.

The first hurdle that had to be overcome was posed by the conceptual toolkit with which anthropologists work, namely the concept of 'culture' (see above). However, instead of disengaging with the notion of 'culture' altogether and letting it be appropriated in the public arena in sometimes very uncomfortable ways, anthropologists have a responsibility to hinder its misconceived usage. Since healing is a form of making whole not only the individual body, the focus of this book is on how concerted efforts are mobilised and techniques implemented to cultivate wholeness, and thereby make 'culture'.

Ultimately, I hope that the Chinese medical routines described will not be reduced solely to the 'illicit sale' of sexual enhancement medicines for an aggressively advertised leisure industry. As we will see, 'Chinese medicine' instigated many different bodily routines, which complemented existent practices – or through minor tweaking, could be made to complement them – alongside some newly evolving, sometimes unsettling reconfigurations of Chinese medical treatment with formula medicines.

My focus is on those (rare) moments of medical treatment and healing that can be perceived as a technology for reconfiguring wholeness. Even though there is strife and competition between different medical actors in urban health markets worldwide, and although there is reason to be cynical about them – after all, not all medical treatment is concerned with healing (Lewis 2021: 187) – this book aims to focus in particular on those processes that were observed to be conducive to the recreation of the relation between self and other. To do so, I researched which medical routines made inroads into which urban spaces, and how they modified them and have been modified by them.

The urban spaces into which the Chinese medical practitioners were trying to insert themselves were not 'empty', even if they looked so, but had distinct textures. One such distinctive texturing had arisen from differences in the histories of the medical profession in the three nation states, Uganda, Kenya and Tanzania. As we will see, these indirectly affected the history of local and regional traditional medical healing practices (e.g. Bruchhausen 2006; Luedke and West 2007; Langwick 2011; Nichols-Belo 2018), and thereby also the ways in which Chinese medicine has been practised in East Africa. Iliffe (1998) highlights with great insight how the different political histories in each of the East African nation states affected their respective medical professions. He does so decidedly indirectly, as his aim has been to focus on the particular, namely the life histories and biographies of East Africa's remarkable health professionals.

## Uganda

Iliffe's (1998) study starts with the achievement of higher medical education in Uganda. My fieldwork, by contrast, started in Tanzania and Kenya; Uganda came last. Following Iliffe, I nevertheless introduce Uganda first. For one thing, the sorrow over Makerere University and its decline that I variously encountered during my fieldwork was palpably painful, and conveyed a sense of loss not only of intellectual life and scientific research, but of humanity. The most recent 'killer' of its once rich, strong and even illustrious scholarship was the commercialisation of higher education (personal communication with an expatriate, December 2007). In late liberalism, 'Money making through short-term masters courses' (Mamdani 2007) and certificate-honoured summer schools had become rampant. Notwithstanding, visually and spatially, the sheer size of the university's territory on Makerere Hill imposed itself on central Kampala, its tall trees throwing long shadows, at dusk in particular, reminiscent of its remarkable history in the colonial past.

At this university, East Africa's first medical school was installed in 1923 with standards that outdid similar institutions in the colonies. With its emphasis on practice alongside theory, it apparently rivalled even London's medical education (Iliffe 1998: 127). 'Its medical students were in general exceptionally gifted . . . [and] experienced a rigorous socialisation which left them with strong group solidarity' (ibid.: 60). After the Second World War, in the 1950s, 'the process of professionalisation became part of decolonisation' (Last 1986: 10, cited in Iliffe 1998: 92). In Uganda, these doctors had a public persona that played a significant role both in bringing about independence in political life and in Africanising the colonial medical institutions. However, with the disintegration of the nation state under Idi Amin in 1971–79, Uganda's visible and strong medical learning, comprising research as well as teaching, which had peaked in the first decade after independence, was shattered. Professionals were divided, internally and in different factions, and a vacuum was created. In the early 2000s, as this vacuum started to be filled and medical institutions were repopulated, there was also an influx of Chinese medical doctors working in private practices in central Kampala.

During my fieldwork in Kampala, I soon became aware of a privately run primary health care station unrivalled in size and significance by others in East Africa. It had been set up about ten years earlier by a Ugandan Western medical physician who had been trained in the PRC. During the five years of his Western medical training in China, he had also received basic training in acupuncture. This had the effect that he became interested in TCM, which he thereupon studied for a further three years in a master's course (shuoshi 硕士) before returning to Kampala. In the mid-2000s Kampala had an urban texture marked by small-to-medium-size enterprises and many Christian NGOs. It was in the spirit of Christian aid that caters to the poor that his Christian NGO clinic was founded, stationed in a popular area close to the main bus station. It combined public health services, comprising family planning, vaccination, paediatrics and other aspects, with treatment through Chinese formula medicines and acupuncture. It was in size and structure both exemplary and unique. No other clinic I visited in East Africa integrated Chinese medicine with primary care as successfully. On the one day that I visited, it was heaving with patients and health personnel (for more detail, see Chapter 7). This large private practice, which evidently relieved suffering among the urban poor, provided a vivid illustration of the importance that TM/CAM assumed in the vacuum in Ugandan health care mentioned by Iliffe (1998).

## *Kenya*

Kenyan doctors were not yet sufficiently numerous to form an influential profession at independence. One important Kenyan development during the following thirty years was the expansion of their numbers through the new medical school in Nairobi. In Kenya, the state did not disintegrate, nor did it crush professional aspirations. Rather, state, society and profession experienced a transition towards capitalism that was already under way in the colonial period, and there was also a proliferation of European and Asian biomedical professionals working in private settings. However, the contrast with private practitioners, who formed the majority, became increasingly marked vis-à-vis the discontented minority of doctors in the neglected state sector. Bringing the two together in united professional action posed real difficulties (Iliffe 1998: 169).

Kenya had been the stronghold of the Allied Forces during and after the Second World War and was only indirectly affected by the waves of world socialism with their epicentre in Beijing. In contrast to Uganda and Tanzania, to which the PRC sent expert medical teams, Kenya was never part of this scheme, although diplomatic relations with Beijing existed from independence in 1963. The history of the Kenyan medical profession directly impacted the way that Chinese medicine was perceived among expatriates as TM/CAM catering primarily to a middle-class clientele. A single renowned Chinese medical doctor was the central figure for creating this understanding of the Chinese medical community. He was a 'gatekeeper' for most Chinese who would later open their own medical practices in Kenya. Gatekeepers are a well-known feature of migration studies (Snyder 1976), which need not mean that they socialise exclusively within the boundaries of national identity (Glick Schiller et al. 1995). Ward boundaries can be protective as well as productively negotiated, as the urban anthropologist Aidan Southall (1956) and his student David Parkin (1969) demonstrated long ago, at a time when social anthropologists tended to each study their 'tribe' in rural areas. Once researchers overcome their methodological nationalism (Wimmer and Glick-Schiller 2003), an immigrant's 'mixed embeddedness' and 'cosmopolitanism' – catering to clients beyond their ethnic group – becomes very apparent. This is relevant particularly for 'business migrants' (e.g. Glick Schiller and Çağlar 2013), among whom the Chinese medical practitioners in East Africa belonged. The cosmopolitan urban textures, which for transculturally oriented entrepreneurs offered ideal 'playing fields' (see Chapter 9), afforded outward and upward mobility, and are perhaps best assessed through an anthropology of scale (Glick Schiller 2005; Glick Schiller and Çağlar 2009).

So, this 'gatekeeper' was one of the first Chinese medical doctors to emigrate to Nairobi, albeit not the very first. In the early 2000s his clinic was thriving and he was in the process of building a factory on African soil to produce Chinese formula medicines. He had also managed to gain recognition in the domain of research and development (R&D), even if only indirectly, by becoming engaged in internationally recognised research. His first widely advertised research project, funded by a respected international funding body, tested a 'herbal tea' that he had developed for treating HIV-infected patients. It involved implementing a double-blind randomised controlled trial (RCT) on a group of women living in Kigera, one of the largest informal settlements of Nairobi. Since the tea would only be effective if the women were adequately nourished, the trial ensured their regular food intake as well. This Chinese medical practitioner had evidently developed his cosmopolitanism to a fine art of health diplomacy, emphasising that business was not actually the motivation of his health enterprise.

## *Tanzania*

By contrast, Tanzania went through what Africanists and historians have called a 'socialist experiment' in 1967/1971–85, initiated by Julius Nyerere (1922–99). 'Tanganyika Territory', which gained independence in 1961, had had this name under British rule (1920–61), after having been part of 'German East Africa' (1880s–1916). Meanwhile, on Zanzibar – which is an archipelago with two main islands, Unguja and Pemba, in the Indian Ocean, not far off the East African coast – independence was obtained in 1963, and a 'socialist revolution' happened early in 1964. The unification of Tanganyika and Zanzibar led to the founding of the United Republic of Tanzania later in 1964.

On Zanzibar, the revolution led to the replacement of an Arab-led government by an African one. Since the medical profession on Zanzibar consisted solely of Arabs, this resulted in the profession's complete annihilation. Zanzibar's medical professionals fled to the African mainland, the Middle East and Britain. Medical and other aid came from communist countries: East Germany, for instance, staffed the hospital in Stone Town on Unguja, and 'the Chinese' built the Abdullah Mzee hospital at Mkoani on Pemba, which was shown to me by Chinese medical team members with pride. Moscow trained medical doctors, one of whom I interviewed during fieldwork. The revolution had apparently abolished private clinics as well as fees at government-funded hospitals, but this was history in the early 2000s when my fieldwork was conducted. Zanzibar still hosted one large Chinese medical team sent by Jiangsu province every two years, which was subdivided into one team stationed at the Mnazi Mnoja hospital in Stone Town and one in Mkoani (Hsu 2007a; Langwick 2011). In regard of some situations observed in Dar es Salaam and Zanzibar, Tanzania was like a post-socialist country: belly up, up for grabs (see e.g. Lindquist 2005), enabling the establishment of unregulated biomedical and TM/CAM businesses.

## More on the History of the Tanzanian Health System

Tanzania, following the Arusha Declaration, had seen a period of socialist orientation and a striving for self-reliance called *ujamaa*. Although the Arusha Declaration prioritised agriculture, industry and education, the medical field was also significantly transformed, particularly in comparison with Uganda, Kenya and elsewhere in Africa.

Health expenditure in rural areas increased from 20 to 42 per cent between 1971 and 1981, and by 1983, apparently, 'Some 93 per cent of the people lived within 10 kilometres of a health facility . . . In 1972 the mainland had 99 health centres and 1,501 dispensaries; the numbers in 1980 were 239 and 2,600 respectively' (Illiffe 1998: 205). These numbers are impressive, and they increased in importance. In the nine years between 1961 and 1970, the number of registered medical doctors had risen from twelve to 123 – and it was to rise to 1,060 by 1982, with 72 per cent being Tanzanian in 1984 (ibid.: 208).

The WHO's primary care programme (declared in 1978 in Alma Ata) was remarkably well implemented in Tanzania's mainland, as it is known to have been also in other socialist states in Africa (Bibeau 1985) and beyond, such as in revolutionary Nicaragua (Garfield and Taboada 1984). In Tanzania, it was focused on mass immunisation, tuberculosis control, and maternal and child health clinics, but nutrition and safe water remained a problem. Nevertheless, life expectancy had risen by about 50 per cent in the first thirty years after independence (Iliffe 1998: 206). However, preventive health care remained insufficient in rural and urban areas. '[I]n 1971, some 60 per cent of medical expenditure was still in Dar es Salaam, only 7 per cent was on prevention, and roughly half of the development expenditure was externally financed, despite commitment to self-reliance' (ibid.: 203). To worsen the situation, the level of medical expertise in these health centres started to be loudly questioned by the World Bank, specifically in 1985. Incidentally, at about the same time, the PRC's barefoot doctors scheme started to be dismantled, also due to apparently insufficient expertise, specifically in 'biomedical literacy' (White 1998). It was as though the revolutionary winds had abated worldwide in health fields.

In Dar es Salaam, the population rose 'between 1967 and 1988 from 272,515 to 1,360,850' (Iliffe 1998: 207), and this rapid urbanisation led to a crowding of underfunded health facilities. Simultaneously, hospital admissions due to malaria increased on the mainland 'between 1968 and 1985 from 13 to 25 per cent' (ibid.: 207). Meanwhile, between 1965 and 1988, 'the GNP per capita had fallen by an average of 0.5 per cent per year' (ibid.: 212). 'Poverty' became a pressing issue. Public complaints became louder. So, in 1985, Julius Nyerere stepped down from the presidency, and the socialist experiment was declared a failure by his successors.

Relevant here are two governmental interventions that left their mark on the post-socialist period (see Chapter 8). One concerned the government's attitude to nonbiomedical knowledge. In socialist-oriented Tanzania, the PRC's institutionalisation of Traditional Chinese Medicine was taken as a model, particularly by high-level politicians (Langwick 2010, 2011). This had the effect that in 1974, the Traditional Medicine Unit at Muhimbili hospital was opened. 'By 1991, it [this unit] had identified over 40,000 healers and tested 3,000 herbs' (Iliffe 1998: 211). Memories of this frantic scientific activity, together with unhappy incidents of bioprospecting in the 1990s, had the effect that in the 2000s many local healers, particularly those between Dar es Salaam and Bagamoyo but also others throughout the Tanzanian hinterland, were extremely reluctant to have any contact with pharmacognosists or ethnobiologists, and also medical anthropologists.

The other socialist-oriented governmental intervention still felt in the early 2000s concerned the opening of private practices (Iliffe 1998: 209–12). The Tanzanian government discouraged the opening of private practices by means of heavy taxation, if not at times by outright prohibition. This remained a thorny issue in the 1990s and 2000s, all the more so as doctors working in government institutions had salaries that were disproportionately low (ibid.: 208). In the 1990s there had been a surge of private practices (ibid.: 218), and it was in this period, the late 1990s, that private Chinese medical enterprises started to be set up all over Dar es Salaam.

In the early 2000s the post-socialist health fields of independent commerce and petty enterprise were anything but well established, and the rapid proliferation of Chinese medical practices was perceived as a phenomenon of 'capitalism'. Several Chinese medical practices were staffed either by Chinese families aiming to build up a new livelihood in Africa (e.g. a Chinese practitioner with spouse, child and grandparents who did the childcare) or by enterprising individuals aiming for high profit margins. Furthermore, there were chains of medical practices; one, for instance, was set up by the daughter firm of a construction firm in the PRC that diversified its production lines by transforming rented office spaces into medical consultation rooms. Health personnel working for this chain had been recruited in the PRC and committed to serve in Africa in these rented spaces for two years in the role of 'Chinese medical doctors'. The firm offered what at the time seemed to suburban and particularly rural Chinese with three years of vocational training a good monthly salary (c. USD 500), in addition to providing transport and boarding facilities.[31] Overall, petty enterprise, even if undertaken in an as-honest-as-possible manner, was often bound to fail due to cut-throat competition, fraud and crime.

At Makerere University, a biomedical profession of respected size and quality had already been built up in colonial times, and its achievements peaked in the 1960s, before political history effected its destruction. It may not be entirely coincidental that in the vacuum that this created in the health field, an NGO that integrated Chinese medicine into primary care received broad support (see Chapter 7). In colonial Kenya, by contrast, the biomedical profession was by comparison insignificant. It gradually grew after independence, both in an underpaid public sector and in a very large and diverse private sector. The successful Chinese medical business person mentioned above accordingly contributed to the diversification of the private sector (see Chapter 5). In Tanzania, socialist orientation from the early 1960s to the mid-1980s had left a legacy that was still starkly felt in the early 2000s, which fostered unease vis-à-vis both private medical and nonbiomedical practices, and Chinese medical enterprises were both private and nonbiomedical (see Chapter 8). As in other post-socialist health fields, the competition in the informal sector was treacherous and cut-throat.

Since the mid-2000s, Africa–China and China–Africa relations have been richly documented, particularly in the political sciences (e.g. Alden et al. 2008; on petty entrepreneurs, see e.g. Chatelard 2018). This literature has expanded extremely quickly, but since it proliferated after the period I spent in the field, I have left it basically untapped, alongside that on health diplomacy. Meanwhile, the history by John Iliffe (1998) provided exactly the foundations I needed for studying the processes by which Chinese medical practitioners treated patients on African soil in the early 2000s.

## The Theoretical Framing: The Texture of Space, and Its Affordances

Heretofore, we have inadvertently reconceptualised a series of cultural exchanges – otherwise presented as a 'technology transfer' – from the PRC to East Africa as a process by which Chinese medical practitioners *emplaced* themselves into the latter's urban textures. By taking account of the textures of the urban spaces in which the African–Chinese clinical encounters happened, this cultural process can be redefined and analysed as a task of accounting for the retexturing of perceived spatial textures. Self and other are thereby implicated into projects that transform urban spaces. Some of those, as I will argue, can generate a sense of wholesomeness among those participating in the efforts of effecting the transformations involved in healing.

As Lefebvre (1991: 57) put it: 'The texture of space affords opportunities'. This spatial texture is a concrete, tangible and material one, and does not merely arise from texts and 'discourse'. We will ask: which 'textures' of East Africa's 'material spaces' were perceived as conducive to the Chinese medical practitioners' emplacement, and that of their patients? What opportunities did these urban textures afford? What do the actors themselves say, what is said about them in their closer and more distant environs, and what can an anthropologist say about the social processes that they are part of and produce?

Lefebvre explains that there are 'acts with no particular place in it [the texture of space] and no particular links with it', and other activities that become 'spatial practices' that 'determine' a person's 'individual or collective use' of space (ibid.). Accordingly, one might ask, was the proliferation of Chinese medical practices in Dar es Salaam, Nairobi and Kampala – and other urban areas of East Africa – a before-the-turn-of-the-millennium, short-lived hype that has since abated? Or have some Chinese medical procedures become enduring and meaningful 'spatial practices', and if so, which ones? To identify the 'spatial practices', it is necessary to break them down into 'acts' and examine any odd 'sequence of acts which embody a signifying practice, even if they cannot be reduced to such practice' (ibid.: 57). What Lefebvre says of 'textured spaces' resonates with practice theory (see also the next section).

Meanwhile, most frameworks used in twentieth-century anthropology, from structuralism to the political economy of health, relate to space as a container, a void filled with people and things. Lefebvre begins his project by criticising this view of space:

> Not so many years ago, the word 'space' had a strictly geometrical meaning: the idea evoked simply that of any empty area. In scholarly use it was generally accompanied by some such epithet as 'Euclidean', 'isotropic', or 'infinite', and the general concept of space was ultimately a mathematical one. (Lefebvre 1991: 1)

This abstract conception of space has been foundational to most of the scholarship of the twentieth century. It is ultimately grounded in a Cartesian understanding of the *cogito* versus the *res extensa* that prevails in the natural sciences, and it is also common in social anthropology. However, space-as-an-empty-container is not merely philosophically flawed and not very practical to think with for the fieldworker, it is also ethically problematic. Lefebvre does not say this as blatantly as I have just expressed, but gestures in this direction in another vocabulary:

> ([F]ormal) content and (material) container are indifferent to each other and so offer no graspable difference. Anything may go in any 'set' of places in the container. Any part of the container can receive anything. This indifference becomes separation, in that contents and container do not impinge on one another in any way. . . . The constitution of such a 'logic of separation' entails and justifies a *strategy* of separation. (Lefebvre 1991: 170)

The subtext to the quote above is xenophobia, hostility against the foreigner, the intruder, the stranger. Implicit consequences are the setting up of walls and boundaries. Needless to say, this subtext is also an important consideration in regard to Chinese medicine practitioners in East Africa. When the media speak of a culture of 'tolerance' and advocate cultural diversity and difference, they allude to a similar space-as-container idiom, where any part of the container can receive anything. However, 'Space is not a pre-existing void, endowed with formal [mathematical] properties alone' (ibid.: 170). This monograph embarks on a project inspired by Lefebvre's approach to reappropriating space, for the humanities and social sciences, as being tangibly textured.

Somewhat paradoxically, Lefebvre's (1991) *The Production of Space* has, in my reading, similar philosophical targets as Ingold's (2009) 'Against Space', which I read as Ingold critiquing Doreen Massey's (2005) *For Space*. However, in this particular piece Ingold somewhat infelicitously conjures up a bucolic *place*, where people live from their *land*, plant their crop in *earth* and harvest it from *fields*, while cattle are grazing in *pastures* (italics added), imagery that links the habits of the organism to a fairly stable, seemingly unchanging ecological habitat.

By contrast, the spaces that interest us here are urban spaces that become implicated in spatial practices. Theoretically, at least, Lefebvre accords seemingly disjointed procedures – say, of distant geographical provenance – the potential to effect a *transformation* of already-given textured spaces (italics added). This view grants Chinese medical procedures the potential to become enduring spatial practices by way of an intricate engagement with East Africa's given urban spaces.

## Spatial Textures and Their Automorphic Symmetries

When Lefebvre speaks of 'spatial practices' that are enduring, Bourdieu's 'structuring structures' and the habitus come to mind. Although Bourdieu (1977) speaks of practice without modifying it as 'spatial', his concept of the habitus is closely linked to a spatial dimension, namely that of the 'field'. Hanks (2005) makes this point very convincingly, in a piece that demonstrates how much Bourdieu owes to Erwin Panofsky (1951). Lefebvre and Bourdieu were contemporary Marxist intellectuals in France during the 1960s and 1970s (e.g. Jenkins 2002). Their discussions of 'the production of space' and 'structuring structures' seem to have more in common than expected. These two analytic concepts both indicate that space is not an empty container but is 'textured', and practice not a voluntary act but a 'structuring' one. Transformations happen not merely within and through, but also with and to those spatial textures and structuring structures. Not everything goes.

As Lefebvre puts it, each living being is space and has its space. As it (re)produces itself in space, it also produces space. This links the body directly to the space surrounding it: 'Can the body, with its capacity for action, and its various energies, be said to create space?' (Lefebvre 1991: 170). Bodies produce space and produce themselves, along with their motions, according to the 'laws of space'. Lefebvre speaks of 'automorphic symmetry', a term he adopted from Herrmann Weyl (1952). Lefebvre, following Weyl, tells us that the spatial body's 'determinants of space' are: 'symmetries, interactions, and reciprocal actions, axes and planes, centres and peripheries, and concrete (spatio-temporal) oppositions' (Lefebvre 1991: 195). Lefebvre stresses, in accord with Weyl, that this is so regardless of scale and domain, regardless of whether the researcher's focus is on crystals or shells, corpuscles or planets, electromagnetic fields or architectural forms. These biologico-spatial realities are 'automorphic', he says, using Weyl's terminology. The spaces that organisms live in and create are not textured in a random way, but in an 'automorphic' way. One is drawn to speak of 'self-symmetrical structuring structures'.

By textured movement, the body creates the spaces around it, and the spaces thereby textured give shape to the body. The signs within these textured spaces may be mutually incomprehensible and multi-layered, but it would be an oxymoron to claim that textures are chaotic or messy. Postmodernism tends to overlook the texture and chunkiness of cultural flows. The acknowledgement that every texture has some sort of symmetry ultimately draws on Lefebvre's engagement with Weyl's 'automorphic symmetry'. It also points towards more recent avant-garde thinking in science studies. Donna Haraway, in particular, has not shied away from engaging with evolutionary biology, in both a critical and creative way, with her thinking about autopoiesis and sympoiesis (Haraway 2016). To a certain extent, this makes her both a follower of Lefebvre, who let his thinking about space be inspired by the symmetries of the life forms of 'more-than-human' organisms, and an innovator who takes this discussion in an entirely different direction (see Chapter 6).

## The Structure of This Book

This book is not an ethnography written in one long summer. Rather, diverse 'situated knowledges' have been reassembled and patched together. The field sites were multiple, as were the conditions under which fieldwork was undertaken. Furthermore, starting to rearrange published work, unpublished field notes and unwritten field experiences in a single book, nine years after my last stay in the field, has not been easy.

My fieldwork findings have been published in ten articles on various themes relating to Chinese medicine in East Africa and in about ten other articles on the herbal antimalarial *qinghao* 青蒿. For the writing of this monograph, some of these pieces have been stripped of their theoretical framing and re-embedded in this book's argument. Each of the nine chapters in this book is divided into three sections, comprising the ethnographic core in the middle, preceded by a section on fieldwork methods and concluded by one on theorists. The ethnographic cores in Chapters 1, 3, 4, 5 and 9 draw heavily on published texts (respectively Hsu 2005a, 2017, 2002, 2012a and 2015), while the ethnographic cores of Chapters 2 and 6 are new, and those of Chapters 7 and 8 (based on Hsu 2009a and 2009b) have been thoroughly renewed. The fabric of the text is thus composite. This will convey a sense of the different spatial textures of multisited ethnographic fieldwork stretched out over eight years. There were tensions, fissures and dissonances that have not been foregrounded, yet an effort was made not to eliminate a sense of their existence in the written-up text. It is important to know that this fieldwork, which was grounded in participant observation, entailed moments of both real friendship and heartfelt joy, alongside a lingering sense of uneasiness and sometimes even outright conflict.[32]

As regards ethnographic fieldwork, some generalities need to be voiced here. For one thing, it cannot disregard number or basic quantitative givens. Thus, it is a misnomer to call the ethnographic methods I used merely 'qualitative methods'. No ethnography can be done without a very basic understanding of number and proportion. Stochastic considerations are so basic to everyday life (Lave 1988) that they will inevitably inform ethnographic research. Even if serendipity is an integral aspect of ethnographic fieldwork, good ethnography is not merely a bunch of 'anecdotes'. Ethnographic

*Introduction*

fieldwork methods are nowadays discussed didactically and systematically in a range of textbooks. However, fieldwork is part of life, and one learns for life in the field (e.g. Laplante et al. 2020). Textbooks on method tend not to include ethnographic accounts of how a method was applied, and tend not to address the emotional dimension (although there are exceptions, e.g. Davies and Spencer 2010; Elliot et al. 2017). Yet feelings and affective states are undeniably part of fieldwork, as my introductory sections on methods will show. These are on: siting, sensing and mapping the field; language learning in the field; conducting semi-structured interviews; working with narrative; tackling prickly issues; bringing the historical dimension into ethnography; and reflecting on one's mistakes as a fieldworker. Those readers interested in just the ethnographic methods, and not so much in Chinese medicine, may endeavour to read in each chapter only the first section on methods. I have taken extra care to write the texts so as to enable a reader to focus on only the experiences of applying fieldwork methods.

The book is structured in three parts. Part I starts with the medical encounter, moving through space and moved by speech. Part II researches the sociality of different configurations of patients, practitioners and 'pots', as well as the 'para-professionals', that is, the interpreters and lab technicians. Part III engages with the materiality and ontology of the medicine *pots* and their affordances. It investigates the hybridity of the Chinese formula medicines as a manifestation of an 'alternative modernity'; explores sensory aspects of Chinese procedures for enhancing fecundity; and compares the 'Chinese antimalarials' *qinghao* 青蒿 (i.e. the plant and 'natural herb' *Artemisia annua* L.) and *qinghaosu* 青蒿素 (the purified chemical substance artemisinin).

The ethnographic core of each chapter, and how it ties in with medical anthropological debates and theory, is discussed at the end of each chapter, in a section called 'Reflections'. Here in the introduction, I merely point to the range of philosophical and anthropological foundations on which this ethnography is based:

The two sections on 'Reflections' in Part I engage with thinkers who emphasised complementarity and cooperation as foundational to cultural and linguistic encounters, such as Alfred Schütz, who foregrounded the *Thou*-relation, or Paul Grice, who developed the concept of the 'cooperative principle'.

The reflections in Part II shift the focus onto techniques of transformation, skills and body techniques, inspired by Marcel Mauss's insistence on the relevance of studying 'concrete' techniques for understanding cultural relatedness (James 1998). I also engage with Michel de Certeau's (1984) differentiation between strategies and tactics. According to de Certeau himself, the latter resonate with the Chinese philosophical understanding of 'power' as given in the 'propensity of things' (*shi*; Jullien 1995). Both thinkers make us attend to the social through the bodily and material aspects of daily life.

Finally, Part III aims to provide an account of the ways in which the materiality of the 'pots', *pots* and pots (as explained in Chapter 6) can explain their bodily felt efficaciousness by investigating the ontologies of caring that they entail. The book ends by pointing out the revolutionary potential for lasting change that is provided by practical knowledge at the grassroots – what Antonio Gramsci (1891–1937) called 'good sense' or 'common sense' (see Crehan 2002, 2016; Robinson 2005).

The final three chapters, which have been inspired by recent social anthropological research into 'ontologies' (e.g. Willerslev 2004a, b; Holbraad 2007; Holbraad and Pedersen 2017), will focus on intersubjective and inter-corporeally negotiated medical-cum-social efficaciousness. Throughout this monograph, a question will be posed regarding the extent to which the body techniques thereby enacted are perceived by 'the self' and 'the other' to reconfigure the refractions of given spatial textures into novel, but nevertheless automorphically symmetric, wholes.

## Notes

1. The ethnographic fieldwork on which this book draws was undertaken in urban areas, specifically urban East Africa (2001–8, *c*. nine months in total), and drew on fieldwork on Chinese medicine conducted in urban China (1988–89, *c*. eighteen months).
2. These are fieldwork-based findings based on interviews with their founders and/or close relatives.
3. Conflicts were multiple, and also existed between socialist-era, pre-socialist and late-liberal Chinese (e.g. Hsu 2007a).
4. 'Slow research' requires reconceptualisations of locality, a sensitivity to 'what is working', the acquisition of knowledge rather than information, and responsiveness to local relevancies (Adams et al. 2014).

*Introduction*

5. It would probably be too pretentious to call these efforts 'patchwork ethnography' (Günel et al. 2020), that is, 'research efforts that maintain [. . .] long-term commitments, language proficiency, contextual knowledge, and slow thinking'.
6. Obrist (2003: 281) notes: 'In health explanations, women emphasised that not only conditions of body and mind but also "living conditions" (*hali ya maisha*) have to be favourable in order to achieve good health.' She explains this in terms of *uzima* as a 'broader conception of well-being, vitality and wholeness'. This holistic notion of well-being contrasted with health through hygiene: '"proper food" (*chakula bora*), "clean water" (*maji safi*), "clean environment" (*mazingira safi*) and "cleanliness" in general (*usafi*)' (ibid.: 283). Yet *usafi* has non-dualist connotations too: clear water signifies both the pure and holy (Obrist 2004).
7. A sense of feeling 'incomplete' is a virtue, Francis Nyamnjoh argued in his seminar on proverbs gathered by Achebe Chinuo (on 4 March 2021, University of Oxford), mentioning this deep-seated sense of incompleteness alongside a commitment to 'mobility/motion, encounter, compositeness, debt and indebtedness, and conviviality'.
8. 'Trying out' is a pragmatist stance; see Whyte (1997), Geissler and Prince (2010a), Cooper and Pratten (2015) and many others.
9. On autochthony as a rootedness balanced by a celebration of a 'fundamental alterity', for instance in myths of strangers as the founders of society, see Ceuppens and Geschiere (2005: 388).
10. The term 'scholarly medicine' is adopted from Bates (1995), as the notion of 'humours' and 'humoral pathologies' is too occidental to be applied cross-culturally (Horden and Hsu 2013). See also Köhle and Kuriyama (2018). These three volumes straddle the boundaries of medical anthropology and, in particular, medical history.
11. The wasting illness *chira* has a regulatory function, as do 'taboos' in early anthropology.
12. Durkheim's (1915) 'society', and the 'collective representations' that make up 'culture', draw on a concept of sameness. However, the homogeneous 'cultural representations' of a disembodied collective, combined with the nationalistic focus on one language, one religion and one territory, render his concept of 'culture' inadequate for this project. As many discerning critics have long noted, it is too static, too bounded, too homogeneous and too idealistic.
13. In fieldwork the 'c' word tended to be mentioned mostly after a preceding miscommunication or a clash of blatantly different assumptions and convictions between people of different class, professional, educational or language backgrounds. Sometimes, it appeared to reinforce differences in 'race', as it had done a century ago. At others, it downplayed the determinism of 'genes'.
14. Mauss is rated one of Durkheim's most creative critiques (e.g. James 1998). Consider also Mauss's two students Leroi-Gourhan (1993) and Haudricourt (1987).

15. Currently, the foundational work on the gift by Mauss ([1925] 1954) is much discussed in contemporary African anthropology that is engaged with ethics (e.g. Neumark 2017, Laws 2019). See also the critique of cash economies and the foregrounding of gift economies (Ferguson 2015). However, the focus for us is on Mauss and technology.
16. 'If it [the forthcoming *Historical Atlas of Civilisation* by O. Spengler] is guided by a priori ideas of *"the* culture" or of a priori defined "such and such cultures", this work will only be full of petitions of principle' (Mauss [1929] 2006a: 66).
17. On South–South relations of China in Africa and Africa in China (CA/AC), see Yoon Jung Park's invaluable e-network, accessible at chinese-in-africa africans-in-china@googlegroups.com (accessed 9 December 2021).
18. On the rapid rise of the field of CA/AC in area studies, see, for instance, Petit and Chatelard (2018).
19. Bräutigam (2011) notes that infrastructure made up 61 per cent of all concessional loans granted by China in a year, not only those for Africa.
20. T/CAM or TM/CAM refers to traditional medicines (considered indigenous or local) and complementary and alternative medicines (professionalised local or transnational TMs; 'popular' or folk practices).
21. E.g. Zimmermann (1987), Langford (2002), Frank (2004), Wujastyk and Smith (2008), Hardiman and Mukharji (2013) and Guenzi (2021).
22. E.g. Bode (2004, 2008), Pordié and Hardon (2015) and Coderey and Pordié (2019).
23. In contrast, the various forms of Chinese medicine in Taiwan are either called *guoyi* 國醫, 'the nation's medicine', or *chuantong yixue* 傳統醫學, 'traditional medicine' (anonymous, personal communication, *Aademia Sinica*, Taiwan, September 1999).
24. The idea of the submergence of the 'self' by the invasion of the 'other' – the nationalist stance of xenophobia – is being expressed ever more loudly in Europe (Banks and Gingrich 2006) and beyond. Even if the 'yellow hordes' of Genghis Khan are now part of the European archive and a memory tinged with legend, the 'hydra' of Chinese aid-cum-business was a repeatedly vocalised threat in East African health fields – 'you cut off their head here, they grow another one there' (hospital physician, personal communication, Dar es Salaam, 2007).
25. The exoticising gaze on 'Far Eastern' art and culture, as cultivated in rarefied circles of a wealthy European elite, may have been an instance of 'Sinophilia' (Russell 1922), but cases of 'Sinophobia' have historically been far more frequent, often seizing wide parts of society. It was not merely in nineteenth-century Hawaii that fears of contagion became the main pillars of Sinophobic governmental legislation, as noted in the foundational medical anthropology article 'Learning to be a Leper' (Waxler 1981); they are arguably perpetuated in US legislation for the sake of TB prevention (e.g. Ho 2001, 2003).
26. A focus on 'im/mobilities of and dis/connectivities' throws light on 'the *patternedness* of flows', 'as well as processes of contestation and fragmenta-

*Introduction*

tion' (Dilger and Mattes 2018: 272–73, italics added). While referring to 'patterns' instead of 'textures', Dilger and Mattes too aim to give the fluid changes more structure and material solidity by speaking of 'figurations'.

27. E.g. Croizier (1968), Unschuld (1973), Kleinman (1976, 1980), Hsu (2001), Scheid (2002), Rogaski (2004), Zhan (2009), Leung and Furth (2010), Andrews (2014), Lei (2014) and Chiang (2015).
28. See Sivin (1987), Ots (1990a), Farquhar (1994), Hsu (1999), Taylor (2005), Scheid (2007) and Zhang (2007).
29. Iliffe no doubt drew here on the classic work by Last and Chavunduka (1986), which changed for medical anthropology the legacy of Evans-Pritchard (1937, whose focus had been on the *why me?* question) in the direction of research undertaken by van der Geest and Whyte (1988), Comaroff and Comaroff (1992), Pool (1994), Dilger and Luig (2010), Langwick (2011), Prince and Marsland (2013), Laplante (2015), Mattes (2019) and many others.
30. For instance, in order to enhance externally applied herbal medications when packing a wound, the powder taken from antibiotics capsules is sprinkled onto it (Bierlich 2007).
31. In 2001–2, the exchange rates for the Tanzanian Shilling ranged between TZS 1,200 and TZS 1,350 per English pound sterling. One thousand TZS was over one US dollar in 2001, and just about equal to one dollar in 2008. In 2001, the salary of a lowest-grade government employee was *c*. TZS 50,000 per month, around GBP 50.
32. Fieldwork was carried out in March–April 2001, December 2001–January 2002, March–April 2002, July 2002, December 2002–January 2003, April 2003, December 2004–January 2005, April 2005 and December 2007–January 2008. All names of my respondents are pseudonyms.

# Part I
## Moving through the Practico-Sensory Realm of Space

# Chapter 1
# Spatial Textures of the Clinical Encounter

## Fieldwork: Siting the Field, Sensing and Mapping

Participant observation starts with the body – the body moving through space. Anthropological fieldwork is supposed to expose the fieldworker's body to the unfamiliar: unfamiliar food; unfamiliar sounds, melodies and music; unfamiliar languages, prosodies and pronunciations; unfamiliar people, dressed unfamiliarly, interacting with each other . . . and also reaching out to me? Gestures, looks, silences, looks again.

My fieldwork began with a tactual alert. A hot blaze seized my body as I stepped out of the aeroplane cabin and, still somewhat sleepy, went down the stairs onto an airport bus in the hazy morning sun. Indoors, the heat soon became sticky and humid. Pearls of sweat formed on my face and back. 'Oh, no, I'm smelly', I thought, slightly embarrassed, while standing in line for passport control. The luggage was already there, and I was able to swiftly leave the premises, which opened onto a taxi stand. This was going to be my first stay in Dar es Salaam, as my fieldwork of the previous two decades had mostly been in China. The accommodation was booked. My first task was to get myself sorted before setting out to explore the city.

Central to the explorations that follow are the insights derived from the gestalt-psychological figure–ground images that underline that perception arises from an active engagement of one's body with one's surroundings. The second part of this methods section will discuss the issue of mapping.

## The Body's Movement through Space: Beyond the Common Notion of Perception

The body is implicated in the texturing of spaces; Lefebvre (1991) is very explicit about this. The movement of the body follows the textures of the surrounding space – the staircases, doors, corridors, border and customs inspection points, and taxi stands. The space through which I moved, however unfamiliar, textured my movement such that I inadvertently became part of it. As Lefebvre (ibid.: 184) put it: 'Space – my space – is not the context of which I constitute the "textuality"'. Rather, 'it is the shifting intersection between that which touches, penetrates, threatens and benefits my body on the one hand and all other bodies on the other'. It is this intermediary that has 'gaps and tensions, contacts and separations' (ibid.). The body, textured by the spaces it projects itself into and texturing them simultaneously, serves as a point of departure for exploring the world (ibid.: 194). Anyone only vaguely familiar with his early writings will recognise in those quotes the thinking of Merleau-Ponty ([1945] 1962, 2012), as developed in the *Phenomenology of Perception*.

Lefebvre does not acknowledge Merleau-Ponty, yet like his contemporary Pierre Bourdieu, who does not acknowledge Merleau-Ponty either, he appears to owe much to the latter's thinking about the body. It was two more decades before Thomas Csordas (e.g. 1990, 1993, 1994a–c, 1999, 2002) brought Merleau-Ponty's philosophically rigorous thinking about the body as the existential grounds of culture into medical anthropology – which he ingeniously did by mobilising Bourdieu's (1977) notions of the 'habitus', the 'field' and 'practice'.

Merleau-Ponty (1945) had famously rejected the empiricist idea of an organism being passively subject to the sensory stimuli of the outside world, which are then decoded in the brain. In line with gestalt psychology (e.g. Köhler 1929), Merleau-Ponty underlined that it was through the actively induced projection of the body into its surroundings that organisms perceived their environment. The body's movement through space was part and parcel of the perceptual process.

In what follows, I first explore the way that the fieldworker's body is implicated in perceptual processes according to a gestalt-psychological approach to perception. Then, I discuss the article on siting the field by Emily Yates-Doerr (2017). This is followed by a comment on the 'embodiment paradigm', which at the time I started fieldwork was on everyone's mind. Finally, some attempts at mapping the field are discussed.

## *Figure–Ground Images: A Gestalt-Psychological Approach to the Phenomenal Field*

Figure–ground images were used by gestalt psychologists to demonstrate that perception is an immediate and unmediated process, so to speak. A lemon is perceived as such, in a holistic way, not by a process of adding up its yellow colour, its fresh feel and its oval shape (Morris 2012: 87). Figures are part of a phenomenal field and their perception requires an active process. Through the perceiver's activity of changing the visual focus, figures or ground are brought to the fore or kept in the background.

Gestalt psychologists brought images like the below into circulation in an effort to highlight that perception is not the sum of different sense perceptions, but an all-attuned-to-one-another or 'holistic' event (or series of events). However, figure–ground images can be read, creatively, in a variety of different ways. Transposed into the discussion entertained here, a figure–ground image can be used to illustrate medical anthropological research that treats the human body as a lone figure in a vacuum, or patient and practitioner as a dyad of disembodied figures in a vacuum on an otherwise untextured ground.

For instance, Figure 1.1 can be seen to capture Aperiçida Vilaça's (2005, 2009) critique of medical anthropological writing on 'embodiment': she noted that although medical anthropologists claim to research embodied cul-

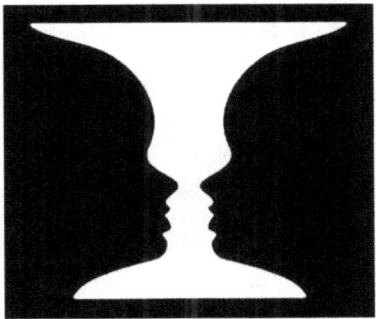

Figure 1.1. A figure–ground image. Gestalt psychology underlined that figure and ground form one single phenomenal field. Perceiving is an active process: by the activity of squinting one's eyes one can either see a white vase or the profile of two human figures in the foreground. Source: Wikimedia Commons, modified by Yuxin Peng, October 2021.

ture, they have mostly focused on the body only, that is, they focused on the clearly contoured black human figures in Figure 1.1 and forgot all about the white ground, as though the body could be studied in detachment from its environment. To emphasise the ontological continuity between a figure or person and their surroundings, which is core to the socialities discussed in this monograph, let us turn to Figures 1.2 a and b:

This modified figure–ground image should account for the textures of a phenomenal field, that is, the urban spaces and architectural structures through which the body moves. It is meant to illustrate Lefebvre's (1974) argument insofar as it can be read as highlighting that both the figure and the surrounding grounds are textured, often in much the same way, as is evident from Figures 1.2 a–b. Spatial textures affect both figure and ground, that is, both the body and its surroundings are textured and texturing. There is a richness of texture to the phenomenal field as a whole, as Katherine Morris underlines in her lucid introduction to Merleau-Ponty:

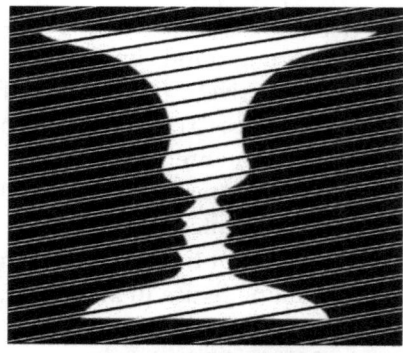

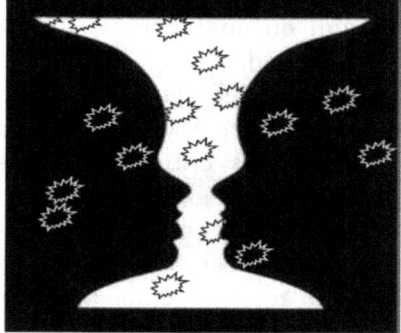

**Figures 1.2 a–b.** A figure–ground image affected by and affecting different textures. A phenomenal field's spatial textures affect both the figures and the ground, and vice versa. What is here vaguely called 'ground' can be seen as 'background', such as for instance the spatial surroundings of a medical encounter between patient and practitioner. Also, what looks like 'a vase in the foreground' can be seen to refer to the medicine pot that is being transacted. Figure and ground, fore- or background, are all textured and also have a texturing capacity. Source: Wikimedia Commons, modified by Yuxin Peng, October 2021.

*Spatial Textures of the Clinical Encounter*

So, the phenomenal field *is* the life-world, shot through with 'lines of force', 'peopled' by demands and resistances, barriers and solicitations. (Morris 2012: 41)

Contrary to the impression that Figure 1.1 may have evoked, the white space of the in-between is not a vacuum but is richly textured, as indicated by Figures 1.2 a–b. These figures should not, however, generate the impression that Lefebvre's understanding of spatial textures was deterministic. On the contrary, just like Bourdieu aimed to account for cultural change in terms of 'structuring structures', which left the future partly undetermined, Lefebvre spoke of sensed 'affordances'. He considered some textures as 'affording' some transformations but not others.

Having said this, Figures 1.2 a–b cannot demonstrate the centrality of the notion of 'affordance' for the sensory, perceptual and experience-texturing processes in focus here (for that, see Chapter 3). Nor do they highlight Lefebvre (1991: 171) drawing on Weyl's (1952: 27) suggestion that transformations within an organism have traits of 'automorphic' symmetries. And they certainly cannot ac-

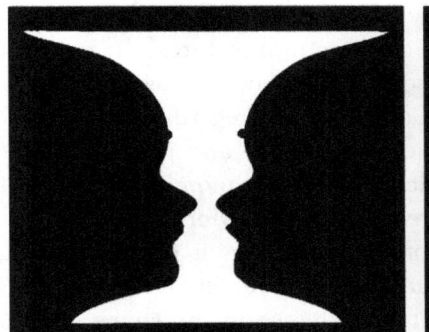 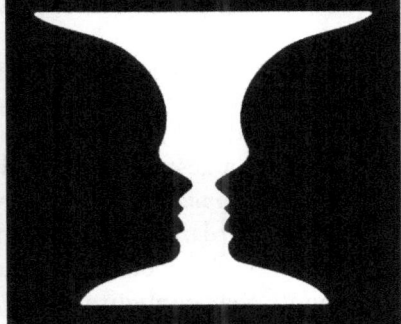

**Figures 1.3 a–b.** The in-between space as pot in a medical encounter. Figures and ground form a single phenomenal field – say, that of patient and practitioner in a medical encounter. Depending on how one approaches the situation, and squints one's eyes, the white in-between space may either be read as depicting a medicine pot (a vase) *in the foreground* or the empty (therapeutic) space *in the background*. Compare Figures 1.3 a and b to the therapeutic process of ingesting a medicine: The changing shape of the white vase (i.e. the materiality of the medicine) instantly effects a change in the profile of the two black human figures. These ideas are further developed in Chapter 6. Source: Wikimedia Commons, modified by Yuxin Peng, October 2021.

count for the complex 'virtual dynamics of ritual',[1] which are intrinsic to ritual transformations that also can affect, according to Kapferer (2004), the habitus and the restorative transformation of a patient from ill to well. So while the interdependency of the *gestalt* of patients, practitioners and pots is key to our investigation, we research it with an understanding that there is a depth to the surface movements. We may be aware of them without being able to spell them out.

Chapters 6–9 in this ethnography will engage extensively with the figure–ground image in yet another way: namely as a phenomenal field where figure and ground are both affected and entwined with one another. Thus, as the shape of the vase that makes up the white space between the two black figures changes, their profiles also change. We emphasise the interdependencies between the texture and materiality of 'the in-between' and the human figures. The ingestion of medical stuff would accordingly transform the profile of a figure – say, of a patient who recovers after ingesting the medicine. This white space of the in-between can be understood either as the medicine 'pots' (in the foreground) that are transacted in the clinic and their bioscientifically described contents, which are to be ingested by the patients, or as the architectural textures, the *pots* (in the background) as they are sensed by the people moving through spaces. 'Pots' are assessed in a Cartesian way regarding 'objective' properties and 'subjective' qualities (Pye 1968) and *pots* are comprehended in a gestalt-psychological and 'physiognomic' way, which emphasises *'immediate practical recognizability'* (Morris 2012: 25).

In other words, this book's ethnographic focus is on the sensed materiality of the medical encounter as it is elicited through the movements that configure it. Just as a change in the shape of the white vase directly affects the shape of the profile of the two black figures, and vice versa, the materialities of the medicine pots and the spaces in which they are transacted have a texturing effect on patient and practitioner, as well as on other people, organisms and things involved in the encounter. Evidently, the impressions, sensations and perceptions of these materialities are 'intersubjectively' produced (Csordas 2008) and may change in different situations, sometimes following bodily interactions and 'intercorporeal' moments (Csordas 2011) that might result in a redefinition of what makes up a medicine, a thing, a structure or a space.

Gestalt psychologists emphasised that perception is an active undertaking – you can squint your eyes and choose to either foreground the two black figures or the white ground (which by being foregrounded becomes a vase or, say, a pot). In other words, contrary to the empiricist view, you are not passively exposed to a world that bombards you with stimuli. Rather, through your own squinting movements of the eye and the locomotion of your whole body, which supports the eyes (Gibson 1979), you elicit certain sensations, impressions and perceptual experiences, and not others. This ultimately leads to a redefinition of the different materialities you engage with, and of what makes up the material world.

## *'Worlds That Come to Matter' by 'Siting the Field'*

A fieldworker arriving in unfamiliar spaces is no longer asked to identify a specific fieldwork locality or to get to know well this bounded cultural entity in order to extrapolate from the particular to the general. The concept of the local and, specifically, the idea of a fieldwork locality that can be located in a bounded Euclidean space has been widely critiqued (e.g. Yates-Doerr 2017). In appreciation of an interconnected world, anthropological knowledge is tied to an (ethical) commitment that is to make the field's production happen. This activity Yates-Doerr calls a 'siting' of the field: 'A practice of *siting* requires paying simultaneous attention to what we study and to the practice of authoring' (ibid.: 382). Accordingly, the fieldworker is tasked with finding respondents whom they can treat as co-authors.

> Siting materialities unsettles the Euro-American concept of perspective suggesting that perspective does not offer a view on a detached world but shapes which worlds come to matter. (Yates-Doerr 2017: 382).

Yates-Doerr's use of the word 'matter' here is intentionally polysemic. I suppose it indicates (a) that the worlds are taking shape in relation to how the fieldworker engages with them; (b) that the material aspects of those worlds matter; and (c) that the materials are not intrinsically given but emerge in relation to the fieldworker.

In a phenomenological vocabulary one would speak, in the case of (a), of an 'affordance' specific to its perceiver and their intention; that is, the perceived world emerges in relation to oneself and one's appetites and wants. In the case of (b) one would say that the material aspects of the world matter for anyone interested in understanding the social. Finally, to better understand (c), Merleau-Ponty's (2012: 103) own words are lucid and compelling:

> With regard to spatiality, which is our present concern, one's own body is the always implied third term of the figure-background structure, and each figure appears perspectivally against the double horizon of external space and bodily space. (Merleau-Ponty [1945] 2012: 103)

Knowledge production is accordingly relational, and taking account of one's own ego-centred positionality is key to perceiving the existence of the other, say, the figure on the figure–background structure. Depending on how one squints, one's eyes will affect 'which worlds come to matter' (Yates-Doerr 2017: 382).

So, here I was. I had finally arrived in the field. I had taken the taxi to the hotel, had a shower and a nap. Rather than demarcating a specific fieldwork locality and staying put there, I was seeking a co-production of knowledge on Chinese medical treatment. I knew that ethnographic knowledge production was co-authored and relational. My findings would depend on how I projected myself into this field, how I squinted my eyes. The light was indeed glaring hot. I found myself moving along spatial textures, following a broad road through a quiet neighbourhood towards the city centre. To my surprise, just a few blocks away, I passed by a Chinese medical practice in the shadow of tropical trees. I would regularly pay visits to it later, but not on that day.

## *Embodiment: Feminist Medical Anthropology in the Early 2000s*

Embodiment as an 'orientation' had its heyday in the 1990s and early 2000s when I was getting prepared for the field. Merleau-Ponty himself did not speak much of 'embodiment', but this term had great traction in medical anthropology at the time. With the 'embodiment paradigm', Csordas (1990, 1994a) hoped to overcome thinking in terms of the Cartesian mind–body dichotomy that continues to frame thinking about the body and disease in medical history, public health and also the medical humanities. Working with an 'embodiment paradigm' promised to provide a transculturally less distorting framework for analysing fieldwork findings.

At the time, the research on nerves as an embodied experience saw a high tide, spurred by a feminist commitment to highlighting the fuzzy boundaries between tiredness due to overwork, emotional irritability and mental health diagnoses of depression or schizophrenia, which could be overly medicalised (e.g. Davis 1988). This was affecting women's lives in particular, many of them migrants (Dunk 1989; Lock 1991; Migliore 1994), others suffering abject poverty and extreme hunger (Scheper-Hughes 1992: Chapter 5, 167–217). This literature came mainly, but not exclusively (e.g. Kohrt and Harper 2008), out of the Americas. So, here I was, on the lookout for whether embodied experiences of 'nerves' were also to be a loudly vocalised issue on the East African coast (they weren't).

The embodiment paradigm also promised to lead us out of the impasse of the cultural relativity debate. Thinking in terms of 'embodiment' provided an alternative to plotting 'incommensurable particulars' against panhuman 'universals'. A much-debated 'universal' in medical anthropology, namely the notion of 'somatisation' and 'somatised affect' (Kleinman 1980, 1986; Obeyesekere 1985), triggered engaged transcultural research on nerves as 'embodied metaphors' (Low 1994; consider also Sobo 1996). The embodiment paradigm opened up a space for attending to 'culturally mediated psychological processes' that would manifest in the physical and material body's intermediate domains of immunology, neurology and endocrinology (Kirmayer 2003). Contrary to the widespread view that implicating the body, and in particular the researcher's own body, into ethnographic research would lead to another navel-gazing exercise, it can be argued, as is done here, that it is precisely the theorising of the body that has made it possible to consider ethnographies of movement, sensory experience and perception relevant to medical anthropology.

However, in the name of embodiment, many texts were written that treated the body as being just as detached from its environs, and its author, as others. Vilaça (2005, 2009), in particular, queried the usefulness of the embodiment paradigm.[2] She was certainly convincing in pointing out that the literatures on embodiment often focused merely on the body-enveloped-by-skin (see Figure 1.1) and rarely on the body with a habitus that was generative of its field and habitat, or the body moving through a textured space that was texturing it while simultaneously being textured by it (see Figures 1.2 a–b). This ethnography takes Vilaça's critique seriously. It is all about embodied suffering, but I will not use those terms. Rather, I aim to emplace the suffering in a socialised space, and ask: which sorts of embodied distress led to these medical encounters, where people from the hosting countries engaged in a commercial transaction with their guests who were medical practitioners selling exotic drugs, and how far would this lead to a therapeutic relation that engendered a renewed sense of wholeness for those implicated into it?

The three sections that follow throw light on the difficulties that the mapping of these socialised spaces involved.

## *Mapping Movement*

When pondering over movement through space, at the interface of which, according to Merleau-Ponty (1945), the body emerges, it occurred to me that one of the first observations of implicating one's own body in reflections about one's fieldwork findings – as 'siting' a field demands – results in a blurring between the 'outsider' and 'insider' view and between 'emic' and 'etic' meanings.[3] Csordas (1993) had already commented on this dissolution between clearly demarcated emic and etic meanings in fieldwork concerned with body work. He thereupon developed the theoretically and methodologically extremely useful concept of 'somatic modes of attention' for documenting the 'cultural elaboration of sensory engagement' (ibid.: 139). This has made possible the non-judgemental documentation of a wide range of differently weighted sensory events (e.g. Hsu 2008).

Alongside the dissolution of emic and etic meanings in fieldwork that implicates the fieldworker's own body in knowledge production comes the dissolution of the spectators of any ritual or medical encounter. Kapferer (2004: 43) emphasises this:

> The notion of ritual gathering embraces what is otherwise referred to as audience or spectators, but these words are far too passive. . . . In much ritual, the ritual gathering (that is, those not directly engaged with the production of the rite) is also participant and vital in the production of rite and its dynamics. . . . I (Kapferer 1984) have shown for Sinhala healing rites how performance sets up a dynamic of exclusion and inclusion for members of the ritual gathering, using them to achieve various transformations in experience and meaning for the central participants.

Since the focus in this book is on those medical encounters that were perceived as healing by (compositionally) establishing wholeness or a sense of wholesomeness, Kapferer's insight that the members of the so-called audience are participants in the ritual transformation is important. Just as the patients in Chinese medical treatment would be affected by the virtual dynamics that successful healing involves, namely a 'slowing down', a 'temporary abeyance of ordinary flows' and 'an engagement with the compositional structurating dynamics of life' (Kapferer 2004: 47), so would be Janzen's (1978) 'therapy managing group'. In this way, the distinction between the emic and etic dissolved and I had to relinquish the idea of being just a member of the audience. My interest in movements through the ritual space of Chinese medical clinics was to implicate me in their transformative (ritual) dynamics. My willy-nilly 'mapping' attempts became efforts at 'siting' the field.

## *From Mapping along Vectors of Time . . .*

Many medical anthropologists who are also medical practitioners have ordered their findings with a view to a timeline rather than to spatialising concerns. This, I suppose, has to do with the centrality of the question of illness causation to the sick person, their social entourage and health systems. Germ theory came in handy, as Latour ([1984] 1988) put it, as it located the pathogen in a single microbe, which was both baffling and convincing due to its simplicity for the nineteenth-century hygienists (whose 'holism' located the pathogenic, as Latour put it, everywhere and nowhere). Monocausal explanations had both an aesthetic elegance and a rational sharpness. Events could be mapped along a timeline. Although monocausal reasoning initially applied primarily to the domain of microbial disease causation, it soon became the hallmark for all biomedical rationales. And this search for the cause of disorders soon became a preoccupation for many medical anthropologists, although there were voices early on reminding us that not all peoples are interested in explaining the occurrence of specific symptoms by attributing them to specific causes (e.g. Lewis 1975). Medical anthropological writing on causality has been rather disjointed, in contrast to the medical historical narratives of progress in controlling 'infectious diseases'. Gilbert Lewis (1975: Chapters 5–6, 154–228; 1995) explicitly linked causal reasoning to questions of perception: what counts as evidence in the course of making a diagnosis? Practitioners are confronted with everyday life problems, yet in their explanations often allude to variables outside everyday life experience. What goes beyond immediate perception is often considered a cause. Anthropologists have been quick, Lewis notes, to interpret as 'causal explanation' evidence recovered through 'divination' or 'diagnosis', which is merely a register of speech that goes beyond that used in daily life. He acknowledged the widespread interest of early medical anthropology in illness causation (e.g. Janzen and Prins 1981), and that of the cognitive sciences (Sperber et al. 1995), but in the case of divination, for instance, causal attribution was best considered a linguistic anthropological problem, a register of speech.

A timeline visualised as a vector that captures the 'before and after' can usefully account for fieldwork-elicited information regarding causal attribution. Lorna Amarasingham Rhodes, in 'Time and the Process of Diagnosis in Sinhalese Ritual Treatment' (1984: 51), made excellent use of such a simple device. She drew what she learned about a woman's enduring misfortune of repeated miscarriages over ten years onto a vector of time. Its cause was located in the very distant past: the day of menarche, when the woman had encountered a demon, an event brought to mind during her pregnancy in a consultative session with an exorcist. At a time when the rationality debate was concerned with causation, Rhodes's ethnography demonstrated that the miscarriages came first, and the explanation for them later, a posteriori.

Rhodes's time vector demonstrated a retrospective allocation of blame, directed at the victim, the afflicted woman. A past event, initially barely considered significant, retrospectively became the cause of misfortune. The final and successful pregnancy had happened in the custody of a biomedical physician but a causal link to biomedicine was not considered. The diagnosis was made during pregnancy, but the ceremony for exorcising the demon was held after successful birthing. When it was finally held three months after the birth, with the infant alive and kicking, the exorcistic ritual became a ceremony simultaneously celebrating life and the woman's achievements. No one else was blamed but the mother of the infant, who by then had just proven her capacity to overcome the evil demonic forces that had caused her previous harm.

The use of time vectors has also been critiqued. In this case, information derived from the ethnographer's observation and from hearsay was treated equally. Each of the events along this vector looked equally valid, but were they? Furthermore, even if one aims to include both outsider and insider perspectives, all mapping along a timeline ultimately represents a device for ordering events as identified by the ethnographer.

As Edwin Ardener (2007: 87) put it, 'an anthropologist as observer is ... required to see himself as a being with a mode of registration'; that is, what we register and temporally order as 'events' ultimately rests on our very own (idiosyncratic) sense for registration. Accordingly, any anthropological account will only reflect what was registered by the eye of the beholder. Ardener comes close here to the insights of Alfred Schütz, whom Csordas (1993: 138) presents as 'the premier methodologist of phenomenological social science'. We will discuss these insights at more length in the third section of this chapter, when reflecting on the foundations of the phenomenological approach that we take in this monograph to spatiality and materiality.

## *Towards a Siting of Spatial Textures*

Mapping is a welcome method to fieldworkers with minimal language competencies, which includes almost all fieldworkers in the initial stages, but it is not discussed in a separate chapter in Bernard's (1994) classic work on anthropological field methods, nor does it figure in the index. Among anthropologists, the drawing of maps appears to be classified among the skills of writing up and knowledge presentation. For instance, they are taught to present their fieldwork locality by zooming in from a bird's-eye view, first of the continent, then of the region and finally of the village or urban neighbourhood (e.g. Coleman and Collins 2006). Mapping, then, tends to be associated with knowledge presentation in a strictly Euclidean space rather than with a fieldwork method.

To co-produce ethnographic knowledge, the objectifying techniques of mapping have to be transformed so as to implicate bodily know-how at the grassroots. Furthermore, the fieldworker's own body is to be crucially implicated in this co-production of knowledge. A siting fieldworker is also committed to sensing the resonances they elicit from the field – the vibes in the room, so to speak – and responding to those with sensitivity. In what follows I will present three moments of fieldwork in which the objectifying technique of mapping was effectively transmuted into practices of siting different fields.

The first instance concerned a neighbourhood of petty enterprise where I became curious about the social entourage of the Chinese medical practice I studied during fieldwork in Kunming in 1988–89. However, walking up and down the street with pen and paper in hand will always make people apprehensive. Drawing maps comes too close to be 'seeing like a state' (Scott 1999).[4] By contrast, setting up a canvas, or simply drawing on a piece of paper the very same street scene that one just wanted to map, is generally acceptable. It transforms the geographer's gaze into that of an artist, and the observer into the person observed – by the crowds of people who then materialise around oneself, coming seemingly out of nowhere. It is then important to be able to interact, speak and joke while drawing, as this sort of mapping may establish rapport.

Second, one may want to turn 'mapping' into a collective and openly performed task. Keen on mapping out the currently inhabited spaces in the old Ming dynasty (1368–1644) mansions of my ancestral village during fieldwork in 2009, I found myself aided by elementary school children who helped me to measure them out. This happened not with a measuring tape, but with our bodies moving through space. If one uses one's own body, for instance by counting one's steps or by timing the period it takes to walk a certain distance, or by stretching out one's fingers, hands or arms to gauge the size of furniture, a window or the width of a door, 'mapping' becomes an ever-present possibility, to hand in situations when nothing other than the proportions of one's own body presents itself as a viable method for the co-production of ethnographic knowledge. In this particular case, the sketching out of how different spaces in centuries-old houses were currently being inhabited, thanks to the children guiding me, also gave me access to more secluded parts of their family's living quarters, such as the kitchen and the storage rooms, into which I myself could not have ventured. As a playful, lively activity, this incident of mapping also acquainted me with the children's parents, thereby opening doors for future conversations and research.

Third, regarding the research presented in this chapter, it was the traffic jams of Nairobi that prompted me to 'map' my field sites. I had hired a taxi driver for several days when interviewing Chinese practitioners in their medical practice, and he drove me from one clinic to the other (they were mostly located in the suburbs, and spread out far from each other).[5] Incidentally, this taxi driver became very interested in my research, with the effect that he remembered the umpteen locations of the Chinese medical clinics I visited. He thereby sped up my research and made it a highly efficient and even fairly comfortable undertaking on every occasion that I stopped by in Nairobi in later years.

Sitting in the car next to the driver, I would amend the written notes taken during the previous interview, but we often got caught in such bad traffic that there was nothing more to add. Given that in traffic jams, small talk never works, it occurred to me that instead of doodling, I might jot down the layout of the clinics I had just visited, as each struck me with its individuality. The spaces I mapped were initially meant to be Euclidean. This changed, however, as I altered my gaze and aimed to follow the movement of the patients through the spatial layout of the Chinese and African medical practices. I was no longer merely aiming to map the functions or symbolic spaces of the clinic (e.g. Bourdieu [1958] 1979). As has been shown in regard to people learning *qigong* practices in Norway, their specific sensory experiences are key to how they will incorporate unknown practices into their own repertoires (Sagli 2017).

Now that I have sketched out how mapping time and space contributes to siting the field and co-producing knowledge with one's respondents, I aim to account for people's experiences of the diagnostic process specific to the spaces through which patients moved in Chinese medical encounters.

## The Ethnographic Focus: How Temporality Textures Spatialities

At the core of this chapter are the spatial textures through which a patient's body moved after entering a Chinese medical practice. In other words, we shall examine the material and spatial textures of the white interstices between the patient and practitioner in a gestalt-psychological figure–ground image, and ask how these spatial textures effected healing through generating a sense of wholeness in patient, practitioner and their surroundings.[6]

First, we follow the patients' movements through the spaces of 'traditional' Chinese medical practices, which were perceived as 'modern' and, sometimes, as (more) 'advanced' medical practices. Second, we visit one of the many different 'traditional' African medical practices on the Swahili-speaking coast north of Dar es Salaam. And third, to avoid becoming too interested in comparing and contrasting the 'African' and 'Chinese' in a culturalising manner, we investigate the layout of a 'modern traditional clinic' (MTC). Between March 2001 and August 2002 (c. four months in four field trips), I worked with Chinese doctors and their patients in Tanzania, Zanzibar (Pemba) and Kenya. In the clinics, I either sat in the waiting rooms with the patients or was permitted to sit in the consultation rooms next to the practitioners, taking notes.

## *'Advanced' Traditional Chinese Medical Practices*

As one entered a consultation room, the table sprang into one's view, with patient, doctor and interpreter (where present) seated around it. Nevertheless, I did not instantly become aware of the table as a texturing principle of Chinese medical encounters during my fieldwork. It was back home, while I reviewed the photos of the Chinese doctors that I had regularly taken with their permission after our informal conversations, that the table struck me as featuring in all of their portraits. Initially, I took the table as an example of the doctors' 'paraphernalia', artefacts that ritual specialists rely on in their ritual practice. The table can certainly be taken as a sign of the Chinese medical doctors' literacy: they write the patient's case record and prescriptions at the table and use it for storing books (not only medical ones, but also books for learning English or Swahili, novels and newspapers, occasionally alongside pamphlets, such as on investment). So, the table was used as a storage place not only for books but also for other openly displayed instruments like those for taking blood-pressure and stethoscopes, as well as calendars (Western-style), plastic Chinese medical models of men with colourful acupuncture channels, packages of so-called formula medicines and the like. In this way, a table could be understood metonymically as an aspect of the doctor's extended body, capabilities and knowledge. Or it could be understood metaphorically, as an emblem of their learning and authority. Yet in this chapter, it will also feature as eliciting a sensory experience in the people who became involved in the diagnostic processes performed in the spaces studied.

The table was usually situated in the centre of the room. It was experienced as the place where conversations and the 'diagnosis' took place. Often, the patient faced the doctor, with the table separating them; or doctor and interpreter sat on opposite sides of the table, but fairly close to each other, and the patient was sat between the two, sometimes at the far end of the table, at a considerable distance. In one very busy practice, the table was built into a tiny consultation room, which was hot and stuffy. In this consultation room the table still marked hierarchical difference, with the practitioner sitting on a large and comfortable chair and the clients on ordinary wooden chairs. However, the size of the space invited quiet conversations marked by closeness and even intimacy.

More often than not, however, the table demarcated difference and distance between practitioner and patient. This asymmetry was sometimes reinforced by the doctor seating themselves on a large padded office chair on the one side of the table, while on the other side, two stools or wooden chairs were offered as seating for the patient and an accompanying family member or friend. In this way the table became part of the spatial texturing during the clinical encounter. In the figure–ground image, it is part of the white space in between, which is not a vacuum but has material contours and textures that can be tactually and otherwise perceived, like a table situated at the centre of a consultation room.

Further exploration of the sensory experience of Chinese medical practices' spatial layout showed that the table was central only in one room among several. As a sketch of a medical practice in Kariakoo, Dar es Salaam (Figure 1.4) shows, and as sketches made at Pangani shopping centre and in the newly established Hurlingham private medical centre in Nairobi also demonstrated, most Chinese medical practices comprised several rooms, each with a specific function.

In general, patients would enter the medical practice via the waiting room. They would be greeted by a woman receptionist, who typically was a local resident and often wore a white coat, like a laboratory assistant. Then, after waiting for a short while – ranging from one to two minutes, to ten, to twenty at most – the patient would enter the consultation room in which the table was the central feature. Many patients left this room within a few moments, with a prescription in hand and a bag full of medicines, without venturing further into the spaces of the practice. Yet without exception, all the Chinese medical practices I visited (about twenty-five in the first two years of fieldwork) had a separate room for a bed, or at least a bed within the same room, often behind white or light blue curtains.

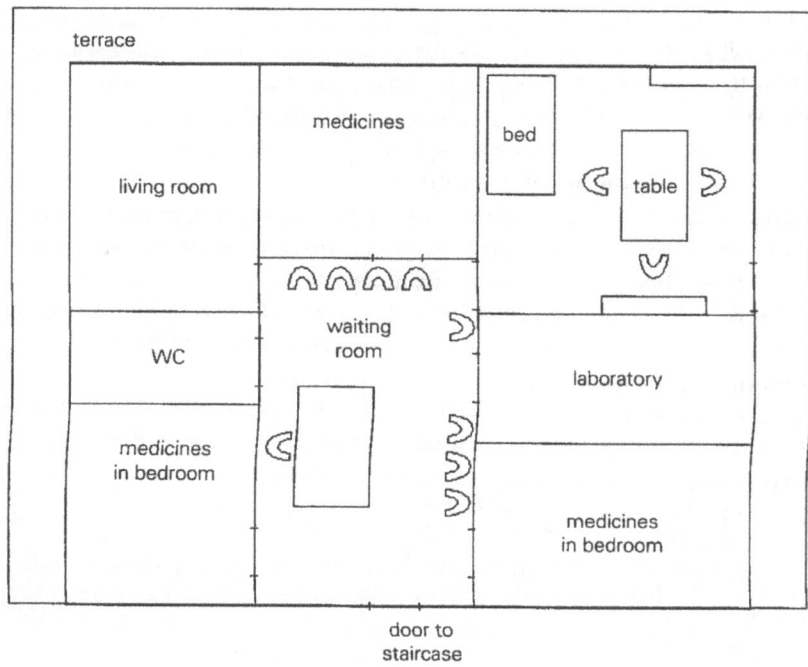

**Figure 1.4.** Chinese medical practice in Kariakoo, Dar es Salaam, 2002. Adapted from Hsu (2005a).

Treatment would typically take place on the bed, and generally was administered to patients lying stretched out in a passive posture. The spatial layout of an 'advanced traditional' Chinese medical practice, which appeared similar to a 'modern' Western medical practice, would thus suggest that the modern scientific ideology – with Phase 1, 'diagnosis', followed by Phase 2, 'treatment' – was indeed adhered to in these separate spaces of table and bed. Table and bed reflected the expectation of a temporal sequencing along a time vector: diagnosis at the table came first and was to be followed by treatment on the bed.

Apart from the consultation room, many Chinese medical practices included a space in which a local laboratory technician would conduct basic Western medical lab tests. They (usually male but not always) had testing equipment to identify malaria, urinary infections, stomach ulcers and, rarely, HIV infection (see Table 1.1).

## Spatial Textures of the Clinical Encounter

**Table 1.1.** Co-opting local expertise: laboratory technicians and their services. Data collected by Elisabeth Hsu, Dar es Salaam, 2001.

| | |
|---|---|
| • B/S for MPS (malaria parasites) | TZS 500 |
| • Stool exam | TZS 500 |
| • Urine R routine | TZS 500 |
| • Urine sugar | TZS 1,000 |
| • Protein 2 albumin | TZS 2,000 |
| • VDRL test (syphilis venereal disease research laboratory) | TZS 2,000 |
| • WIDAL test (for typhoid) | TZS 1,500 |
| • FBP (full blood pressure) | TZS 10,000 |
| • UPT (urinary pregnancy test) | TZS 2,000 |
| • Haemoglobin (iron and protein Hb) | TZS 500 |
| • Gram stain (bacteria gram +/ gram –) | TZS 2,000 |
| • Occult blood (intestinal ulcers) | TZS 3,000 |
| • Fasting blood sugar (Type I and Type II diabetes mellitus) | TZS 2,000 |

The importance of the laboratory in a Chinese medical practice cannot be overemphasised, as it produced rapid results – that is, in less than half an hour – and these results were considered reliable (by Chinese doctors, by their mostly African clientele and by most, but not all, European and North American medical professionals whom I consulted).[7] This 'ritual space' of the biomedical laboratory in Chinese medical practices was one space that the patients generally would not enter (except if blood had to be drawn). Similarly, the inner sanctum in a religious setting is often closed to the public. Yet precisely the activities undertaken in those spaces make them important in medical and religious terms.

As I gathered from various remarks, the Chinese medical entrepreneurs met the desire of patients who were determined to work through the nuisance of a medical procedure as quickly and as efficiently as possible. Western medical services were known for 'red-tapism', and were said to be 'a waste of time', because they provided each of the above services in separate spaces, often in different buildings, and they required patients to queue for each. 'And at last, we are given prescriptions for medicines that cannot be purchased in any pharmacy because they ran out of stock', an exasperated patient in a Chinese clinic in Nairobi explained. One of the main reasons that he and other African patients sought Chinese doctors was that they provided the services of consultation, lab testing, and the handing out of the relevant medicines all in one space. Clearly, it was not primarily the Chinese medical rationale or the Chinese philosophy of life that was deemed attractive, but the entrepreneurial structure of these practices.

It is the case that every Chinese medical practice I visited featured not only a table (for diagnostics) but also a bed (for treatment). However, while in the acupuncture clinics of the People's Republic of China, where I had done extended fieldwork previously, beds were regularly used, in East Africa's private Chinese medical clinics treatment on the bed was frequently omitted, despite the spatial arrangements provided. At one clinic in Dar es Salaam, I never saw a patient treated on the bed in the three weeks that I spent every day there; the bed was in the consultation room but was used as a storage place for the telephone, telephone books and newspapers. So although the spatial arrangement seemed to hint at it, Phase 2 of a clinical encounter, consisting of 'treatment on the bed', did not really feature in many Chinese medical encounters on the Swahili-speaking coast of East Africa. Instead, Phase 2 consisted mostly of the purchase of drugs.

This is most obvious from the spatial texturing of one of the busiest medical practices I visited in East Africa. In that practice, the room with the bed was tiny, situated next to the toilet in the back of the practice, and was used for storing cleaning utensils. Meanwhile, most of the space of the medical practice was occupied by a pharmacy: shelves and shelves of Chinese formula medicines. In this practice, many patients very evidently skipped Phase 1, that is, the diagnosis at the table with the doctor, and entered the practice solely for the purchase of medicines dispensed by two intelligent receptionists. Phase 2 took place not at the bedside, but in front of the counter with formula medicines on display. In those instances, the clinic had primarily the function of a drugstore and pharmacy. On one afternoon, which was in fact the first I spent at that clinic, I saw mainly men going to the large glass counter, purchasing, as far as could be made out from the other side of the room, the bright red cartons of sexual performance-enhancing formula medicines.[8]

In other Chinese medical practices there was a separate storage room for medicines, which like the biomedical laboratory space was closed to the public. This storage room was always locked and veiled in secrecy, even more so than the laboratory. Chinese medical doctors were permitted to sell so-called 'herbal' or 'natural' products, but not Western pharmaceuticals. Nevertheless, it was an open secret that they did so, although the health authorities probably overestimated the frequency of their purchase. Furthermore, the health authorities considered some of the Chinese formula medicines highly controversial, as they were seen as hybrid and inauthentic, if not impure (Douglas 1966, see Chapter 7). However, their ambiguous status as hybrids that combined traditional and modern substances in one also made them attractive (see Chapter 8).

To summarise, the spatial texture of Chinese medical practices generally included a table for diagnosis and a bed for treatment. In this way, the ideal of a clinical encounter that consisted of two separate 'before and after' phases had textured the spaces through which patients were expected to move, namely from table to bed. As cause precedes effect, so diagnosis precedes treatment. Having said this, the spaces of a Chinese medical practice afforded variations in movement: sometimes clients would go directly to the counter and purchase medication, as in a drugstore, sometimes nipping in and out of the practice, and at others, exploring at length their options with the receptionists or the practitioners themselves.

## *'Traditional' African Practices*

There was no bed in the healers' practices that I visited on the Swahili-speaking coast (c. twenty). I understood this to indicate that treatment on a passive physical body that lies flat in front of the healer does not feature prominently in their practices. Nor were tables a prominent feature, although most healers had a basic degree of literacy, and some possessed scholarly medical books. Did this indicate that the principle 'diagnosis comes first, and treatment second' is not central to all healing?

Even more striking than the absence or presence of any particular item, like tables and beds, was the great variation between the spatial textures of different African practices. The African practitioners whom I visited on the Swahili-speaking coast between Dar es Salaam and Tanga worked in spaces that were far less similar in structure to each other than were those of the Chinese practitioners. I took this to indicate that TCM had been subject to more rigorous standardisation than so-called 'traditional African' medical practices.

The visits to all these healers and diviners included some shared features. To access some of these practices, for instance, one entered first into a space where people waited – the courtyard or some chairs on a terrace. This space was separate from the diviner's consultation room. At other practices the patients waiting for treatment formed an audience and were to participate in the healing performances that took place within that very ritual space. Sometimes the diagnostic conversations and healing procedures occurred in different places in a sprawling complex of buildings, at others in a single tiny room. The variation was remarkable. Overall, it is fair to say that the ritual space for most of the 'traditional African' healing did not reflect a division of the medical encounter into the two temporal phases 'diagnosis first, treatment second'.

However, medical practices on the Swahili-speaking coast did feature one recurrent motif: not a bed, nor a table, but a fireplace. Most healers had a fairly clearly defined fireplace, even though it was often small and portable (Figure 1.5). The healer was usually seated close to the fire, but I never observed him (woman healers were rare) seated directly in front of it, as though the fireplace were the central place in the practice, more central to it than the healer himself, who accordingly appeared to be its steward. He could handle the fire while remaining seated; he could light it, add incense to it and feed it with various kinds of resin and wood, thereby generating smoke or

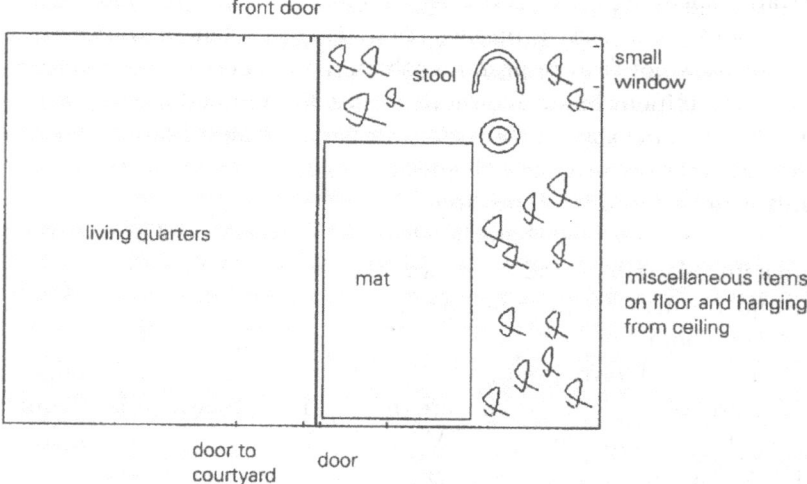

Figure 1.5. Spatial textures of a traditional African healer's practice in Bagamoyo, 2002. Adapted from Hsu (2005a).

scents of various kinds. It was difficult to know what meanings people were prepared to attribute to the fire and the incense burning, as people did not volunteer to comment on this. To me, the ethnographer, the scent was always pleasant, sometimes almost intoxicating, and I assumed that the patients of these healers might experience it as pleasant and intoxicating too, as the scents enveloped us all in a blurry indistinctness.

Sensuous moments of this kind are typically shared with others present in the same space, be they human, divine or otherwise. Blacking (1977a: 13), drawing on his experience of performing chamber music, spoke of the experience of 'a generalized state of fellow-feeling that can be perceived through the sensations of individual organisms'. Csordas (1993: 139) speaks of 'somatic modes of attention'. The nausea that the rich aromatic scent of incense can cause would accordingly be 'a phenomenon of embodied intersubjectivity that is performatively elaborated in certain societies' (ibid.: 146). These 'somatic modes of attention' capture the congruent feelings arising within the spaces of the in-between. They have much in common with the 'moments of meeting' in psychoanalytical jargon (e.g. Stern et al. 1998), yet appear to foreground the embodiment aspect more. Csordas (1993) makes this contribution to anthropological theory in anticipation of a sceptical, cynical, or empiricist position that considers these 'moments of meeting' an illusion or deceit, cunningly brought about by a skilled trickster.

Meanwhile, in the hot, stuffy room, next to the healer who was handling the fire, the rising smoke would suddenly become white and quite thick, but just like a spirit being, it remained intangible as it ascended and accumulated underneath the iron sheet roof or dissipated into the foliage of a tree or through a window in the wall. It felt as though the fire, the scent and the smoke made present spiritual forces.

As it would appear from the above, diagnosis is treatment, or – as, based on fieldwork in north-eastern Tanzania, Steven Feierman (1981) long noted – treatment is diagnosis. In other words, diagnosis and treatment happen in one single, undifferentiated space. Susan Whyte (1997), in her study of Nyole divination, underlines this by emphasising that the practice of divination is governed by several 'principles of uncertainty'. First, the patient is supposed not to know the cause of their illness or misfortune; second, the healer is also expected not to know any details of the case in question. Uncertainty, Whyte emphasises, is the point of departure for a Nyole seance: 'this uncertainty is not simply "there". It is constructed and emphasized' (ibid. 68). The foremost principle of this constructed uncertainty between the healer and his clientele is, in Whyte's analysis, the 'relative privacy' of a seance. The divination hut as the space of the ritual setting contributes, no doubt, to the construction of such 'relative privacy' and uncertainty.

Parkin (1991) too underlined such socially constructed uncertainty in his linguistic anthropological account of Giriama diviners. Uncertainty was created by 'oracular speech' that conveyed 'jumbled ideas and metaphors that suggest various possible interpretations', but ultimately this oracular speech would be 'superseded by an unambiguous classification of the causes of the sickness and the material to cure it' (ibid.: 183). Uncertainty was in this social process caused by what Parkin, with a view to C. G. Jung, called 'simultaneity' (Jung 1968, cited in Parkin 1991). In those moments of uncertainty, Parkin asked, were certain modes of thought other than the scientific one prevailing? He suggested there were, namely *bricolage*, 'the schizophrenic' and 'art' 'thought processes', all three in one, which each contained within it a creative potential.

Several of the healers I visited worked in ritual spaces marked by a certain closeness or intimacy. More than once I found myself cramped into a very small space, together with my Swahili teacher, friend and colleague who was interested in how traditional healers dealt with psychiatric problems. With 'stuff' lying about or hanging from the roof, the room was filled with ritual paraphernalia to the extent that one barely found space to put one's legs; sometimes, ventilation, or just breathing, became a problem. In one practice, the healer turned on an electric fan to alleviate the suffocating atmosphere during the majority of the medical encounter, except for the phase of fumigation that featured in almost all the treatments he performed. Then he turned off the fan, allowing the intoxicating smoke to envelope us all.

Having said this, it is important to bear in mind that there was great variation in spatial arrangements among the healers on the Swahili-speaking East African coast, and not every healer cramped his patients into tiny rooms. Nevertheless, the textured spaces in many practices emphasised what I propose to call a sense of 'syn-

Spatial Textures of the Clinical Encounter

chronicity'. They were produced by carefully attuned body techniques, such as for instance instigating that the healer was seated close beside the patient rather than facing them on the opposite side of a table. This spatial nearness no doubt created an affective closeness. Table and bed, on the other hand, rather than emphasising synchronicity, divided the medical encounter into two phases, one of diagnosis followed by one of treatment; and, rather than enhancing solidarity, both the table and the bed instituted a distance between doctor and patient, accentuating their asymmetry and in this way enhancing the doctor's authority.

## 'Modern Traditional' Clinics (MTC)

Before committing the fallacy of working out a clear-cut contrast between the spatial texturing of 'traditional' African and 'advanced' Chinese practices, let us once again be reminded of the great variety of the African practices. Among those belonged also a 'modern traditional clinic', which advertised itself with the acronym MTC, no doubt playfully echoing that of TCM. The MTC's spaces were textured into two rooms and a corridor between them. One room was furnished with a large table, with an enormous office chair behind it and two small wooden stools in front of it. The other room was closed to the public, except for a decoratively sculpted hole in the wall that opened into the corridor between the two rooms. This second room stored the medicines, which were dispensed through the hole in the wall just like goods were sold in local grocery shops or kiosks. Modernity was widely associated with anonymous economic transactions, and the corridor made it possible that neither the practitioner nor the drug seller would easily see who might furtively nip in for an over-the-counter transaction. In this MTC, the rooms played on a contrast between words and herbs, open and closed doors, the modern and the traditional. The spatial textures furthermore allowed for a temporally staged procedure, not from table to bed, but from table to till.

The layout of this 'modern traditional clinic' demonstrates that it would be misguided to plot an essentialised 'Chinese' against an 'African' culture of healing. Rather, the spatial arrangements reflected a kaleidoscopic refracturing of material culture, like the fireplace, bed and table. The patient's movement from a diagnosis at the table to a treatment on the bed might have reflected an idealised scientific medical intervention, where diagnosis precedes treatment. However, based on the above ethnographic moments, we can say that no such movement took place in any of these 'traditional', 'modern traditional' and 'advanced' Chinese and African practices.

In this context one wonders whether Chinese medical encounters also took place in spaces – without a table and bed – that generated synchronicity before they were Westernised and modernised? In ancient China, diagnosis took place on a mat (Sivin 1995), much the same, we may surmise, as is illustrated in depictions of pulse diagnostics in 'traditional Japan' (Kuriyama 1999: 58–59, Figures 7 and 8). On the mat, it appears, spatial closeness and 'simultaneity' were perhaps not primarily created by schizophrenic talk, stuffy heat or the sweet scent of incense, as in a Giriama diviner's hut, but by a gesture: the physician's touch to examine the patient's *mai* 脉 ('vessel' or 'pulse').

The gesture of touching the *mai* certainly involved being attentive to the pulse as felt at the wrist, which was a body part that could be stretched out as far away as possible in observance of propriety, an issue particularly for women in Late Imperial China (Furth 1999). However, it is difficult to be certain which body parts ancient Chinese physicians touched and what exactly they attended to – the pulse, the body's temperature, the smoothness of the skin's surface or swellings in the subcutaneous tissue (Hsu 2005c). Regardless, the pulse diagnostic touch has great potential to generate a sense of synchronicity between the patient and practitioner. Furthermore, touching can cause a 'presence' that affects everyone in the space in which it happens (Hsu 2010a: 10–14). One feels compelled to suggest that pulse diagnostics enjoyed recognition for millennia and in many different parts of the world precisely due to this empowering tactile sensory event of synchronicity, and not merely for the cognitive insights of pulse diagnosis.[9]

In Late Imperial China, by contrast, as illustrations of the Ming and Qing dynasties (1368–1644 and 1644–1911) show, pulse diagnostics took place at a table, with physician and patient seated on either side. The chair had been introduced into China through Buddhism, as early as the sixth century CE, to ease the strains of meditation (Kieschnick 2003: 241).[10]

We need not go into the history of Chinese furniture, however, in order to show that the exhortation to do 'diagnosis by the table first, treatment by the bedside second' need not necessarily be an intrinsic aspect of Chinese medical practice since antiquity. Rather, it reflects an ideological claim about the 'modern scientific' as opposed to the 'traditional and artful'. To show this, the linguistically inept ethnographer's attentiveness to spatial textures is insufficient. It now becomes necessary to make use of Chinese language skills.

## The 'Synchronicity' of Diagnosis and Treatment in Acupuncture

In the acupuncture clinics I studied in the PRC, it was common practice for a patient to sit in Phase 1 at a table, opposite the doctor, and have their tongue-and-complexion, smell-and-voice, verbal explanation and pulse examined (fieldwork, 1988–89). These four modes of examination (*sizhen* 四诊) allowed the physician to identify so-called 'distinguishing patterns' (*bianzheng* 辨证), which are specific to the occasion and person (*Zhongyi zhenduanxue* 1984, Farquhar 1994). The patient would then see the doctor jot a 'diagnosis' into the case history booklet (which typically was in the client's care), and would then move onto a bed where the doctor would work with acupuncture needles on the body. When I read such case records, I found that most 'diagnoses' were fairly similar, often reading: 'Liver and kidney blood is depleted' (*ganshen xue xu* 肝肾血虚).[11] The sameness of 'diagnosis' contradicted the acupuncturists' doings at the bedside, where on every patient different acupuncture points would be needled. This suggests that it was at the bedside, in the process of deciding which acupuncture point was to be needled, in which way and with which method of the hand (*shoufa* 手法), that the doctor differentiated the patient's particular condition from others. However, no one would be explicit about this. In this context we are reminded that biomedical practice also makes use of the bed for diagnostic purposes, particularly for the manual examinations that through their touching effect a co-presence between patient and practitioner. Accordingly, rather than reflecting a lived experience, the table and bed were indicative more of a claim to modern scientific ideology, according to which diagnosis in Phase 1 and treatment in Phase 2 should happen one after the other, in separate spaces.

No TCM doctor would agree with me that 'diagnoses' are made at the bedside and not at the table, because no TCM doctor would consider the silent procedures of the acupuncturist at the bedside to be 'diagnosis'. The diagnosis was the verbally expressed statement, made at the table and written into the case records. However, it is evident that what was written down at the table was far too general to have a great bearing on the choice of acupuncture points, which differed between patients. From an observer's point of view, individual diagnosis and treatment took place in one and the same space, at the bedside, synchronously.

TCM colleagues who wrote prescriptions for their patients – so-called formulas (*fangji* 方剂) grounded in historically developed, complex reasoning – often made fun of acupuncturists for treating just one condition, namely 'liver kidney blood depletion', and barely any others; they felt superior on the grounds that they considered acupuncture to involve 'just treatment' (*liaozhi* 疗治). However, they were evidently overly literacy-minded, and could not see that the acupuncturist engaged in diagnosis at the bedside, and that good acupuncturists gave each patient a different treatment, even if the 'diagnosis' in the notebook was much the same. Furthermore, TCM-trained acupuncturists themselves spoke of the procedure of choosing acupuncture points as a 'therapeutic skill' (*liaofa* 疗法) rather than as 'diagnostics' (*zhenduan* 诊断). They placed it in the domain of what sociologists of science call 'tacit knowledge'. They adhered to what an anthropologist might call the 'actor's claim', which reflects a standpoint diametrically opposed to that of an outside observer, who sees in the procedures at the bedside a 'diagnostic' process, or more precisely, a simultaneous 'diagnosis-cum-treatment', that is, a matter of 'generating synchronicity'.

## Concluding Remarks

Earlier research into pulse diagnostics, and my question as to why this particular diagnostic method has been so popular in so many places for over two thousand years, suggest that it was perhaps the 'therapeutic touch' given in the process of diagnosis, not unlike the king's healing touch, and experienced as empowering for patient and physician alike, that made this 'diagnostic' method so successful. Alongside the learning surrounding the identification of the patient's pulse qualities, this tactile technique of taking the pulse would produce an affective co-presence and a sense of wholeness. This is said not to belittle pulse diagnostic learning but to query the claim that diagnostic procedures must ideally be separated from therapeutic ones. African or Chinese traditional healing appears to require the opposite, namely 'making whole' through 'generating synchronicity'.

At this point, one could of course point to the importance of the fireplace and the capacity it has to instantiate the co-presence of spirits through rising smoke, which characteristically has an intoxicating scent (Parkin 2007). One could argue that this synchronous sensory engagement is a 'typical' feature of 'premodern' and 'traditional' medical practice, which is absent in more secular 'advanced traditional', 'modern' and 'modern traditional' medicines. However, one would thereby disregard moments of synchronicity that persist even in 'modern' biomedical practice, for instance when the biomedical diagnostic process initiated at the table is continued, if necessary, at the bedside. Furthermore, one would perpetuate the highly problematic presumption that 'traditional' and 'modern' knowledge production is grounded in fundamentally different rationales. This first ethnographic chapter shows quite the contrary: techniques that refine one's sense for the other's bodily co-presence are key for healing that makes whole – in Africa, in China and in Europe.

## Reflections: Contra Solipsism

As the method of mapping showed, a medical anthropologist interested in problematising the issue of causal attribution was well served by mapping the narrative of past events onto a time vector. Meanwhile, a medical anthropologist interested in how healing is effected through 'making whole' resorted to mapping the textures of the white spaces between the figures of practitioner and patient, and in doing so stumbled upon the table and the bed. This socialised-materiality-oriented gaze had her identify other textures in the in-between spaces that seemed to indicate that healing consisted of an effort of 'generating synchronicity'. Only then did I realise that these findings spoke to long-standing and ongoing anthropological and philosophical debates.

### *Shared Somatic States and Somatic Modes of Attention*

We are reminded here of the busiest Chinese medical practice on the East African coast, where a tiny consultation room, accordingly hot and stuffy, invited quiet conversations marked by closeness and even intimacy. Or we might remember the Swahili-speaking 'traditional

African' healer's fire and fireplace whence would rise, at intervals, thick clouds that were almost tangible, yet ever elusive, as is the spirit world. To make sense of these ethnographic events, 'embodiment as an orientation' proved illuminating (Csordas 1990, 1993, 1994a, 1994b). Intense sensuous moments were found to be shared with others present in the same space, be they human, divine or otherwise. John Blacking (1977a) spoke of 'fellow-feelings' and 'shared somatic states', which happened in moments when in the course of performing chamber music participants felt completely in tune.[12] This was well before the embodiment paradigm came into circulation.

Importantly, moments of such 'a generalized state of fellow-feeling' (Blacking 1977a: 13), were infused with a general sense of elation. This positive affective dimension may explain why, once one is on the lookout for them, many healing techniques appear to be geared towards producing such highly charged moments of what might be called an 'elated co-presence'. We are not speaking of 'altered states of consciousness' nor of 'trances', two terms that due to their ethnocentrism are best not used for anthropological analysis. It is a floating, intermediary state, too indistinct to be called a perception: the fumigation with resins intoxicating everyone in a divination hut, the heat and stuffiness of a consultation room prone to eliciting intimate information, the subtle pulse diagnostic touch in ancient China, affecting practitioner and patient sitting on a mat; and there are many more. Moments of such indeterminacy are culturally produced and intentional, and as argued here, are key to processes of healing through reconfiguring wholeness.

According to Blacking, these 'shared somatic states' and 'fellow-feelings' belong among 'the basic condition of human society', underlining that 'non-verbal forms of interaction are fundamental' to anthropology, and in particular, to the field he proposed to call 'the anthropology of the body' (Blacking 1977a: 13).[13] Disregard for these fellow feelings between self and other predisposes people to disease: 'The discourse of non-verbal communication is precisely concerned with matters of relationship – love, hate, respect, fear, dependency, etc. – between self and vis-a-vis or between self and environment and . . . the nature of human society is such that falsification of this discourse rapidly becomes pathogenic' (ibid., citing Bateson 1973b: 388). This makes these non-verbal and sensuous, yet notoriously indeterminate, moments rather important social events. It may therefore not be surprising that techniques for instigating wholesomeness and health – in both preventive and therapeutic ways – are geared precisely towards generating such moments of 'synchronicity'.

Csordas (1993: 139) speaks of 'somatic modes of attention', as noted above. Take the nauseating scent of incense as an 'embodied intersubjectivity that is performatively elaborated in certain societies' (ibid.: 146). It would accordingly induce a moment of mutual heightened somatic attention. It is marked by 'indeterminacy' (ibid.: 150), an indeterminacy that is both existential and methodological, best comprehended as 'an inevitable background condition of our analyses' (ibid.). Csordas is explicit in pointing out the importance of outlining a methodological toolkit that can accurately account for such highly charged, yet indeterminate sensuous moments. He notes: 'We operate with categories of cognition and affect, neither one of which alone can do justice to these phenomena' (ibid.: 147).

Csordas thus proposed considering 'somatic modes of attention' as a theoretical analytic 'construct', which can account for 'culturally elaborated attention to and with the body in the immediacy of an intersubjective milieu' (ibid.: 139). 'Somatic modes of attention' referred not only to instantaneous experiences felt to be visceral and unreflected; he presented them also as a theoretical analytic 'construct'. Csordas tasked anthropology with finding a way to theorise such heightened feelings of co-presence. He did so, not least, in anticipation of 'solipsism' as interpretation that would render them as moments of romanticised self-deception.

Alfred Schütz (1971: 23 ff.) specifically addresses 'solipsism', which evidently arises from a theoretical position that cannot easily accept the idea of 'shared somatic states' (Blacking 1977a) nor of an 'intersubjective milieu' (Csordas 1993). In the section on the 'Social Reality Within Reach of Direct Experience', Schütz speaks of the 'face-to-face situation and the "pure" we-relation'. He continues: 'The temporal and spatial immediacy' – for instance, as relevant here, as experienced in the hot and stuffy divination hut – 'are essential characteristics of the face-to-face situation'. The face-to-face situation becomes constituted through what he defines as *Thou*-orientation: 'The *Thou*-orientation is a prepredicative experience of a fellow being. In this experience I grasp the existence of a fellow-man in the actuality of a particular person who must be present here and now.'[14]

Schütz (1971: 25) continues, 'If you and I observe a bird in flight my "bird-flight observations" are a sequence of experiences, in my own mind just as your "bird-flight observations" are experiences in your mind. Neither you nor I, nor any other person, can say whether my experiences are identical with yours since no one can have direct access to another man's mind.' Any student of twentieth-century thinking will be familiar with this sceptical position, but Schütz continues here with a 'nevertheless', followed by a meticulous step-by-step philosophical argument (not reproduced here).

Schütz's main point is that the we-relation is the starting point of anyone's direct experience, and in the we-relation the I is not preoccupied primarily with itself but busy attending to the *Thou*: 'my partner is given to me more vividly, and in a sense more "directly" than I apprehend myself' (1971: 29). To think about the self requires breaking out of the we-relationship, and if it happens, Schütz claims, it always happens in a second step. Strathern's (1988) identification of 'dividuals' making up 'Melanesian sociality' can be interpreted as an ethnographic instantiation of this self that understands itself always as part of a we-relation. The we comes first, and only in a second step comes differentiation. Importantly, in Schütz's philosophy 'solipsism' has no place: there may be actual instances where you do not understand me, which superficially look like cases of solipsism, but on a more basic level, whatever I experience is critically dependent on the you and how I experience you. Schütz underlines that the self experiences itself primarily through the other.[15]

Merleau-Ponty (1962: 186, cited in Blacking 1977a: 1) seemingly takes up a contrary stance when he says: 'It is through my body that I understand other people; just as it is through my body that I perceive "things"'. The body has intentionality and is orientated towards the world, projecting itself into the surrounding space. However, on a par with Alfred Schütz's argument above, Merleau-Ponty finds that the spatial extension that is 'my body' is secondary to the space surrounding it: 'It is of it'. 'To be a body is to be tied to a certain world, our body is not primarily in space; it is of it' (1962: 148). Merleau-Ponty highlights an existential interdependence between the body and its spatial surroundings, just like Schütz underlines such interdependence between the you and the I. Both posit a continuity between self and other (Schütz) or between the body and its spatial surroundings (Merleau-Ponty), as do the notions of 'shared somatic state' (Blacking) or 'intersubjective milieu' (Csordas).

## Generating Synchronicity

There is a literature in cognitive anthropology (e.g. Cohen et al. 2010) that investigates the bonding of healthy individuals through synchronous activities such as rowing, dancing and singing. These activities, which evidently are governed by rhythm, have been found to enhance both so-called group cohesion and individual performance and self esteem. However, it would appear that these studies are ultimately grounded in an understanding of culture through sameness, that is, the same rhythm.

There is no doubt that the techniques that 'generate synchronicity' in healing processes can and often will be marked by an identical rhythmical beat. However, rather than insisting on sameness in beat, the techniques for 'generating synchronicity' have been seen above to be more complex. They appear to envelop self and other into a variety of wholeness-generating processes specific to the situation. It is not surprising, then, that none other than Confucius (in Ott's interpretation) spoke of 'generating peace/harmony' (*he* 和), rather than insisting on sameness as conducive to sociability.

> The exemplary person harmonizes, and does not make identical; the small person makes identical, but does not harmonize 君子和而不同，小人同而不和. (See *Analects* 13.23, as translated by Ott n.d.: 104)

I came across this saying by Confucius by chance. It is not quoted here to emphasise the difference in moral standing between the exemplary and the small person, nor to plot the modern Western cognitive sciences against ancient Confucian Chinese socio-moral thinking. Rather, my aim is to highlight that *he* 和, which means 'peace' and 'harmony' and can also be pronounced as *huo*, 'mixing', is a form of creating a harmonious wholeness other than by equalising, standardising and seeking sameness. In this context, 'to harmonise', *he*, can be interpreted as an effort to reconfigure ontologically disparate social events such that they nevertheless form a whole. What this requires is a shift, primarily in one's aesthetics of appreciating what constitutes wholeness.

Here, Bruce Kapferer's (2004) theorising of how the 'virtual of ritual' can result in ontologically disparate social events that are being mixed (so-called *huo*) and creating a newly emergent wholeness, becomes interesting:

> The general point ... is that the force of much ritual may be in the dynamics of the rite qua dynamics, in the way sensory perception is dynamically organized [to create 'illusions', which are independent of the cultural meanings placed upon then], which then simultaneously becomes the ground and the force behind the meaningful constructions that are woven into the dynamics. (Kapferer 2004: 41)

This quotation is difficult to understand on its own, yet it has been formulated on the basis of a concern that Kapferer shares with Csordas. They both emphasise that it is important to theorise the indeterminate heightened feelings of co-presence discussed throughout this chapter, the so-called 'somatic modes of attention' marked by indeterminacy and generated by synchronicity. Csordas anticipated that empiricists would dismiss these as 'moments of romanticized self deception' and Kapferer indeed refers to them as '"illusions"', but in quotation marks, because they are not actually illusions. Kapferer shows, by recounting Steven Friedson's (1996) ethnomusicological analysis of the specifics of Vimbuza dancing, that such a sensory 'illusion' – say, of being penetrated by a hard object – can be intentionally created, for instance through a particular technique of drumming. Kapferer does not use Csordas's word 'indeterminate', but gestures in the same direction when he proposes to differentiate these sensory 'illusions' from more solidified 'cultural perceptions'. Both for Csordas and Kapferer these moments that a solipsist would put down to self-deception are key to the structuring of perception and the composite transformation effected through these ritual dynamics.

> The features of rites that for some scholars make them inappropriate to contemporary actualities disguise the crucial potencies of their dynamics that an attention to them as virtualities highlights. (Kapferer 2004: 50)

Kapferer ends his exposition on the note that the ritual-specific 'dynamics of rite qua dynamics' have crucial potencies that are relevant for understanding social developments today, but are completely underestimated by contemporary scholarship. As he seems to imply, it is probably due to their having features typical of the rite as a genre that they are mistakenly reduced to routines of reproducing 'tradition'.

Michael Jackson's (1983a: 339) account of 'lighting a fire' is precisely about such a shift in one's aesthetics and conveys an appreciation of how specific bodily micro-techniques can 'make whole', again in a domain whose relevance for anthropological analysis is undervalued. These micro-techniques of everyday life, which generate a sense of being in sync with the surrounding world, no doubt originate in the long histories of peoples' efforts towards generating figurations of wholeness. As micro-activities performed in what Lefebvre called the practico-sensory realm, they can also be seen to originate in what Antonio Gramsci called 'common sense', or the 'good sense', specifically located in the domain of the practical probing of daily chores (Gramsci 1971; Robinson 2005), as for instance 'lighting a fire'.

Jackson tells us that he initially regarded lighting a fire as a 'mundane chore' that had little bearing on his field research, 'a task to get done quickly so that I could get on with what I took to be more important things' (Jackson 1983a: 340). But once he 'took the pains' to light a fire as Kuranko women did, he found himself 'suddenly aware' of 'the intelligence of their technique'. He noted that 'it maximized the scarce fire wood . . . , produced exactly the amount of heat required for cooking and enabled instant control of the flame'. He mentioned economic ('people economized both fuel and human energy') and aesthetic aspects (an 'economy of effort and grace of movement') (ibid.).

Jackson discussed a mundane skill, a body technique. He thereby made an excellent case 'against undue abstraction in ethnographical analysis' and for 'anthropological understanding to be first and foremost a way of acquiring social and practical skills without any a priori assumptions of their significance or function' (Jackson 1983a: 339). Once he attended to the specifics of the technique, he was struck by what one might call 'deep learning' and an immediate comprehension of the entwining between self and other, women and wood, Kuranko and their natural environment as a whole.

Jackson's insight of studying an everyday technique in order to appreciate the aesthetics involved in configuring wholeness applies also to this ethnography. Rather than being transfixed by (traditional) medical treatment and its efficacy in regard to an assumed *homo rationalis*, the exploration in this chapter – of how the textured spaces of 'traditional' medicine practices facilitated the enactment of certain therapeutic techniques, such as those for generating synchronicity or creating a heightened 'co-presence' between self and other – speaks to a *homo ritualis* (as outlined in Hsu 2011). Techniques that heal – say, through generating synchronicity, 'moments of meeting' or co-presence – affect spatial textures in ways that can be comprehended by a *homo ritualis* rather than a *homo rationalis*. This chapter emphasises how the texturing of spatialities works towards a healing that makes whole.

# Notes

1. Important for us here is that the 'virtual of ritual' structures perception and cognition, as it is neither a representation of external reality nor an alternative reality. 'It bears a connection to ordinary, lived realities, as depth to surface' (Kapferer 2004: 37). Ritual dynamics are composite and hybrid, and they also follow internally given textures and temporalities.
2. Vilaça's critique is accurate regarding how the term 'embodiment' has been applied in medical anthropology among a wide range of authors, rather than being a theoretically valid critique. A much-delayed response is in preparation.
3. As one of the architects of linguistic anthropology and ethnoscience, Kenneth Pike (1967) proposed to differentiate 'etic' and 'emic' meaning analogously to the way that sound was documented either phonetically (through mechanistic sound recordings) or phonemically (according to the hearing of the spoken sounds among people who were linguistically competent).
4. Naturally, there is always the possibility of drawing a map from memory, in the evenings while writing one's diary, and memorising daily the next store adjacent to the ones already recorded. However, this method made me feel like a thief, since I knew it rendered uneasy the people I worked with. It was clandestine knowledge production and not the ethnographic co-production of knowledge to which anthropologists commit.
5. Being thinly spread out is a well-known Chinese migration pattern (*yige Zhongguo ren shi tiao long, sange Zhongguo ren yiqun chong* 一个中国人是条龙，三个中国人一群虫), as I was to learn later (Haugen and Carling 2005 and personal communication, Oxford, 2007).
6. This section elaborates on an earlier version of Elisabeth Hsu. 2005a. 'Time Inscribed in Space, and the Process of Diagnosis in African and Chinese Medical Practices', in Wendy James and David W. Mills (eds), *The Qualities of Time: Anthropological Approaches*. Oxford: Berg, pp. 155–70.
7. One of the latter explained that there was scope for improving further education for paramedical staff in East Africa, and that currently, lab technicians who might start seeing plasmodia where there was just an impurity of the blood sample had no opportunity to correct and improve their professional performance.

*Spatial Textures of the Clinical Encounter*

8. This was a brief interval, but it was not entirely unrepresentative (see Chapter 8). On the advert for the range of disorders that this practice treated, consisting of blue script on a glass door, 'impotence' was the only handwritten item. It was likely added at a later stage due to the clientele that this Chinese practitioner eventually attracted.
9. According to Csordas (1993: 143–44), the Sinhalese pulse diagnostics that Daniel (1984) described in terms of Peircean semiotics is best understood as a 'somatic mode of attention' (further explained below). It highlighted iconicity as central to the Sinhalese technique. By contrast, in some realms of Chinese pulse diagnostics the indexicality of the tactile sign mattered too (Hsu 2010a: 347–57). Regardless of whether an iconic confluence of pulse rhythms is sought or merely an indexical sign, the pulse-taking hand's touch causes a 'co-presence' between practitioner and patient.
10. Tables with long legs are widely known from illustrations dating to the Song dynasty (960–1279), but not the Tang dynasty (618–907); they must represent an adjustment in height required by the long-legged chair.
11. Blood, kidneys and liver all have specific Chinese medical meanings, and should not be mistaken for what these words designate in biomedicine. Depletion is a typical sign of old age, and the liver that stores blood dries out in old age. Acupuncture wards took on the functions of a day-care centre for the elderly (Ots 1990a), mostly for women but also for men (fieldwork in Chengdu, 1985, and in Kunming, 1988–89).
12. What Blacking (1977a: 147–48) calls 'sensations', Csordas (1993) refers to as 'somatic modes of attention'. Other anthropologists may speak of 'intuition' and 'imagination', 'perceptions' or 'experiences'.
13. Of interest for the history of medical anthropology in the UK is that the ASA volume on the anthropology of the *body* was edited by an ethnomusicologist, John Blacking (1977b), one year after *Social Anthropology & Medicine,* edited by the medic J. B. Loudon (1976). Gilbert Lewis and Murray Last published in both volumes, which have since become foundational for a broadly conceived medical anthropology in the UK. For an outline of medical anthropology's history in Europe, see Hsu and Potter ([2012] 2015) and Hsu (2012c).
14. What Schütz calls the 'prepredicative experience' I understand to refer to an experience that arises from an engagement with surrounding spaces before the textures of these spaces are perceived and classified, that is, it refers to what Csordas (1994b) calls the 'pre-objective'. There is always some 'indeterminacy' in our experience of the world. Or, as Schütz put it, the *Thou*-orientation is 'actualized in different degrees of concreteness and specificity' (1971: 24). If the *Thou*-orientation is reciprocal, a 'social relation becomes constituted' (ibid.).
15. He underlines that in a face-to-face situation it comes naturally to the self to be oriented to the other.

# Chapter 2
# Misunderstandings, and the Spaces They Create

## Fieldwork: Language-Learning as an Ethnographic Method

How do you learn a language? As adults we are encouraged to learn other languages by learning their grammar in class or by repeating idiomatic phrases in the language laboratory (or both). I did the latter while preparing for my second field trip to East Africa. Every Saturday morning I spent two hours in the language lab. However, I found it very hard to keep up this practice. I looked for a conversation partner. Surprisingly, many people in Oxford knew Swahili, but life was too hectic to arrange regular sessions.

### Basics

I have always learned spoken languages best in the places they are spoken, perhaps because language learning is for me an embodied process that almost 'comes naturally', like swimming in the water. One is immersed in a language's phonemic sounds and prosodic rhythm. For my first field trip I had bought *Teach Yourself Swahili*, and I got through to Lesson 2. As usual for a new field site, for which one has to obtain permits and licenses, I spent long hours waiting for the completion of bureaucratic procedures, and while sitting on the benches in corridors I memorised vocabulary and practised how to greet and thank with willing respondents who were also waiting. However, the Great Leap Forward in language learning happened during the second field trip.

First, I found an excellent teacher. I had by then already made friends with a local researcher interested in how local healers treated mental health problems. She not only introduced me to several local healers, but would also spend one hour of every other day in conversation with me, reviewing the contents of said book for an agreed sum. She had a genuine interest in language and linguistics, was lots of fun to be with and was very patient; she targeted me with new sentence structures at exactly the level of language learning that I was at. This resulted in a wonderful and edifying experience for me, and I hope for us both.

Second, during this fieldwork period I was involved in daily semi-structured interviews with patients, some of whom spoke to me only in Swahili (see Chapter 4). This gave me the opportunity to repeat the same questions over and over again. Nevertheless, my Swahili was so rudimentary that I often had to rely on family members who acted as interpreters or, occasionally, on the taxi driver who had driven me to the patient's home. He spoke but a smattering of English, but as days and weeks progressed, he became very knowledgeable of my linguistic competencies, and was able to translate the interviewees' Swahili into a Swahili I understood. In cases when I did not understand a sentence that appeared key to me, I had it written into my notebook and in the evening asked my teacher what it meant.

Third, the conversational training and the interviewing would not have progressed as rapidly if I had not spent another hour or two daily on my own, generally after dinner, by my tiny desk lamp (not available in the entire city of Dar es Salaam but bought in England), memorising words and reading aloud idiomatic phrases and sentences. In order to hold a conversation about life, misfortune and luck, one has to know the language quite well, not least to understand the implicit and pick up on the unsaid. However, to collect the basic sociological information needed at the beginning of an interview, one can progress quite far with a limited vocabulary.

What is your name, your age, your gender, your religion, your place of birth, your current residence, your profession, your education? Why did you go to see the Chinese doctor? Which medications did they give you? Which practitioners did you visit and whose counsel have you sought, before seeing the Chinese doctor? I would also ask about the care situation: are you single, married, divorced? Do you have help in the household?

When, in this context, I asked, *kabila gani* (which 'tribe'/ethnic group do you belong to?), Tanzanians would usually smile and turn their head to the side in embarrassment, or laugh out loud and make clear that this was not a question to ask. Tribal conflict was a problem that President Julius Nyerere recognised early on as a pandemic hindering the development of a modern nation state. For this reason, I suppose, the Tanzanian interview partners shied away from answering this question. I spoke rudimentary Swahili, but was instantly reminded to consider history. For the same reason, I suppose, the Natural History Museum in Dar es Salaam, which in 2001 was both run-down and deserted, did not exhibit the material culture of different 'tribes', but merely indicated items' places of manufacture, and presented them, like the Pitt Rivers in Oxford, in terms of function and applicability. The question *kabila gani?* also caused slight discomfort in Kenya, where 'tribal conflict' was flaring up again and again during the presidential elections during and after the period of my research. For some, it lay at the root of Africa's poverty.

The intonation of an utterance is of course important, often more so than the pronunciation. In Chinese specifically, the proper *shengdiao* 声调 (the tone of a word) is considered more conducive to communication than the accurate *fayin* 发音 (pronunciation), and although Swahili does not have tones, it has melodic rhythms, like any language. Therefore, I found that time is well spent if it is just used for producing new and unusual sounds, both when learning Chinese in the PRC when I was 19 years old and when learning Swahili in Dar es Salaam at more than double that age.

## *Walking Rhythms*

I felt I made great progress in language learning while walking, as walking bundles body and mind into its rhythm. I walked the city, as does Ingold's (2011) 'wayfarer', long before I became aware that wayfaring was being theorised as an ethnographic method (e.g. Lee and Ingold 2008). On my first field trip I had stationed myself at the Swiss Garden Hotel. In many ways this place provided an ideal entry point into a new field site, as the hotel residents included many aid workers, university-based researchers, and UN and NGO staff, some of whom had 'known' Tanzania for decades. I had the privilege to have interesting conversations with them, usually over breakfast. Yet all too soon they left, one by one, as they were called to work. Usually, a chauffeur in a fancy Land Rover came first to fetch the WHO officer. Then, a slightly smaller four-wheel-drive vehicle called for the FAO representative. Then, a taxi came for the medical researcher, and thereafter an old NGO jeep for our newest arrival: a computer troubleshooter, an East German (he spent just a few days with us; it was his first visit to Africa, and he marvelled at the region's lush greenness, which completely toppled his idea – instilled by the media – of this continent as a hunger-ridden desert zone). Finally, after everyone had left, the gardener would open a side gate for me, as I slipped out into the blazing sun and half a mile up the hill to Muhimbili hospital, just in time to be there when the staff had their coffee break after seeing their early-morning patients.

On these walks I was occasionally joined by mostly male youths. They sometimes walked for miles with me, sometimes chaperoning me through difficult territory (e.g. some neighbourhoods of informal settlements), more often just providing me with company (some were keen to practise their English). I had learned early on, as a tourist in the Maghreb in my twenties, that seeing a woman walking unencumbered on her own in public places makes men feel uneasy not only about her, but also about themselves not offering her protection. So I let myself be accompanied by whoever wished to do so, except the very obnoxious, who were mostly quite easy to shake off because of their single-mindedness (about selling things or having sex). Having said this, I was well aware that it was risky to walk with any man through unknown terrain. One of the principles I adhered to very consequentially was that however interesting our conversation turned out to be and however enticing a cold drink at a friend's *shamba* was, I would not let myself be diverted from the destination I had when starting to walk: the hospital, the Sheraton with its ATM, the ruins of a mosque (as mentioned in the *Lonely Planet*) or the recently-set-up tourist resort and nature reserve, which demonstrated that the late-liberal Ethnicity Inc. (Comaroff and Comaroff 2009) had made impressive inroads even into one of the still quite rural townships of Dar es Salaam's hinterland, which was on the cusp of turning into a suburb. One could say that walking with someone else creates co-presence (Lee and Ingold 2008), and without having to be in step as lovers can be, one inadvertently relates to another's movement in ways that resonate with one's own.

Rhythm was key to my field experience of language learning, and walking, in the company of another person or alone, reinforced rhythmicity. Language is generally associated with symbolisation, imagination, cognition and what André Leroi-Gourhan (1993: 359) calls 'figurative life', an idea not unrelated to that of his senior contemporary Merleau-Ponty (1962: 194), who commented on language's 'figurative significance'. Yet language learning throws us back onto very basic sensory and rhythmic aspects of speaking. This makes speaking a body technique, an embodied experience and even a sense perception, as it is recognised among some peoples such as the Anlo-Ewe of West Africa (e.g. Geurts 2002: 58–61). Speech as a sense perception is indeed a lived experience when one is in the course of learning a language; it is as though one has to learn to perceive how to fit oneself linguistically into an existent rhythm of verbal exchanges. I still remember vividly today how I was told off by my host as one evening we were walking past the fields of local Zaramo farmers, and one of them politely greeted me: 'Shikamoo'. The rhythm of the words exchanged in a greeting would have required me to say: 'Marahaba', but I had been lost in my own thoughts and had not speech-perceived (i.e. 'heard' in English) and responded to the man greeting me.[1]

I speak here of perception in Leroi-Gourhan's (1993: 282) sense, as when he noted: 'Broadly speaking, individual perception intervenes between external rhythms and an individual's motor responses to them.' If speech was a sensory modality of perception, *shikamoo* was the external rhythm and *marahaba* would have been my motor response to it. I suppose I did not perceive the farmer's greeting because I considered myself as being invited for supper at my host's family home in a suburb of Dar es Salaam, and I was cued into performing the kind of non-responsiveness to external rhythms that makes possible the anonymity of life in the city. Historically, Dar es Salaam became very rapidly urbanised (see introduction), but what this rapid urbanisation implied is rarely spelled out in the social science literature. This is that Dar es Salaam's 'sprawling suburbs' were often more rural than urban in their physical aspect, atmosphere and rhythm, and this evidently had a direct impact on the above episode of inappropriate sociolinguistic conduct. In the countryside one greets passers-by, but not in the city.

In *Gesture and Speech*, Leroi-Gourhan (1993: 281), describes rhythm as constitutive of 'physiological aesthetics':

> In animals, the simplest forms of behaviour can, from the sensory point of view, be reduced to three levels: that of feeding behaviour, which ensures the functioning of the body by processing materials assimible by the or-

ganism; that of physical affectivity, which ensures the genetic survival of the species; and that of integration in space, which makes the two others possible. . . . The aesthetic implications of these three levels are still observable in humans; we could describe them as 'physiological aesthetics'. They bring into play, in varying proportions, all the instruments of the sensory apparatus: Visceral sensitivity, muscular sensitivity, taste, smell, touch, hearing and balance, and sight. (Ibid.: 282)

Leroi-Gourhan links the 'sensory equipment' of human beings to that of animals – '[T]he human is not known to have any organ of perception not shared with the rest of the mammals' – and he sees rhythm as a basic organising principle of perception more generally: 'We obey the rhythms of our digestion, we feed at fixed times, in a crowd, we obey the collective rhythm like a sheep, . . . , our muscles flex and relax without our consciousness coming into play.' It follows logically that: 'Rhythms are creators of time and space, at least for the individual. Space and time do not enter lived experience until they are materialized within a rhythmic frame' (ibid.: 309).

Leroi-Gourhan then proceeds to differentiate between musical rhythms and technical rhythms: 'Musical rhythm generates behavior that symbolically marks the frontier between the natural world and humanized space, while technical rhythm materially transforms untamed nature into instruments of humanization' (ibid.: 310). Leroi-Gourhan links the 'rhythmicity of walking' to 'musical rhythm', and this does not appear to have been contested since. Meanwhile, he says of the latter: 'Technical rhythm [like hammering] has no imagination, it does not humanize behaviour but only raw matter' (ibid.: 310). Needless to say, recent research into material culture has revised this viewpoint (e.g. Ingold 2013). Language learning often feels like the engagement in a technical rhythm, as though one were in the process of transforming 'untamed nature', that is, the tongue, lips and throat, into an 'instrument of humanization', namely speaking. Language learning surely partakes in both 'technical rhythm' and 'musical rhythm'. It would appear that both rhythms are reinforced by the 'rhythmicity of walking', and their distinctiveness is thereby dissolved and rendered irrelevant to our analysis.

In summary, we owe much to Leroi-Gourhan for enabling us to see sensory perception as being sensitive to the external universe's rhythms, which can be circadian, lunar or seasonal, or can arise out of the rhythmicity of the action itself, like walking on one's legs (posterior limbs) or hammering with one's arms (anterior limbs). Leroi-Gourhan recognised this connection. He underlined that sensory perception was intricately linked to the sensing of rhythms external to the organism and to the adjusting to these external rhythms with the organism's muscular responsiveness. In this way he was able to comprehend sense perception and muscular action as part of a continuum that enabled the organism to partake in the rhythmic changes of the environs into which it projected itself. Leroi-Gourhan thought of human beings and animals not in opposition to each other, as did scholars of the humanist tradition, but as organisms that are part of a continuum of different life forms that to a certain degree share a common aesthetics. The physical activity of walking, no doubt, provided a rhythmic co-presence that enhanced my language learning.

## *When in Suspense, Do Small Talk*

Walks brought with them waits as well. In the space of suspension while waiting for the bus, ferry, *dalla dalla* or *matatu* minibus, when one did not know whether or when one would meet the other again in future, I learned so much from my respondents that I could never have learned in a formal interview.[2]

If waiting times were protracted, they sometimes turned into useful occasions for language learning, particularly if a group of people was involved. These episodes of protracted waiting made me think about the history of our discipline and social anthropology's predilection for recording genealogies. British social anthropology, as we know (Kuper 2015), was interested in government and researched social structure. However – who knows – perhaps some more mundane and more practical reasons played a role in early social anthropologists' reliance on the genealogical method as well? A very basic linguistic repertoire is required to ask: Is this your sister? How many do you have? Is that your brother? Is he elder or younger? Before long, I found that detailed branches of family trees were being drawn in the sand as I was jotting new vocabulary into my notebook. Combined with other fieldwork goals, this minimal linguistic effort no doubt produced maximal sociopolitical insight. The youth, or sometimes just elementary school children, enjoyed it. They were competitive between each other too. If I made inquiries into his family, I had to ask after hers too. They were fascinated by how I tried to pronounce the most mundane words, and they spelled them out for me, patiently repeating their pronunciations. And then, suddenly, they swarmed off. Or, finally, my ship or my bus had arrived.

## *Speaking, Reading and Writing Chinese*

When I started fieldwork in March 2001, I spoke fluent Chinese and had spoken it for over twenty years. I had also received Chinese medical training in the PRC. I received it in Chinese, in the classroom and the clinic, while conducting fieldwork for eighteen months (Hsu 1999), and I had just edited a volume on recent and pre-twentieth-century Chinese medical history (Hsu 2001). I could read Chinese medical textbooks quite effortlessly, and once I was familiar with the doctors' handwriting, I could decipher the Chinese of their patient records. My sponsor in Tanzania was a medical anthropologist who had a doctorate in ethnomedicine from the University of Vienna and worked at the Traditional Medicine Unit in Muhimbili hospital. It was Muhimbili hospital's HIV/AIDS clinic that had brought me to Tanzania. Yet the research permit I obtained in December 2001 specified that I was not to conduct research into Chinese medical treatment of HIV/AIDS.

This meant that I was left to study Chinese medicine as offered in the urban spaces of the emergent global health markets burgeoning mostly in the informal sector. People with whom I discussed this research option were ambivalent, yet their comments revealed that it was a poorly understood phenomenon: 'The problem with Chinese treatment is the language, their medicines are in the Chinese language.' Why was I interested in researching Chinese medicine, I was then asked, and how did I think it was possible to converse with the practitioners? 'They are so secretive'[3] and 'their treatment is very expensive'.[4] An intellectual who said of himself, 'I am a modern man and a law student at university', queried my motives: 'Are you making some research [on them], on which grounds?' I was then told: 'TCM centres on the towns, most are not doctors, they are businessmen.' I was predicted to encounter deviousness, in the same breath as I was told: 'I know some are very good doctors'. The heterogeneity of comments that Tanzanian contacts and friends volunteered presaged a difficult terrain. My Chinese language skills would be key to opening that aspect of my research field.

An unabated interest in 'traditional healing' led me, during my first four field trips in the first two years, along the coast to Bagamoyo, to a TM/CAM specialist 'from the inland' who was incredibly syncretic and synthetic in his practice; to Manzese, where a nurse at Muhimbili hospital regularly went into a state of speaking in a high voice with the spirits for divinatory purposes; to a Sukuma healer 'who had *tunguli*' and hence 'did the real thing'; and to officials who worked in medical bureaucracies but spent most of their time treating private patients in their office hours. I went past Bagamoyo to the 'Tanga AIDS group', to representatives of herbalist medical associations, to Lushoto's architectural heritage of colonial science and pre-Second World War medical innovation and finally back to the South Asian healer who lived just round the corner in Ilala, on the fifth floor, not far from the hotel I stayed at from my second fieldwork period onwards. This healer had not advertised himself loudly but depended entirely on word of mouth within the Indian community.

> You have to make yourself small, then traditional healers will teach you. If you do not know how he is harvesting, when, how he prepares the medicines, boil or chew them . . . If you go there as the boss and want to teach him, he will not teach you. 90% of the people speak Swahili. If you know Swahili, they will like it. And Swahili is not a difficult language. (April 2001, small notebook, p. 11).

In summary, by treating language learning as an ethnographic method or technique, I experienced it as a sensory process that involved both the modification of existent and the acquisition of new body techniques, their refinement and their mutual attunement. I mentioned specifically the experience of turn-taking and rhythm in sociolinguistic interaction, walking and waiting, and the alternations between goal-directed movement and periods of being in suspense, where languish can turn into languaging.

# The Ethnographic Focus: Thriving on Misunderstandings

In a hot and stuffy consultation room, Dr Ming sat on one side, with me sitting next to him, while the patient and their carer were seated on the opposite side of the table. The tape recorder was on the table, and patients who had just entered the room were asked whether they would mind to be recorded, to which only some objected. Meanwhile, each and every patient closed the door firmly after they en-

*Misunderstandings, and the Spaces They Create*

tered this tiny room. This heightened the heat and stuffiness, and created an atmosphere of intimacy. In this clinic, which was one of the busiest on the East African coast, the doctor saw around fifteen to forty patients a day, which meant that he usually spent no longer than ten minutes on each consultation, and often less.[5]

The patients would hand their records to the doctor, who then glanced at the notes that he had taken on their medical history. The patient's records each had a number and the recorded name, age and gender of the patient. In this clinic, the records were kept deep within a very large brown folder, demonstrating very tactually the doctor's absolute discreetness. The receptionist stacked them up, ordered according to number, on the shelves behind her counter, stationed just in front of the consultation room's door. The openly displayed bureaucratic meticulousness of well over seven hundred records no doubt inspired confidence in Dr Ming's medical prowess (see also Street 2012).

This was the only clinic in which I could tape-record the medical consultations (by the end of my fieldwork I had seen well over 400–800 overall, but had recorded only about forty consultation interviews). Yet I also took handwritten notes in my notebook on several hundred patients. Central to what follows are the conversations held during the clinical encounter. One could characterise them as being marked by a probing rapprochement where both sides were well aware that image-making, trickery, and stealing and deceiving were daily concerns. Patients entered the sphere of the Chinese medical practice with curiosity, and sometimes also with a sense of honour, masculinity and hope, probing the possibility perhaps of appropriating into their own repertoire what was newly on offer.

Dr Ming's notes contained professional TCM jargon, but not exclusively. The language in which they were written was quite heterogeneous. It contained phrases and words that much like the script on the Chinese medical formula medicines' packaging were used to colloquially express complaints (e.g. 'headache' or 'stomach ache' in Chinese). It sometimes also contained specific Chinese and Swahili folk-medical terms (e.g. *gesi* meaning 'gas' or 'heartburn'), alongside remarks made in standard TCM terminology, Western biomedical terminology (in Chinese) and folk-medicalised biomedical vocabulary (e.g. 'sugar' for diabetes or 'pressure' for hypertension). Dr Ming was not a TCM doctor who had graduated from a TCM university after five years of medical study. Rather, he was a young man who had once aspired to study history at his province's prestigious university. After participating in a major student movement and failing university entry exams, he started applying for a passport to emigrate, while attending evening classes in TCM alongside others in Chinese cooking. These were the Chinese arts and technologies, he said, that Western audiences had learned to appreciate. His English was unusually good; he had learned it in high school. It was thanks to his language skills that he was approached at short notice to work as an interpreter for a semi-governmental firm in Uganda. He seized the opportunity.

Dr Ming explained that he had been learning on the job, well aware of his shortcomings in medicine. He was a fast learner. He apprenticed himself with the only Chinese medical doctor in East Africa who had, in addition to the required regular five-year training (*benke* 本科), completed a three-year master's course (*shuoshi* 硕士) in TCM. However, by the time I got to know Dr Ming, the two had fallen out with each other. The former said of the latter that he was a cheater and not a professional medic in any case; the latter of the former that he smoked and spat, did not keep records, and was lazy and impolite such that many patients would not buy the medicines he prescribed, and the business declined. Worse still, he apparently interfered with matters regarding Dr Ming's employees.

## *Good Attire, a Good Business*

Dr Ming's complaint about his former teacher and confidant contained the secret to his business: Dr Ming had immaculate professional attire; he was always friendly, always polite and never rough. He told me that establishing this social persona was the most important thing for being a good doctor: he made sure his clothes were ironed and clean, which was an important task for one of the several part-time housekeepers he employed, and he always came to work by car. In 2002, when I visited his practice for the first time, his car was second-hand, but thereafter he had on every visit a fancier car. Not that he was a car fetishist; he upgraded the brand of his cars on a calculated basis, for his business. He also converted to Christianity shortly after setting foot in Kenya, attending a church populated mostly by Chinese. So as would be expected of a Chinese businessman, his practice was open daily, except on Sunday mornings when he went to church.

While I worked in Dr Ming's practice, the elder of the two receptionists, who was of impressive stature and very loyal to him, made sure that I complied with the standards of the business: 'I don't believe you dress like this in Oxford. Why don't you give us the respect you give your colleagues and dress as you do in England?' I told her that I wore natural fabric, always, everywhere. The nylon dresses that she proposed I wear, the fashionable and stylish choices, had never been mine. But she was right, of course. I was not complying with the rules of the business. Nor did I dress like a tourist. Rather, I savoured the opportunity to wear colourful clothes, the kitenges I had bought in West Africa years earlier. I was well aware that in East Africa, women dress in this way only at home for doing housework in the compound, but I felt uncomfortable in a *kanga* when I very obviously was not assuming one of the local feminine roles.⁶ However, I did take extra care to cover my shoulders and legs in order not to be indecent, well aware that the sight of bare legs can exert erotic attraction. 'And look at your shoes!', the receptionist exclaimed. So I did. They were made of the finest black leather, but they were old and worn out, covered in mud and dust. It was obvious that I walked long distances with them (see previous section). 'Get yourself some high heels!'

## Brokers Brokering with Brokers

Dr Ming knew that his business depended on the reputation that local brokers, like his receptionists, gave it. He made sure that he paid them a good salary and occasionally gave them bonuses. Some doctors also gave the friends and family members of their employees treatment at a special rate. In this case, the two receptionists enjoyed each other's company, and Dr Ming supported that. He also had a lab assistant on his premises on and off, and sometimes a third receptionist, in addition to the cleaning personnel that he hired by the hour from the business next door.

After working in Mombasa for several years, Dr Ming also opened a restaurant, or more accurately, as he insisted, his wife did so. Other TCM practitioners also had second and third businesses on the side; the wife of one was embarrassed when during the medical practice's opening times, a customer made inquiries about sofa transportation (6 December 2005, diary entry), revealing a furniture business, in addition to their second-hand car business. So when Ming and I were comfortably seated in the car, driving between work and his house where I would lodge with him and his wife, I took advantage of this comfortable and enclosed space to ask him uncomfortable questions. For instance, I would ask whether petty theft was an issue with his employees. He answered, as the sovereign businessman would, that he would rather trust them than supervise them too closely.

> I ask him whether his employees steal, and he says not his, they know he is too intelligent. How many times has his staff changed [at the restaurant]? One big loss was the cook who had worked for the former Korean restaurant owner. This was because he knew the taste[s] of the locals well. Then, he and his wife [who was the owner of the restaurant] had called a Sichuanese cook over, for six months, but they did not prolong the visa; Ming did not say why. He had currently four cooks; 'all are Africans' (*dou shi heiren* 都是黑人), he said. He had had two waiters who fought each other over the tips; so, he fired them both. The drawback was that they had been experienced waiters. He also sacked the first bar man because he had cheated, but he, Ming, instantly found out. There were actually many changes in personnel but Ming did not want to acknowledge that. He avoided further questions and said repeatedly that he trusted his employees fully, rather than supervising them too closely. (9 December 2005, diary entry, slightly modified)

In December 2005, Dr Ming's phone rang incessantly during the medical consultations in his hot and stuffy consultation room. He answered every call. In most cases he spoke in Chinese, often saying that he would ring back later. In other cases, he left the room and went outside onto the street to talk, sometimes for up to five minutes. When he came back, he continued his conversations with his clientele, as though he had not been interrupted. All practitioners in East Africa found themselves encumbered by telephone calls, and some ingeniously wove them into their medical practice (Parkin 2011). Thus, some local Swahili-speaking healers went centre-stage, sonically talking on the phone in front of the crowd of patients waiting to consult them. They engaged in long discussions, publicly displaying their privileged connection to some distant other. This made present the other, who was disembodied and not seen in person, yet powerful and directly spoken to, like a deity or spirit. However, in Ming's case, some of his patients, whom I later interviewed in their homes, considered the many phone calls rather disruptive.

## Trusting, Yet Probing

Trust is a tricky issue. How does one instil trust in one's patients, employees and business partners? How were 'African' patients and 'Chinese' doctors brought into conversation, and ultimately, how would spatial textures enable them to collaborate in ways that would co-produce wholesomeness and health? Dr Ming, with a twinkle in his eye, chirped the Chinese Communist Party line: 'Soft touch', he said, 'light touch.' It seemed that for him, there was no difference between the art of gaining wealth through commerce and that of repairing health through medicine. In both cases, he implied, one was interacting with living beings who had internal dynamics of their own.

Is the probing attitude of 'trying out' a desperate search on the part of the patient in urban spaces, where ignorance and greed multiply with suffering and poverty, and where 'suggestions and counter-suggestions come from all directions – you do not know whom to trust' (Das and Das 2005: 80)? Or is it part of everyday life to probe resistances, to probingly push one's horizons and to be basically trusting, yet curious about the uncertain (Whyte 1997; Geissler and Prince 2010b)? Healers can only 'try their best'; but what happens if the treatment is not successful (Parkin 2011)? Some invoke God's blessing, others compliance, that is, the patient's willingness to participate in the process of treatment. Some speak of witchcraft and curses. Either can entail long therapeutic journeys, across religious boundaries too (Rhodes 1980; Beckerleg 1994; Beckmann 2012). Patients may have the courage to transgress into an other and unfamiliar terrain temporarily, but how is more enduring trust generated? Why should anyone trust the promised, or what is heard or viewed as being promised? Lewis (2021: 188) points to Pierre Janet's (1859–1947) 'outstanding work on psychological healing' and his finding that 'moral persuasion' mattered perhaps more than 'verbal technique'.[7] Inner moral strength inspires trust, no doubt, and nurturing personal relationships can grow from it. This is an important insight. However, how will the fieldworker be able to recognise inner moral strength? Let us consider techniques not merely as superficial externalities but as part of the texturing forces of the non-Euclidean space that provides a matrix for all living beings. Let us ask, accordingly: How is the trust generated that causes people to return, to commit, to comply, to be willing to consider moral persuasion and feelings of a concern for a whole to arise? The soft touch that Dr Ming alluded to can be put forward as a superficial strategy or technique, a deviously gentle trigger, but perhaps it is to be understood not merely in a mechanistic way but as a disposition that directs the patient into a cascade of events once they have entered the spatial textures of a Chinese medical practice and followed its flow. Trust is then no longer psychological capital that builds up within a clearly bounded individual, but an aspect of the interdependencies between self and other. Getting to trust someone, and their healing efforts, is then a configurative process that one can let gradually happen, and learning to live with the tensions of being part of this process might eventually reconfigure or even dissolve seemingly diametrically opposed dimensions of the self, such as 'gut feeling' and 'moral persuasion'.

## *Semiotics of the Body and Its Parts*

Social and medical anthropological studies of the medical encounter and research into the history of the body have often centred on metaphors of the body (e.g. Lévi-Strauss 1963; Tambiah 1969; Lloyd 1983; Martin 1987; Kirmayer 1992) and the semiotics of cultural difference (Duden 1991; Kuriyama 1999; King 2013). My field research in Chinese medical clinics certainly led to the recording of instances of a semiotics of the body: a Swahili-speaking patient's understanding of the body often differed from that of biomedicine, that is, a body in terms of *homo rationalis*. I present two excerpts in the following that I recorded in the consultation room of Dr Ming's clinic to convey a flavour of these. The semiotics of body parts is, however, not the main theme of this chapter. Rather, this chapter, in line with the theme adhered to throughout the book, will work with the concept of a *homo ritualis*: it will attempt to find out how the self and the other can become closely engaged by becoming part of a ritual dynamic that leads towards the production of the patient's health, and in this way engenders a renewed sense of wholeness among those people involved in the process.

> A. 52-year-old man, driver, speaks English; no file with handwritten notes on him could be retrieved, but he has receipts of several previous lab tests in this clinic; No. 672 (17 December 2005).

Doctor: What about you?

Patient: The bladder?

D: Gall bladder?

P: Prostatitis?

D: Ah, the stomach. [searches in the drawer of his desk for leaflet on prostatitis]

P: Yes, the stomach [*tumbo*], I feel it moving.

D: What's the problem of the stomach?

P: It grumbles . . . *gesi* ['gas']

D: You should test [for] typhoid.

P: I tested two years ago.

D: The stool is a bit hard, the stomach grumbling, it is likely you have it. You are a driver . . .

A woman laboratory technician is called to assist as an interpreter between English and Swahili. The patient does not mention prostatitis in her presence, but after she leaves the room, he asks to see the practice's leaflet about prostatitis treatment.

D: This [prostatitis] is not your problem.

P: How do you know you have it?

D: You urinate a lot at night.

P: That is sugar . . .

D: How old are you? . . .

This brief exchange between doctor and patient is interesting in at least three respects: first, the main criteria by which the Chinese doctor hazards a diagnostic guess; second, the patient's disposition towards and expectations of this Chinese medical practice; and third, the attribution of a felt experience of discomfort to dysfunctions of a body part.

First, the above excerpt makes blatantly clear that Dr Ming tried to diagnose the patient's condition on the basis of sociological criteria, namely the patient's profession, gender and age. He explained to me in Chinese that taxi drivers, who were mostly men, often presented with typhoid because they could not predict the volume of either traffic or clientele, and therefore ate irregularly, often from food stalls where drinking water was contaminated or food was prepared in unhygienic ways. The doctor framed the problem here as irregular food intake, based on the natural philosophy tenets of Chinese antiquity that gave rise to a 'medicine of moderation', as was the case also in other stratified societies of antiquity (Bates 1995; Horden and Hsu 2013; Köhle and Kuriyama 2018), but otherwise, there was not much specifically related to Chinese medicine in his diagnostics. While the movement in the stomach, the grumbling and the 'gas' were noted, the Chinese practitioner's medical gaze, like that of a general practitioner in the UK, was primarily epidemiological in orientation, based on the statistics of prevalent complaints. The third diagnostic maxim in TCM, *wen* 闻, which means both 'to listen' and 'to smell', hints at the importance of eliciting such population-specific information during a medical encounter.

Second, the patient himself raised the question of whether he might be suffering from prostatitis, although he did not raise the issue in front of the female interpreter. He likely felt too embarrassed. It is necessary to know in this context that Dr Ming often praised himself for having developed a Chinese medical formula that successfully treated prostatitis; he was known for it citywide. His prostatitis treatment was the trademark of his medical practice and attracted a sometimes quite wealthy clientele. His final question to the patient referenced the statistical prevalence of prostatitis in the elderly. A 52-year-old man would belong among the elderly in urban East Africa, and in the patient's age group some men had likely been diagnosed with prostatitis and perhaps satisfactorily treated by Dr Ming. After the consultation, the client bought a deworming medication, although he had not complained of intestinal worms. This was much less costly than a typhoid test and the antibiotics that Dr Ming prescribed for treating typhoid, alongside the Chinese herbal preparations. The patient had however mentioned 'movement' in the stomach, a 'grumbling' and 'gas', which among many traditional medical practitioners would be taken as a sign of intestinal worms. It was a pragmatic move to buy an inexpensive medicine first. The fact that he purchased anything at all signalled an interest in keeping in contact, while demonstrating the limitations of his spending powers.

Third, this excerpt contains some interesting hints about the semiotics of the body. The bladder, gall bladder and stomach were mentioned in close succession to identify the body part to which the patient attributed his complaint. All three have a bag-like structure according to Western biomedicine, the layperson's common knowledge and Chinese medicine (Hsu 2010a: 216–20). *Gesi* meant 'gas', an undefined condition of malaise often associated with bloating, and sometimes, as already mentioned, with intestinal worms. Some patients complained of reduced libido due to *gesi*, thus conceptualising it as affecting the urogenital system (the bladder?). The word *tumbo* in Swahili meant stomach, but it too had a wide semantic stretch, and when adversely affected could signal an existential loss of vitality (Schmoll 1993). Regardless of the precise diagnosis of the above patient's suffering, a semiotics of the body would be interested in the 'ethnophysiology' of the three different body-internal 'bags' recognised by three unrelated medical knowledge systems.

A similar kind of semiotic uncertainty about the internal body parts can be observed in the following excerpt:

> B. A couple. They have been married for five years, with no children; no. 683 (seen on 17 December 2005).
>
> P: My wife has problems too . . . in the liver?
>
> D: [silence]
>
> P: Not the ovaries . . . ?
>
> D: The kidneys?
>
> P: Yes, the kidneys, there are two kidneys, right?

This excerpt, like the previous one, highlights an uncertainty among Swahili-speaking people regarding the functions of internal organs in a biomedical body. In Chinese medicine, the liver is often considered the female reproductive organ (e.g. Bray 1995; Despeux 1996; Furth 1999; Wilms 2002; Wu 2010; Valussi 2014). The liver stores blood, and the woman's menses are related to fertility. Thus, the liver in Chinese medicine has been associated with fertility problems in women (Wilms 2005), particularly since the Song dynasty (Furth 1999). By contrast, biomedical physicians would initially check the ovaries in women and the testicles in men. Dr Ming spoke of the kidneys, presumably because in Chinese medicine fertility problems in men are mostly relegated to the so-called 'kidneys', for which, as in the case of the liver and other internal organs, the Chinese medical concept is much wider than the biomedical one and includes many functions of reproduction. The above excerpt shows that even a fairly well-educated clientele is not very familiar with biomedical understandings of the internal organs – the couple had told Dr Ming earlier that they had been to the Aga Khan, a private hospital, which had identified the problem to be with the man and given ART (artificial reproductive treatment). In this excerpt too the semiotics of the body highlight difference: gender differences and cultural differences. While it is important to acknowledge such differences, which implicitly celebrate the rationality of the biomedical sciences, let us take a more decolonising attitude to our observations below.

## *Phonemic Misperceptions*

However enticing research into the semiotics of the body would have been, I did not pursue it systematically. Rather, the question in focus was: how do patients and practitioners become engaged with each other through their linguistic exchanges in a process of producing wholesomeness when expending efforts towards healing? For this reason, I took what might be called a phenomenological approach to language, in that I paid particular attention to instances that had in common the patient's sensory experience of the sound of a word that to the observer appeared to be a mishearing or misunderstanding. This form of (mis)communication was fairly frequent in my notes, but I could not make out why. Nevertheless, I felt that it would be worth further exploration. Admittedly, some of the misunderstandings were intentional, as in the following excerpt (C), but this was not the norm.

> C. A man makes inquiries for his brother who apparently has prostatitis.
>
> P: His legs are hot.
>
> D: How many times a night [does he urinate]?
>
> P: Four times.
>
> D: He should come and take a test on Monday, before breakfast.
>
> The doctor overhears a question regarding the costs of the treatment, and misunderstands it:
>
> P: How much does it cost?
>
> D: 1,600 KES [c. GBP 16]

In this case, Dr Ming clearly did not wish to understand the question. He gave a figure that I knew related to just one week's expenses, but the inquirer went away under the impression that the entire treatment would cost this much. Dr Ming's treatment of prostatitis took at least one entire month, that is, 4 x 1,600 = KES 6,400 (*c*. GBP 64). The doctor's motive for misunderstanding the inquiry regarding the basic expenses of the treatment seemed clear to me. He did not wish to jeopardise the recruitment of a potential patient. There is little doubt that this was an intentional misunderstanding. However, in my notes, there are further instances that were not as evidently intentional 'mishearings'. As we will see, they mostly involved phonemics (the language-specific pronunciation of a word).[8]

> D. Woman, no age given; she is a nurse and has joint pains. The BP (blood pressure) is measured: 138/100 mm Hg; no. 20 (seen on 19 December 2005).
>
> P: Still not yet quite good.
>
> D: But better. . . . Are you going back home [for Christmas]?
>
> P: My home is actually here, I'm going to see my parents.
>
> D: Well, that's what I mean by going home. . . . to be happy, . . . **less thought**.
>
> P: yeah, **less salt**.
>
> D: [does not correct her, continues talking] . . . Take exercise. We try our best with herbal medicines.
>
> P: [to me] I was with this doctor Kiswahili *kizungu*, [i.e. a foreign doctor – a biomedical doctor] but I thought I come to this herbal one.
>
> The blood pressure records in her file are:
> 24.8; 30.8; 11.11 BP: 165/90;
> 19.11: BP: 145/105;
> 8.12: 80/60;
> 19.12: 138/100.

In this case, neither doctor nor patient were native English speakers, and both spoke with a strong accent. This was the patient's sixth treatment. Apparently, the three treatments in the summer had had no visible effect; they had been delivered by Dr Ming's former teacher, who had sold Dr Ming the clinic several years earlier and who stepped in to substitute him the summer before while Dr Ming was in China due to a family emergency. Dr Ming thus considered only the three latter BP readings to reflect his treatment. 'Less salt' was advice relating to a biomedically comprehended body, and the patient, who was a practising nurse, evidently anticipated that the Chinese doctor would give advice in line with modern biomedical rationales of treating hypertension. When the Chinese practitioner, in non-idiomatic English, said that the patient should not worry too much – 'less thought' – the advice was well meant and appealed to good sense. The doctor seemed to be guided by a Western 'folk model' according to which stress, worry and anxiety increase blood pressure. Simultaneously, his comment may have been motivated by a Chinese medical concern, within the paradigm of the *wuxing* (five phases or five agents; Porkert 1974; Sivin 1987). In this, emotional qualities are inherent to physiological and somatic processes (Ots 1990a, 1990b), and thinking and feeling are considered a single bodily process (Zhang 2007; Hsu 2013a). Worry and ratiocination are an aspect of the spleen, but TCM practitioners would usually associate hypertension with an anxious heart or an angry liver, and mention these *bodily organs* to speak about *emotional* irritability; this would be rendered in both colloquial English and colloquial Chinese as '*thinking* too much' (*ni xiang tai duo* 你想太多). However, in biomedical circles, 'thinking in circles' (i.e. unproductively) is not an aspect of the spleen, heart or liver, which are all 'of the body', but is attributed to the mind. As a Chinese medical doctor who spoke English, Dr Ming was not expected to allude to the Cartesian mind, and the patient inferred that he was speaking about the Cartesian body: 'less salt'.

> E. A 26-year-old woman, accompanied by her father; no. 672 (seen on 16 December 2005).
>
> P's father: It is not that the lump gets worse during her periods [as she said before in response to D's questioning]. She played with her brother [brother-in-law, from the shipping company] and he hit her . . . .
>
> D: Wants me to do a manual investigation. I refuse.
>
> D [taps on her chest]
>
> D: Is it the rib?
>
> P: . . . [has not understood question, is silent].
>
> D: I do not believe in Mombasa hospitals. My wife was [accurately] diagnosed in China.
>
> P's father: My daughter has a headache.
>
> D: One side or both **sides**?
>
> P's father: **Sight** is fine. I first thought it is the spectacles.

*Misunderstandings, and the Spaces They Create*

Notably, the father spoke for the daughter as a carer, a well-known phenomenon (e.g. Good and Good 1994). In this case, the doctor would have reasoned in terms of a Chinese medical body if he had asked whether the headache was lateral or not, as headaches presenting with lateral pain are usually attributed to the minor *yang* 少阳 gall bladder channel (*Zhenjiuxue* 1985: 101–4). However, the question was whether the headache was unilateral or bilateral, which is a question likely motivated by a Western medical concern with migraines. Unilateral pain tends to be diagnosed as a migraine. The patient's father by contrast seemed to associate headaches with dizziness or nausea, and hence spoke of 'sight'. The consultation was over before any further questions were asked.

F. A 28-year-old man; no. 683 (seen on 17 December 2005).

D: You have taken the *dawa* [medicine] for one week now. How is it? The *taste*?

P: The *test*? It is OK. I'm travelling on the 29th to Saudi Arabia. Kuwait.

D: . . . [no response]

P: Kuwait.

D: But Kuwait is not Saudi Arabia.

P: I see so many Chinese there, I see Chinese restaurants, you have no connection there?

D: [Prescribes two weeks of medication]

Two misunderstandings happened in this short exchange, but the second about the doctor's comment on Kuwait, I cannot explain (it is possible that the doctor did not misunderstand the patient's comment, but that they were both testing me, the anthropologist, and my linguistic knowledge). The first misunderstanding, however, is phonemic and of the kind investigated here. As in the previous cases, the doctor does not correct the patient when it occurs. He knows that the ingestion of Chinese herbal decoctions can be very unpleasant. They are often bitter, even very bitter, but the patient obviously did not expect to be asked something as trivial as whether or not the medicine was palatable. The client's question, 'The test?', is telling, as it gives a very faint hint that the patient is facing a risk of infection. STDs (sexually transmitted diseases) are associated with the consumption of the medicines he bought for the business trip abroad.

G. Mathilda, a 50-year-old woman from South America; she is on Chinese formula medicines. She shows the package: 妇科千金片 'Gynaecological tablets worth a thousand gold [ounces]' (seen in December 2005).

D: [reads aloud text on the packaging]: 千金片 *qianjinpian*

P: **Changing?**

D: The fibroid is 2 cm, not so big, not a big problem, you still can get pregnant. One eye is bigger than the other, one testicle bigger than the other. [It meant: we all have blemishes, don't worry.]

P: My doctor in 1990 wanted to do an operation but my cousin said it is not necessary. Recently I had heavy bleeding and pain during the first two days. They said: take away the uterus. This is very expensive. My cousin is in Kenyatta hospital, I could have done it for free.

D: I suggest you finish this [medicine package] first, come next week. [talks about successful Chinese medical treatment of fibroids]

This is clearly another phonemic misunderstanding. The doctor reads aloud a Chinese term and Mathilda hears an English word. The doctor does not clarify the misunderstanding, as the word 'changing' is clearly conducive to the treatment in that it expresses the positive and hopeful attitude of the patient. This is the fifth instance of a phonemic mishearing presented here, but there were many more. My aim is not to record them all but to try to understand why they happened fairly frequently and what their purpose was.

## *Grice's Cooperative Principle*

These phonemically motivated misunderstandings were quite frequent during the consultations that I witnessed throughout the two or three weeks in December 2005 that I spent seated next to Dr Ming in a small and stuffy consultation room.[9] Of course, one will ask how to make sense of the above findings. They clearly do not lend themselves to the semiotics of the body. Interpreting them as instances of misunderstanding presupposes that it is possible to contrast them with cases of mutual understanding.

Much in the sense of the *Thou*-orientation of Alfred Schütz, briefly introduced in Chapter 1, which posits that the 'I' is naturally inclined and oriented towards the 'you', the philosopher Paul Grice suggested that people who converse with each other submit to a 'cooperative principle', which is that they wish to understand the other and make themselves understood by them. As seen above, this cooperative principle need not apply to every linguistic event, as for instance when a Chinese medical doctor does not want to understand a query regarding how much a course of a particular medical treatment costs (Case C, above). However, Grice posited that everyday life conversations were usually grounded in a cooperative principle: 'Make your contribution such as is required, at the stage at which it occurs, by the accepted purpose or direction of talk exchange in which you are engaged' (Grice [1967] 1989: 26–27; see also Levinson 1983: 101).

This definition of the cooperative principle clearly demonstrates Grice's view that conversations have a processual character. Depending on the stage at which they occur, the requirements for one's contribution to the conversation differ. At the time, leading scholars of conversation analysis, such as Harvey Sacks, Emanuel Schegloff and Gail Jefferson (1974), identified the openings and closings of conversation and wrote about turn-taking. They noted the rhythmic and processual character of conversations without making explicit allusions to a musical rhythm or a ritual interaction. Their research can easily be applied to an embodied interpretation of language, speech and gesture.

Meanwhile, Grice formulated four maxims of conversation, which jointly should express the cooperative principle, and he also identified genres of speech brought about by flouting these maxims (see Table 2.1):

Can we assume that Grice's principle of cooperation applies also to the medical encounters recorded in the stuffy, divination hut-like Chinese medical consultation room? Indeed, only a quick glance at the field notes taken makes it possible to find excerpts of talk that indicate that speakers were, against all odds, engaging in a conversation that can be interpreted as testifying to a commitment to Grice's principle of cooperation, such as in the following excerpt:

> H. The same male patient as in the couple mentioned in excerpt B. This 28-year-old patient had undergone many biomedical tests, and his testicles were biopsied, as they apparently do not produce sperm; no. 683 (seen on 17 December 2005).
>
> P: I went to so many hospitals. It is . . . .
>
> D: Yes, it is **genic**.
>
> P: Yes, yes . . .
>
> P: Can you help?
>
> D: For one month, then see.

**Table 2.1.** Grice's four maxims for the principle of cooperation (*and their flouting*). Adapted from Levinson (1983: 101–2 and 109–13).

| |
|---|
| 1. Maxim of quality:<br>Try to make your contribution one that is true:<br>a) Do not say what you believe to be false<br>b) Do not say that for which you lack adequate evidence<br>*If you blatantly flout it, it is a case of irony.* |
| 2. Maxim of quantity:<br>a) make your contribution as informative as is required for the current purposes of exchange<br>b) do not make your contribution more informative than is required<br>*If you blatantly flout it, it is a case of politeness or of embarrassment.* |
| 3. Maxim of relevance:<br>a) make your contributions relevant<br>*If you blatantly flout it, is it cultural ignorance?* |
| 4. Maxim of manner:<br>be perspicuous<br>a) avoid obscurity<br>b) avoid ambiguity<br>c) be brief<br>d) be orderly<br>*You blatantly flout it in order to create 'simultaneity'.* |

In this case, neither doctor nor patient seems to know the correct biomedical word, but both know the concept. Neither corrects what the other says, and both understand each other. It is a 'genetic' problem. I propose to read this excerpt as an example in which one can see how both speakers were committed to trying to understand each other in an honourable, honest and cooperative way.

## *Flouting Grice's Maxim of Manner*

Based on instances like H, then, we can assume that the conversations in the clinic were undertaken in a cooperative way. If Grice's cooperative principle is applied to the above conversations, which maxim was being flouted in a 'sound-based' way by 'phonemic misunderstandings'? Was the maxim of quality, quantity, relevance or manner being flouted?

With the materials at hand, it would appear that the maxim of manner was flouted. First, the above excerpts D–G can be interpreted as enhancing *obscurity*, all the more so as none of the speakers undertook an effort at clarification. In this way they also promoted *ambiguity*. They were furthermore slightly *chaotic* (I had to give considerable background information, particularly on the different medical frameworks implicitly alluded to, to make sense of the excerpts). Admittedly, the excerpts were rarely *lengthy*, as they were snippets of longer conversations. However, it is reasonable to suggest that the maxim of manner was flouted. Accordingly, the phonemic misunderstandings I recorded would have created a sort of 'simultaneity'.

If we look at the speech situation as a whole, we note that ambiguity and obscurity can create moments in which the patient in particular experiences socially produced moments of uncertainty. The final excerpt presented below reveals an intentionality on the side of the practitioner that, in the previous excerpts, I was not able to detect. This excerpt, however, assured me, the probing ethnographer, that I may have picked up on a non-arbitrary feature and pattern of the conversations held during clinical encounters:

I. A 26-year-old man of South Asian descent.

P: I have an erectile problem. . . .

D: You are still with your wife?

P: She is in India now . . .

D: Do you have any other problem? . . . What about your appetite? . . . This *dawa* [medicine] you take one hour before intercourse. It is a Tibetan medicine. Tibet. You do not know Tibet? . . . You know **Himalaya**?

P: Ah, yes, . . . **Malaya**?

D: On the other side of the mountain is Tibet. [prescribes the medicine]

[silence]

Receptionist: It is out of stock.

I cannot say why, but as I was sitting next to Dr Ming during the consultation and recorded this conversation in my notebook, I sensed something unusual; as usual, however, time did not allow for raising any questions, and I soon forgot about it. I recorded the word *malaya* without understanding its meanings, but when, seven years later, I presented the above excerpts at a conference on narrative in medical anthropology, I had not entirely forgotten about the charged atmosphere that this verbal exchange evoked at the time. Some colleagues in the audience, fluent in Swahili, understood the pun but kept quiet, cognisant of the fact that other conference delegates may have found the doctor's implicit recommendation ethically problematic. Indeed, Dr Ming had pronounced the word 'Himalaya' with a certain pathos and with what might have been an imperceptible sideways glance:[10] *malaya* is the common word for prostitute in Swahili.

This final excerpt demonstrates unambiguously that the phenomenology of sound in linguistic exchanges that produced 'phonemic misunderstandings' during medical conversations was sometimes intentionally presented as unintentional. It asks for a linguistic-cum-medical anthropological analysis. The suggestion made in what follows is that the flouting of what Grice called the 'maxim of manner' caused 'simultaneity'. To understand the therapeutic potential of this sort of simultaneity, we have to interpret the speech during the diagnostic conversations as a social interaction within which dimensions of *homo ritualis*, rather than *homo rationalis*, become important.[11] Evidently, these conversations were about something other than merely factual information exchange. If we look at these conversational excerpts as part of a procedure of healing, they may contribute to what Kapferer (e.g. 2004: 41, 50) referred to as 'the virtual dynamics of ritual' (and not merely as what Turner (1969) had earlier called the 'ritual process'). As already suggested earlier, medical treatment and healing can be seen as triggering virtualities that involve ritual transformation to some degree.

# Reflections: Towards a Phenomenology of Speaking

Traditional medical treatment can be understood as a process in which different techniques effect different bodily processes, and studies of its medical efficaciousness should account for the different stages of treatment through a 'sensory semantics' (or so-called 'material semiotics'). This entails a move away from studying 'traditional' medicine in terms of an assumed *homo rationalis* and a move towards research on procedures involving a *homo ritualis*. How self and other are implicated in a healing process and expend effort towards re-establishing the patient as whole and healthy, and whether and how this may be relevant for reconfiguring sociality more generally, accordingly becomes a question regarding dimensions of *homo ritualis*, who takes part in 'ritual dynamics' (as outlined in Kapferer 2004).

Participant observation did yield observations that lent themselves to a semiotics of the body (excerpts A and B), but I chose to focus on those instances (D–G and I) that were recurrent, distinctively textured and not directly comprehensible to me: they arose from an auditory (mis)perception that in the conversational excerpts recorded was not further commented upon, neither by the practitioner nor by the patient. What was happening here?

The idea of applying Grice's maxim of manner to make sense of these excerpts, and seeing it flouted, came to me years later during the preparation of a conference paper. It suggested that these phonemic (mis)understandings created moments of enhanced obscurity and ambiguity, which were however usually quite brief and, while they were not neatly ordered, were not entirely disordered. According to Grice, the flouting of the maxim would produce moments of 'simultaneity'. This instantly brings us back to what we discussed in the Reflections section in Chapter 1, on 'generating synchronicity'!

In Chapter 1, the body's motility and spatiality were foregrounded, along with the way that self and other, together with the relevant furniture in the spaces of the medical practice, namely the fireplace or the table and bed, produced moments of synchronicity or did not. Meanwhile, in this chapter, we are trying to make sense of speech events in the divination hut-like stuffiness of Dr Ming's consultation room, which, with reference to the flouting of the maxim of manner in conversation, were found to be best interpreted as producing 'simultaneity'. This interpretation goes far beyond my fieldwork recordings.

Merleau-Ponty (1962: 174–99), in Chapter 6, titled 'The Body as Expression, and Speech', clearly signals that the body, which has spatiality and motility, is not to be opposed to the mind. Rather, Merleau-Ponty relates to the body and speech as a process, one of 'aesthetic expression', which he considers to have a particular peculiarity: 'Aesthetic expression confers on what it expresses an existence in itself, installs it in nature as a thing perceived and accessible to all' (ibid.: 183). His premise is: 'This process of expression . . . brings meaning into existence as a thing' (ibid.: 182). In other words, although aesthetic expression is a process, be it expressed by a moving body or a speaking person, it is experienced as a thing.

Accordingly, Merleau-Ponty says of 'thought', which people tend to conceive of as an internal thing, as opposed to external speech and 'language', that 'Thought is no internal thing, and does not exist independently of the world, and of words' (1962: 183). 'Thought' is not a thing that exists independently inside the person, and language is not 'but an external accompaniment of thought' (ibid.: 177).[12] In *The Absent Body*, Drew Leder (1990) elaborates on this insight of Merleau-Ponty's, which entails that a bodily experience, like thinking as an internal thing, becomes the cornerstone of an ontology. The body knows of its existence only when its functioning becomes dysfunctional, and the person experiences pain.

Merleau-Ponty's philosophy evidently goes diametrically against the Saussurean distinction between sign and signified, and between word form and word meaning (de Saussure 1916). In my view, his critique is able to outline a way of how best to engage with and make sense of the fieldwork observations presented above. This is, ultimately, one might say, by emphasising that speech has 'gestural meaning' (Merleau-Ponty 1962: 179): 'The spoken word is a genuine gesture' (ibid.: 183). Merleau-Ponty associated speech with gesture as a way of engaging with the world, where speaker and listener made use of the word, as of an instrument: 'The word could be identified as an instrument of action' (ibid.: 175); he herewith pre-empted John Austin's ([1955] 1962) *How to Do Things with Words*. The history of humanity is sedimented in the linguistic repertoire, in words, Merleau-Ponty claimed, but the way one uses words is always particular to the situation: 'And the meaning of speech is nothing other than the way . . . in which it plays modulations on the keyboard of acquired meanings' (ibid.: 186). Merleau-Ponty very consequentially applies his understanding of sedimentation to bodies and spoken words (which have a materiality, namely in the sonic resonances that speech generates).

In this chapter, I did not seriously engage with semiotics. I only indicated that I had materials worthy of semiotic analysis in my field notes, thereby aiming to signal to future fieldworkers that research on metaphors and semiotics of the body remains worthwhile. For patients – and for practitioners (as stressed by Das and Das 2005) – it is very difficult to extract from the twenty-first century's information overload those information bites that are accurate and fit together.

In many urban neighbourhoods, half-knowledge, ignorance, exaggeration, indifference and intentional deception were quotidian, resulting in a semiotics of bodies as presented above in cases A and B. To recapitulate, the above phonemic misperceptions are difficult to explain from a structural linguistic point of view. Therefore, I made recourse to Merleau-Ponty's *Phenomenology of Perception*, which treats speech events as generated by body parts moving through space. My field research attended to the rhythmicity of speaking and turn-taking. I recorded sound perceptions and interpreted my findings in terms of linguistic pragmatics, namely Grice's cooperative principle. A subfield pertaining to the 'phenomenology of speaking' in order to make sense of ethnographic findings, like the above, has already provided invaluable insights for a medical anthropology interested in how healing is conceptualised and done, and what makes it efficacious.

In de Saussure's *Cours* (1916), *langue* is the ideal system and *parole* is the always-incomplete and messy expression of it. This reproduces a view, ascribed to the ancient Greeks and Plato, of the 'idea' as perfect, and of the sense-perceived and the bodily as imperfect. It also instils the Christian religious sentiment that the otherworldly is perfect and the this-worldly is imperfect. Furthermore, it reflects, in oversimplified form, the Cartesian view that mindful cogitation resulting in theory is elegant and beautiful, but manual practice is always incomplete and messy.

However, in several of the above quotations, Merleau-Ponty takes a different approach to the spatially experienced materialities that are supposedly messy and incomplete. Accordingly, a phenomenology of speaking would be interested in *parole* but would evaluate instances of it in an aesthetically compelling way.

Mauss's (2006b) unfinished lines of thought, collated and commentated by Nathan Schlanger, incidentally also seem to be concerned more with *parole* than with *langue*. In particular, he seems to see speech as a craft that can be developed to an art by the masterful interplay of voice, prosody, pronunciation, speed and rhythm, alongside the judicious choice of words for the construction of sentences. A speech can be moving and can grip an audience even if it is ungrammatical in many places. Why? Because it is a matter of craftsmanship, and what matters to the appreciation of a craft is the wholeness of its making.

If human beings engage with the world through speaking and gesturing in a process of aesthetic expression, they value speaking not merely for its informative qualities of communication. The above 'phonemic' misperceptions, based on a Gricean flouting of the principle of manner, are perhaps best interpreted as generating moments of 'simultaneity'. They are best comprehended as giving verbal expression to ambivalences and ambiguities of the situation: should a patient try out and trust Chinese medical treatment?

## More on Trust

Let us here turn to my own earlier medical anthropological research undertaken in the late 1980s in the PRC's urban spaces, where petty enterprise thrived. Questions prevailed as to whether or not the treatment in question, called *qigong* 气功, would be efficacious, and whether or not the healer could be trusted. In that context I pointed to concrete stages of treatment as part of a 'ritual dynamics'. I suggested that healer and patient became enthralled with each other in a process of healing with different stages. I identified five. The first involved different 'forms of recruitment': 'Clients were given time, in the very beginning, to decide what chances they themselves gave this unusual treatment. The outcome of the treatment was thus largely determined before the treatment had begun' (Hsu 1999: 61). As thus outlined, the *qigong* healer engaged in a variety of strategies to subtly instil trust in their healing techniques.

In this initial phase, potential clients deliberated on their 'choices of treatment', or rather the choices they perceived themselves to have. Once a patient decided to embark on a specific treatment, patient and healer were considered to enter into a phase of 'mutual commitment', as treatment was delivered and paid for in cycles, say of ten *qigong* sessions. These treatment cycles could be repeated several times. Whether or not the treatment 'worked' was in cases of chronic ailments a prolonged matter of 'reaching consensus'. Sometimes, the criteria of what was considered recovery was repeatedly reconceptualised. Finally, in a fifth stage of the treatment during which patients maintained or periodically renewed their relations with the healer as a friend, they would stop by occasionally, send gifts for his wedding or his son's first anniversary, or recommend him by word of mouth to potential future clients. Thanks to his healing techniques the *qigong* healer was able to build up a circle of friends

(Hsu 1999: 58–67). In this way, the *qigong* healer resembled a shaman, whose healing seances tend to give rise to a sense of wholeness not only in the patient but also among the participants partaking in the ritual (e.g. Desjarlais 1996).

In urban East Africa, the Chinese practitioners also built up patient communities around themselves – networks of patients, one might say – but nowhere were they as embedded into the locality as was the *qigong* healer or were the Yolmö shamans that Desjarlais worked with, whose healing efforts were also geared towards enhancing their own standing in the places they inhabited. Meanwhile, not all Chinese practitioners lived on the premises of their practices, as their practices were often located, at least in Kenya, in the shopping centres of suburbia. Some of these were popular shopping centres, particularly for car-wheeled middle classes, but in the evenings they were closed and looked deserted.

In most cases, trust evolves over time, and it was expressed differently in the different stages of *qigong* treatment. Likewise, negotiations over a treatment's efficaciousness were marked by a variety of concerns, some of which had an intrinsically given rhythm (e.g. period pains, seasonal allergies, monthly payment difficulties, etc.). Patients performed deeds of social obligation that expressed trust in the healer's practice, generally after their treatment had been successfully terminated. However, as intimated above, it was in the early phases, before the patient embarked on treatment, that its potential outcome was gauged. Perhaps, the simultaneity that was generated through a flouting of Grice's maxim of manner was a 'form of recruitment', in so far as it gave the patient a space for being ambivalent and hesitant before committing to the unusual Chinese medical treatments on offer?

## Spaces Generated for Overcoming Social Distance

There are of course very different qualities of trust and commitment, of care and friendship, and what follows is an afterthought. Regarding the argument just made, it highlights that there was a social distance for local nationals to become friendly and familiar with Chinese medical practitioners. In Kenya, it certainly was easier to relate to them as business people. I knew of many Chinese medical doctors, particularly men, who had become 'friends' with African business partners. Dr Ming had one such friendship with a local journalist who was building up a local radio station. Obviously, both benefited from the other's intelligent initiative. Ming's weekly session on Chinese medical advice both attracted new listeners to his friend's private radio programme and simultaneously provided an advertisement opportunity for his medical clinic. Both young men were sparkling, enterprising and working towards a better future, and they hoped to reach out beyond the fairly affluent local communities they physically moved in. Furthermore, the friendship they had struck up also enabled them to help each other out in other ways.

While East Africa's urban spaces in the early 2000s were favourable to petty entrepreneurship and 'mixed embeddedness', there was a widely perceived 'cultural' difference that made it difficult for 'African' patients to become friends with their 'Chinese' medical doctors. Some of the elderly Chinese doctors in particular, and also some very young practitioners from rural China, who had minimal school education and were ignorant of world affairs, might make comments that sounded rather 'racist'. Yet I also observed Chinese medical practitioners treat their patients with great commitment and responsibility. They would readily nurse and treat a patient over long periods of time, sometimes for minimal payment. They might have said, 'it is my duty as a doctor' (*yinggai zuode* 应该做的), but they clearly had a commitment to doing good to fellow human beings regardless of their social background. However, the idea of 'making friends' with locals and being at leisure with them (*wan'er wan'er* 玩儿玩儿), let alone getting married to 'an African' (*heiren* 黑人), was unthinkable for most of them at the turn of the millennium.

In this context, an inner-city Chinese medical practice comes to mind, staffed by a female doctor who was a trained TCM practitioner, a mother of a toddler whom she had left with her spouse in China and a member of a group of Chinese employees contracted for two years to work for a semi-private firm in Dar es Salaam. In the waiting room of that practice I retrospectively noted that I had encountered a certain retired engineer more frequently than any other patient. He was a widower who readily accepted being interviewed as a patient of Chinese medicine (see Chapter 4). His home, which I visited for the interview, was a bungalow in a northern suburb, which overlooked his sheep grazing on a meadow while the dark blue sea glittered in the background. On one level, the scene that he had created was paradise on earth. He had lived and worked for many years in Canada but returned to Tanzania after retirement. He seemed to know what mattered in life for him. If he felt lonely, he said, downtown was less than half an hour's trip away by *dalla dalla*.

Did he, in his retirement, perhaps feel deprived of intellectual conversation and exchanges? I did not ask him that question at the time, but reading through my notes it came to mind. He was one of the only Tanzanians to articulate a felt affinity between Chinese and Africans: 'The Chinese', he said, 'are just like the Africans'; they could accommodate to less-than-ideal conditions, which 'the white man cannot do'. Years later, that female doctor got in touch with me over email; she had retrained as a psychologist. Surely, her professional trajectory testified to China's current psycho-boom (Kleinman 2011; Huang 2014; Bram 2020), but one wonders whether she had also turned to the study of psychology for unacknowledged, subdued and more subtle – perhaps even unwanted – feelings, possibly of friendship and trust between a Chinese practitioner and a Tanzanian client? The social distance was not unsurmountable, but it was present. Considering social distance, might the phonemic mishearings, here interpreted as causing moments of indeterminate 'simultaneity', have been a therapeutic technique of creating space for reflection before committing to seeking health through Chinese medical treatment?

# Notes

1. The shock this episode caused is still so very present, and has me cringe today when I think of it – I need no diary entry of it.
2. This point is also forcefully made by Gonçalves Martín (2016), about what is said among the Yanomami in the minutes before the helicopter lands and departs.
3. Yan et al. (2019), however, query the implications and accuracy of this dictum.
4. Kadetz and Hood (2017: 350) interviewed informants who did not consider Chinese medical treatment and acupuncture expensive. Were we interviewing members of comparable socio-economic groups? I doubt it. The respondent who said this to me was a low-ranking hospital employee (salary *c*. TZS 30,000 per month, equivalent to *c*. GBP 30 at the time).
5. This section is based on a paper presented at 'Revisiting Narrative in Medical Anthropology', held at the School of Anthropology and Museum Ethnography, University of Oxford, in December 2012, organised by Kristine Krause, Elisabeth Hsu and David Parkin, funded by the MPI Goettingen and Green Templeton College, Oxford.

6. On the *kanga* and the feminine worlds of Zanzibar, see e.g. Larsen (2008).
7. 'He [Pierre Janet] laid great stress on rapport in moral influence; it depended on a direct personal relationship between healer and the sick person in which the healer himself was perhaps more important than his method' (Lewis 2021: 190). This has become a widely appreciated insight in medical anthropology.
8. In the following five cases, my interpretation of possible TCM and biomedical diagnoses was checked for accuracy in discussion with Dr Xin Sun (in summer 2019).
9. This may seem a very short period, but it was a long-term achievement; it was only on my fifth visit to this clinic that I was granted this privilege.
10. Methodologically, this episode highlights that it is vital for a medical anthropology fieldworker not to belittle participant observation as too time consuming a fieldwork method and delegate so-called 'primary data' collection to research assistants.
11. On *homo ritualis*, see Hsu (2011), building on Kapferer (2004).
12. Merleau-Ponty (1962: 183) explains: 'What misleads us in the connection, and causes us to believe in a thought which exists for itself, prior to expression, is thought already constituted and expressed, which we can silently recall to ourselves, and through which we acquire the illusion of an inner life. But in reality . . . this inner life is an inner language.'

# Part II
*Emplacement, Emplotment, 'Empotment'*

## Chapter 3
# Patients, Practitioners and Their *Pots*

## Fieldwork: A Multisited Meshwork

Multisited fieldwork meant repeatedly returning to the same neighbourhoods, shopping malls, high streets and back streets. I initially tried to undertake multi-levelled fieldwork (van der Geest et al. 1990), but the doors to the Chinese Embassy, the Ministry of Health, the National Institute for Medical Research and hospital authorities remained shut after a first superficial contact, despite repeated attempts on my part to renew contact. So I undertook fieldwork in multiple sites with Chinese practitioners and their clientele, taxi drivers, NGO workers, expatriates, and many many friends in Tanzania, Zanzibar (Unguja and Pemba), Kenya and Uganda (on 'friends' in field research, see Löffler 2012: 24 ff.), thereby co-producing a 'meshwork' (Ingold 2009: 34, drawing on Lefebvre 1991: 117–18).

> I borrow the term meshwork from the philosopher Henri Lefebvre, who speaks of 'the reticular patterns left by animals, both wild and domestic, and by people (in and around the houses of village or small town, as in the town's immediate environs)', whose movements weave an environment that is more 'archi-textural' than architectural. (Ingold 2007a: 80)

Unlike a disembodied 'network', generally comprehended as 'subordinated to the frameworks of politics', Lefebvre (1991: 116–17) tells us that a 'meshwork' emerges through 'the spatio-temporal rhythms of nature [say, in the field] as transformed by social practice [say, of the fieldworker and their respondents]'. The researcher is implicated in a 'meshwork' in ways that an observer is not. Indeed, before long, my meshwork of friends extended also into Oxford: one of my Zanzibari friends had a daughter and a son at a British high school, and stopped over in Oxford on his way to the Midlands. Another one, who had consulted the Chinese almanac, believed that I would bring him luck and sent me monthly letters for many years. Yet others reached me by phone in my office on the Banbury Road and had me instigate emergency cash transfers from George Street or send packages full of medication from Walton Street. And there was one journalist on his way from the USA to Tanzania whom I even treated to tea, tuna and cucumber sandwiches on the High Street. He had very charmingly managed to cheat me for well over a year. He had offered to photocopy, if I paid him in advance, any article on Chinese medical doctors that he chanced upon while working on archived newspapers in the library . . . and then there were so many articles on the topic! I was constantly back at the Western Union making yet another cash transfer. Despite whatever means I might have wanted to use to draw boundaries with 'informants' in a faraway 'field', the meshwork I co-produced came skin-close, and sometimes closer than I felt was comfortable.

Since my fieldwork was multisited, it involved staying in low-budget hotels, mostly in urban but also in rural and remote areas. However, it soon became very apparent that sharing the premises of my hosts was ethnographically infinitely more valuable. Whenever I could I accepted invitations to stay with the families of the people I worked with. This included a Chinese restaurant owner, a Chinese Western medical technician, a Chinese medical doctor, a Nyamwezi Chinese medicine patient's mother on the border with Zambia, her relatives in a village that was a full day's walk away, a Bukoba healer living among the Zaramo, a Tanzanian healer's client, a half-Arab nurse, an Arab shopkeeper on the archipelago of Lamu, a Kojani herbalist, a Pentecostal woman preacher and her daughter on the Tanzanian–Kenyan border, a Ugandan apothecary and several British expatriates. In most cases, I was on the move and grateful for a bed, but in some places I stayed well over a fortnight.

Fieldwork was undertaken mostly during the short rainy periods in December–January, but also during the rainy season in March–April and the dry season in July–August. The destinations I travelled to were Dar es Salaam, Bagamoyo, Tanga, Arusha, Moshi and Mbeya in Tanzania; Stone Town, Chake Chake and Kojani in Zanzibar; Nairobi, Mombasa, Malindi and Lamu in Kenya; and Kampala and Jinja in Uganda. During the first few fieldwork periods I was keen to visit as many Tanzanian, Kenyan and Zanzibari healers as possible, and was introduced to as many as twenty or more, whom I either interviewed or watched while they were treating patients. However, in later years, my research in the Chinese medical practices became more interesting and absorbing. I went wherever people told me there was a Chinese medical practice – clinics opened and closed quickly, and practitioners were constantly on the move. I believe I visited almost all those who were then in operation, but I know that I missed one practitioner in Eldoret in Kenya, one or two in Kisumu, two in Mwanza and one in Dodoma in Tanzania. I also missed several Chinese medical clinics in Kampala.

At the time of fieldwork, there were permanent tensions in national politics and turmoil in world history. In Tanzania, Benjamin Mkapa was president between 1995 and 2005, followed by Jakaya Kikwete from 2005 to 2015. Julius Nyerere and his era was still often referred to, although his name was rarely mentioned. In Zanzibar, and particularly on Pemba, there were repeated violent outbreaks in the early 2000s, one outbreak having happened just weeks before I started my fieldwork in March 2001. In Kenya, Daniel arap Moi (1978–2002) stepped down after twenty-four years of presidency in 2002, and the election of Mwai Kibaki (2002–13) was accompanied by violence, particularly in the coastal areas, where I did fieldwork not long after it abated. In Uganda, Yoweri Kaguta Museveni had been in power since 1986, and the first elections were held in 1996, in 2001 and again in 2006. When I undertook fieldwork in Kampala, there was general disquiet about him having just won a third re-election . . . and he is still in office today, in 2021.

One evening, returning just before dusk from interviews with patients in the sprawling suburbs of Dar es Salaam, I found a crowd of men in the lounge of the hotel at which I was staying, standing tightly side by side in utter silence. They all looked in the same direction. I looked too, and I saw in that very moment a much celebrated and intensely hated figure emerging out of a dark rectangular structure. Sky TV was on. I felt embarrassed to stand there in a crowd of men, but decided not to assume the gender role, and stayed put. The next image on TV was a mouth inspection; then hair was cut, hairs in the nostrils; a hand pushed the former head of state's head to one side, then to the other. Everyone in the room was still; no words, no motion. Then, the next news item was shown. I stayed for a minute or two, then walked up the stairs to my hotel room. Later that evening I passed through the same lounge on the ground floor to have my supper in an eatery nearby; it was empty but for the usual few who were sitting on the sofa. There was not a trace of the silent violence just witnessed.

Anthropological fieldwork depends on serendipity, and walking into situations like the above reminds us of both its strengths and limitations. It also made me aware of the outlandishness of my research theme, if not its utter irrelevance for my Muslim hosts at a time of military aggression and humiliation. I had entered the country on a tourist visa in 2001, having left too little time to obtain a research permit while still in the UK. I had learned about a Chinese–Tanzanian HIV/AIDS clinic at Muhimbili hospital, Dar es Salaam, and hoped to focus on it in my study; this topic would have been of direct interest to my Tanzanian hosts.

Twice weekly, said HIV/AIDS clinic offered treatment to patients willing to sign up to a Chinese medical treatment regime. It was an initiative of the Tanzanian state and the Ministry of Health in Beijing, set up in the highest echelons in 1990. This was years before treatment with ARVs became a possibility for Tanzanians. The Tanzanian doctor in charge, who had trained in Western medicine in the PRC and spoke Chinese, took great care to uphold a professional cheerfulness in the consultation room as I found her wedged between two TCM doctors, behind a tall tower of patients' consultation records. After over ten years of the project, renowned senior doctors had been replaced by postdocs, each wearing a plastic glove on their right hand with which they would take the pulse at the patients' wrists. They knew how to diagnose distinguishing patterns and write personally tailored prescriptions, or formulas. The Chinese *materia medica* (*zhongyao* 中药) they had access to (in a large air-conditioned annex) had been imported from a prestigious Chinese medical pharmacy, the Tongren Tang 同仁堂 (discussed in Cochran 2006: 16–37). This was exciting, high-profile research. However, when I finally obtained the research permit from Tanzania's Commission for Science and Technology (COSTECH), I was explicitly told not to work with HIV/AIDS patients.[1]

The few informal exploratory visits I made to this Chinese–Tanzanian clinic were suggestive of some patients having obtained stunning results; some had regained weight and the occasional smile had returned to their faces. A lively 5-year-old toddler was proudly shown to patients over and over again; she had been transformed from an anaemic little worm to a lovely little girl. Other patients had survived for over a decade (the secret, one menopausal woman said, was not to have sex, as her condition had massively improved immediately after she gained control over her sexuality; the doctor nodded). This HIV/AIDS programme was well worth researching, and in some Chinese circles, as I learned during a visit to Beijing in 2005, the programme's treatment results were considered legendary in the early 1990s.

So, I conducted participant observation of medical encounters in private medical practices whenever possible, and, like Mei Zhan (2009), saw them as a constitutive part of the whirl of 'worlding' practices. While the whirl of late-liberal health markets that Zhan studied was on the northern Pacific Rim, stretching from China's east coast to California and back again, the spatial dimensions that started to attract my attention in East Africa were in themselves quite notably and distinctively patterned by architectural and agricultural structures, testifying to local and transregional histories and politics. Evidently, these urban spaces were part of the whirl that was instigating and instigated by worldwide mobilities and commerce, entangled in a back and forth between Africa and China, and feeding into global health and trade flows.

As emerges from the above reflections on the multisited meshworks that I co-produced, the ripples of the late-liberal health markets that I researched were clearly beyond the regulatory grip of the state. Perfectly honourable and otherwise honest people were relegated to the informal sector, and even into grey zones on the edge of legality, due to health regulations that made little sense and criminalised them due to the medicines they dispensed (as already noted for the USA by Adams 2002). Similarly, even the most helpful research-regulating bureaucrats were at a loss on how to issue a permit for carrying out multisited, transnational ethnographic fieldwork over eight years on non-nationals (the practitioners) and floating populations (some of the patients).

My fieldwork was multisited; my visits were sporadic, yet they lasted for years. My friends and I became familiar with each other; children grew and parents greyed. Patients recognised me on the street; we would chat, share a coke, suffer the same cough, help each other get a ticket, a takeaway or a haircut. Our social relations in this meshwork included the handling of multiple *pots*.

## The Ethnographic Focus: Patients and Practitioners Probing Pots

### Beyond the Dyad of Patient and Practitioner

The medical encounter has a long tradition of being analysed in terms of the patient–practitioner dyad, especially in medical sociology. However, medical anthropologists have from the very start critiqued this dyadic focus as too narrow. John Janzen's (1978) monograph on 'medical pluralism', which became foundational to medical anthropology emphasised that decisions regarding treatment were not usually taken by the patient and practitioner in a medical consultation and that a focus on the patient–practitioner dyad was misplaced. Rather, medical decision-making involved a wide range of different people, a so-called 'therapy-managing group'. Janzen, who worked as a general practitioner in a dispensary in central Africa, had noted that his medical intervention was but one in a long series of consultations with diviners and herbalists, friends and relatives, and large meetings held by prophets or village elders. He recorded the stories that his clientele told him and found that each was different, thereby suggesting that the therapeutic field was one of 'medical pluralism', where patients opted for different treatments in an unpredictable and arbitrary fashion.[2]

### . . . to Plurified Practitioners in Medical Anthropology

Janzen presents six case histories in separate chapters. As Figure 17 in his monograph's appendix, which provides an excellent visualised summary of each of his chapters, highlights, the six patients he studied all consulted with several decision-making bodies, and the sequence of medical authorities sought does not follow a particular pattern (Janzen 1978: 220). Rather, it comes across as fairly random, demonstrating that people engaged in a highly individualistic search for therapy. This may have been a covert critique of the rather rigid formula of 'hierarchies of resort' identified earlier by Romanucci-Schwartz (1969). In line with the tenor of his time, Janzen advanced a notion of 'medical pluralism' that aimed to overcome the then-prevailing dichotomous view of the medical field, with medical professionals on the one hand and Indigenous healers and exorcists on the other. This idea of medical pluralism was to be taken further to emphasise the multiplicity of choice, situational decision-making and probing attitudes of experimentation. Byron Good and Mary-Jo DelVecchio Good (1994) would later speak of a 'subjunctive mode' in illness narratives, and Susan Whyte (1997) of a pragmatist 'trying out'. The zigzags in Janzen's Figure 17 illustrate nicely how medical anthropologists have conceived of patients seeking health, the notion being that in the case of illness, everything is tried out and probed, even by otherwise most principled and 'rational' people.

The concept of medical pluralism became prominent in debates that pitted 'pragmatic' over 'rational' choice. However, the concept lends itself also to another long-standing anthropological problem, that of the medical 'culture' (Last 1981). Inquiry into the theme of medical pluralism can be used to counter the widespread idea that in a crisis event, which a serious sickness generally is, 'culture' provides its members with a normative set of behaviours. However, in the medical field this has been shown not to be the case. Rather, ever-changing reconfigurations of patients, practitioners and *pots* arise, as argued here, out of a probing of place. Despite the exasperation and desperation that can accompany the search for therapy, it is possible to discern in this probing a sometimes almost playful bricolage and experimenting, spurred by an attitudinal shift into which human beings are propelled in the event of a crisis: a subjunctive, curiosity-driven, explorative, sometimes even hopeful, yet probing mood.

Although in the face of suffering, the word 'play' seems inappropriate to our modern sensibilities, an anthropological concept of play may frame the therapeutic endeavour in a productive way, as it comments on configurations created by multiple actors' mutually attuned yet testing attentiveness (Huizinga 1980). Importantly, the 'as if' attitude, which makes play possible among animals and humans (Bateson 1973a), arises from the ability to recognise and adhere to certain – if only temporary – patterns of conduct. Play and ritual cannot be reduced to sincerity (Seligman et al. 2008); the 'as if' attitude and its probing flair would seem to define them. Not 'everything goes', as the postmodernist would have it; there are so-called 'internal dynamics' to ritual, as Kapferer (2004) noted, and likewise, it would seem, to those crisis situations in which there is a patient seeking therapy.

## *Multifaceted Patients*

Lorna Amarasingham Rhodes (1980) went a step further. Yes, she put one single patient centre stage, and the patient's health-seeking was probing. However, it was also textured, and not arbitrary. The event in focus was that of a girl who suffered from an attack of *pissu* (madness) while preparing for her high school exams. Rhodes depicted the consultations that the father, who was the main caretaker, arranged for his daughter as mutually constitutive parts in an extended journey, until finally, the girl was sent to the psychiatric ward on which Rhodes worked, and was there successfully treated with anti-psychotic medication. However, what some biomedical professionals might have called a 'six-month delay' is, on the basis of post-hoc interviews with the father and other carers, put in a different light: for them the movement among healers constituted an integral part of the girl's recovery. The stars and planets (which prompted consultation of two astrologers), the demons and gods (warranting exorcism and, later, pilgrimage to a holy shrine) and the bodily juices and humours (and the according medication, Ayurvedic and biomedical) were seen to complement each other. The consultations undertaken outside the biomedical establishment were not merely 'a waste of time', delaying the patient's access to 'urgently needed treatment', but paved the way for making it successful and efficacious. Although the ethnographer Rhodes does not make a point of it, it goes without saying that the health-seeking involved a probing attitude.[3] We note the testing, the 'trying out', the 'what if' attitude that is so characteristic of play. This probing exploration was not considered an entirely random zigzag, but a patterned or perhaps even a textured one. It was textured insofar as the ethnographer accounted for historically given dynamics specific to the landscape populated by the human and non-human actors to whom the patient presented herself in the course of health-seeking, willing to heed or at least negotiate their demands.

Rhodes saw herself as attending to different 'epistemologies' and 'world views', but she can be read as having implicated the 'things' that mattered in Sri Lanka's medical landscapes as well: demons and gods, stars and humours, the physicality of overwork and the emotionality of excessive happiness. In our own common parlance, on which materialist philosophies have left their mark, we would not call demons or overwork 'things', although they could be interpreted to qualify as what Bruno Latour (1988) called the *tertium quid*.[4] Insofar as they became entwined into the patient's journey, the stars and demons that are tangible might even be viewed as *pots*. The search for therapy involved the navigation of a universe of different 'players', each with their own 'internal dynamics' (cf. Kapferer 2004), affecting multiple, mutually interdependent levels of the patient's well-being.

## *Pluripotent Pots*

Where Janzen highlighted that there was a multiplicity of medical authorities and Rhodes that patients had a plurality of different issues demanding attention, the pluripotent *pot* is here added as the third player in the medical encounter, thereby transposing the gaze from the patient–practitioner dyad onto an analytically relevant triad. By *pot* I mean the materialities that are perceived by the researcher and their respondents as constitutive of the medical encounter. The *pots* are 'pluripotent' insofar as different perceptions of the materialities are brought into play during a medical encounter depending on the particular situation in question. The medical encounter is no longer merely a dyadic event between patient and practitioner, but involves the triad of patients, *pots* and practitioners.

Mark Nichter ([1980] 1996) long ago stressed the importance of focusing on the material aspects of the medical encounter. In the patient's perception, the practitioner's learning was not as salient as the equipment on display: the medicines' coating, the flashy medical apparatus, the practitioner's white coat. The patient inferred from these perceived *pots* the practitioner's powers. Nichter discussed the taste and colour of capsules, pills and tablets, their packaging, their brands and the place of manufacture of instruments like stethoscopes. These *things* mattered, alongside the more recent, richly documented *sense perceptions* (Nichter 2008). However, Nichter's focus was mostly on the meanings of these sense perceptions. Packaging (for instance) was conceptualised as a carrier of meaning for the patient about the quality of the practitioner's medical provision.

The interpretive focus on symbolic meanings of appearance and make has since been updated with what seems to me to be more attuned research on doing, sensing and handling materialities. *Pots* that have become constitutive of a medical encounter comprise more than the biochemical substance of the medicines on offer in medicine pots. It would be wrong to speak of 'pots' as the objectively given and 'real' thing, and of *pots* as the intersubjective experience of the thing. Warnier (2007) has long made this point, for instance in his eye-opening monograph *The Pot King*. Pots are everywhere; apart from the obvious cooking pots, he considers rooms, houses, palaces and dwellings as pots. Nevertheless, the pots that Warnier refers to are those of a Euclidean space, and the things he attends to are material in a good Marxist materialist sense.

By contrast, the *pots* referred to here are not to be understood as randomly distributed things stacked up in a Euclidean space conceptualised as a three-dimensional container. As we will see in Part III, the pots (I consistently refer to pots in the plural) will be used as a superordinate term comprising both 'pots' as they exist in a Euclidean space (Chapter 7) and *pots*, which are part of interpersonally sensed texturing and textured spaces (Chapter 8).

With the monosyllabic word *pot* I propose to refer to a complex and dynamic configuration of 'things-implicated-into-techniques'. 'Things-implicated-into-techniques' become *pots* through the intercorporeality of two people engaged in one action (Csordas 2008) and the interactions and practices of which they are constitutive. Where 'emplotment' is a matter of intersubjectivity (Mattingly 1998, 2010), 'empotment' adds to it the dimension of intercorporeality. So, *pots* are intersubjectively perceived materials, things, atmospheres or beings that have become part of a triadic intercorporeal relationship that they form with patients and practitioners.

The notion of 'affordance' is important to understanding the concept of the *pot* that I propose to work with. It is a concept generally associated with James Gibson (e.g. 1979), whose work on it as 'demand character' currently enjoys a career in biological and evolutionary theory, in the cognitive sciences and in complementary and alternative medical considerations. However, Gibson's notion of affordance has a static aspect (Morris 2012: 156, fn. 24), which earlier notions of 'affordance' that had long been in use did not have. Phenomenologists, like Erwin Straus (1963), emphasised that sense perception is always oriented towards the perceiver, and the perceived affordances of a thing or material are always modulated by the affective responses that it elicits from the perceiver.

It is in this non-Cartesian understanding of the world that a certain configuration's affordances play into the sense perception of *pots*. At stake is a practical efficacy that emerges out of peoples' practical engagement with the world. This may explain why in different cultural settings different people might adopt comparable techniques on one level, even if they differ on another. As we have seen, this happens with and through their bodies, bodies that move and share certain propensities for locomotion.

Affordances are not a priori given but arise in a social relation. They have a directionality. Accordingly, *pots* can be repellent or attractive to the people who become engaged with them. 'Fierce' and 'violent' Chinese medical herbs are repulsive to a person with a 'weak' constitution. So, in addition to the materialist understanding of matter, as given in an 'objective' description of its 'properties' and in an empiricist bioscientific identification of chemical composition, the ethnographer studying *pots* needs to find a way of accounting for their sensed and relational efficaciousness. Perhaps this can be achieved through attending to their affordances?

## *Interlude*

In summary, the patient–practitioner dyad as an analytic unit has always posed problems to medical anthropologists. Janzen's seminal study of medical pluralism highlighted that a doctor was not actually dealing with a single patient, but also with a multiplicity of relatives and friends (the 'therapy managing group'), as well as with multiple competing practitioners. Rhodes (1980), based on comparable case materials, multiplied the facets of well-being that matter to a patient, and this allowed her to place the practitioners into a therapeutic landscape where they were not merely competing with each other, but mutually complementary. Taking exorcism measures, ensuring 'good fortune' and renewing the blessing of the gods, together with balancing out one's humoral make-up and getting one's brain chemistry right, were depicted not merely as matters of belief, but as intrinsic to the multifaceted aspects of well-being. Rhodes discussed both the epistemologies of the practitioners and the perceived physicalities that motivated the patient's carer's actions, but her focus was not on things and their affordances, let alone their agency.

Many medical anthropologists are modernists whose thinking is affected by what Whitehead (1920: 30) called 'the bifurcation of nature', by which he meant that there was a dichotomy between research into questions posed by a reflective 'sense awareness' of matter on the one hand, and into the unreflectively or one-dimensionally sensed, that is, sense-perceived matter, on the other. Latour (2000b) accordingly suggested that social scientists were studying disembodied social relations and natural scientists were researching decontextualised things.

Actor–network theory (ANT) has to be credited for giving things an agency of their own and not merely treating them as a medium through which patient and practitioner communicate, as the term 'paraphernalia' (meaning 'that which is brought along') would appear to imply. ANT reconnected decontextualised things by making them into independent actors or 'actants' in a network, some human and some non-human (Woolgar and Lezaun 2015). However, by locating agency in the actor or actant, rather than in the interaction, a Cartesian understanding of personhood and its mind–body dichotomy is perpetuated.[5]

Latour's *tertium quid* and Mol's (2002) hospital technology worked towards a bridging of the bifurcation, as the microbes and materials were implicated in the description of the social. In a similar vein, a sensory account of the medical encounter, which aims to overcome this bifurcation, aims to pay attention to material aspects of the encounter. We will see that materialities come into play in as specific ways as the practitioners were, and on as multiple levels as the different facets of the patient's well-being demanded.

In this way, Whitehead's insights are also relevant for the sensory anthropologist aiming to overcome the gap between the bodily sense perception of matter and the mindful sense awareness that modernity posits. As we will see, ecological thinking becomes important here, as it emphasises relations and relationalities that are interdependent and heterogeneous (Ingold 2007b). The affordance of a thing treats its intended or unintended use as constitutive, if not defining, of what it is; what constitutes a thing thus emerges from its interrelations.

So rather than imbuing the practitioner, the patient and the *pot* each with ego-centred self-interest and agency, I consider their dynamics of mutual involvement to derive from their interactions. I challenge the ego-centred sense of agency intrinsic to each actor that appears to underly otherwise convincing pragmatically oriented research and many actor–network analyses. Instead, I appeal to the automorphic symmetries and kaleidoscopic refractions that happen during a medical encounter: rhythms, patterned interdependencies and textured transformations.

'Empotment' underlines the intercorporeal aspects of the different dynamics that a medical procedure tends to have in the textured spaces thereby brought into focus. As body techniques and skills are involved, practitioners, in conjunction with their patients, are turned into craftsmen, and those, by definition, will always strive for the concrete perfection of their craft (Mauss 2006b). Accordingly, a practitioner's practice is far from messy, but due to the involvement of bodily skill, always textured.

## *Injections for Syphilis, or: Why an Anthropology of Substances Matters*

A Chinese medical doctor once allowed me to observe his treatment of a syphilis patient, who regularly travelled from Dar es Salaam all the way to Zanzibar island just to receive this doctor's treatment. So I was told by the practitioner and the patient in the former's presence. The Chinese practitioner was proud of his newly invented technique, and he had told me several times that it attracted syphilis sufferers from far away. His treatment involved injecting a fluid into the acupuncture point *guanyuan* 关元 that is located three inches (*cun* 寸) below the navel. The treatment was over in five minutes. 'What is so special about this?!', I asked. I had seen other Chinese medical practitioners in East Africa treat syphilis patients by needling the *guanyuan*, as stimulation of that acupuncture point is known to enhance one's most essential life forces and bolster the *jing* 精 ('semen', 'distilled and refined fluids'). He retorted that I had seen others needle the *guanyuan* point with acupuncture needles; he, however, injected a fluid, a medicine, a substance. 'And I will not tell you what it is as this is my secret.' He knew it was unlawful for a Chinese practitioner to use purified chemical substances such as penicillin or other antibiotics, and being secretive was for that reason well advised. His treatment was not the first I had seen of a syphilis patient. I already knew by then – several years into my fieldwork – that for the treatment of syphilis, Chinese medical practitioners would give a combined treatment of a penicillin injection in the thigh and an acupuncture session of about ten to twenty minutes during which they needled the *guanyuan*. This doctor's hybrid method was ingenious in that it collapsed the two techniques into one. It also had distinctive sensory effects: there was a brief phase of very unusual and acute pain as the syringe pierced the subcutaneous tissue (injections hurt more than fine acupuncture needles), and this in the lower abdomen, which for most people is an extremely intimate and sensitive bodily region.[6] Furthermore, it shortened the duration of the treatment and exerted power through brevity.

Such a rather painful injection of medicines by syringe facilitates the absorption of substances into the body, as does the widespread method in Africa of making razor-blade cuttings, which also are meant to hurt briefly, as fresh-plant preparations are rubbed into the bloodstream.[7] These forms of pain infliction that generate a synchronicity between practitioner and patient may be warranted, as are the feelings of sourness (*suan* 酸), cribbling (*ma* 麻) and swelling (*zhang* 胀) elicited by acupuncture needling, which are considered crucial for its efficaciousness in China (Hsu 2005b). Warnier (2007) describes how the spit of the Fon king, mixed with raffia wine, is sprayed over his assembled community, which seeks to absorb his blessings in front of his palace; I imagine how each and every individual in the crowd feels the barely perceptible prickling on the skin that cooling water droplets effect, and that this heightens the participants' presence in an event that by this sensed prickling is made into an intercorporeal one. Taylor (1988) emphasises, in a similar vein, that in sexual union the exchange of fluids matters and that well-being, more generally, derives from an experience of being connected through substances. In this context it is noteworthy that Africanist medical anthropologists stress the absorption of substances as a mode of emplacing people into a locality.

Geissler and Prince (2010b) highlight that among the Luo in Kisumu, Kenya, the daily herbal baths for fortifying toddlers involve not only splashing water and banter, which evoke a multilayered presence among adults and children alike, but also fresh plants that grow on the ancestral land of the paternal grandmother. The children who are washed with these plant substances absorb them through their skin, and those who, like the grandmother, drink them are in this way made consubstantial with the patriline's lands. Whatever the chemistry of the fresh leaf bathwater may be, this daily procedure strengthens their lineage identity, and ultimately also their health and well-being. Likewise, Kelly (2014) noted in the forests of Oku in northern Cameroon that the ingestion and absorption of herbal medications connects the patient to the ancestors, who typically dwell in the region of the roots of the plant, underground. This relation to the ground and earth in Oku in turn resonates well with observations in other places where earths are sacred.

Fayers-Kerr (2013) describes, among the agro-pastoralist Mursi (or Mun) in the Lower Omo valley, 'body painting' that involves what appears to us to be an application of colourful clays onto one's skin. Why should this be healthful? One might endeavour to argue in terms of the clay's pharmacology and the patient's physiology, given that fungi in the soil have produced substances that are antibiotic. A more culturally attuned explanation would be that such procedures of emplacement are meant to strengthen one's lineage identity, and thereby one's health. Finally, according to the phenomenological approach taken here, which foregrounds the significance of the materiality of the *pots* implemented during a therapeutic encounter, the application of clay all over the face and body can be interpreted as a preventive medical measure, specifically a body technique effecting, in a physical way, an 'empotment' into the Mursi's ancestral lands, which makes them consubstantial with their ancestors and soils. The small lumps of clay that they carry with them in the folds of their tunics, each with its specific hue, they take from their lineage's sacred clay pits, which they tend to visit, discretely, in passing. These procedures, causing the absorption of colourful mineral-rich clays through the skin, are said to involve an 'eating' of the clay, a word that is best understood in a 'physiognomic', practical and immediately recognisable way (Morris 2012: 25).

In other words, one 'eats' the clay to become consubstantial with one's ancestral lands. An auspicious dream might prompt a young man to grace his favourite cow and himself with the clay from the ancestral clay pit. It may look as though this is a protective measure, but simultaneously it might be an ornamentation for celebrating the dream and strengthening the presence of the moment. More recently, tourists have been filmed and observed (e.g. Turton 2004; Silvester 2009) prompting young Mursi to decorate their bodies through the offer of cash for photography. These encounters are marked by a discomforting irony, as they make living people into objects of art.

Meanwhile, the play with clay initiated by a monetary economy in the encounter between the culturally distant Mursi and tourists does not appear to be about emplacement, or if so, only in a hyper-ironic way. Likewise, as the familiar was mixed with the foreign in Chinese medical clinics, it sometimes transgressed the limits of what was felt to be acceptable for a self-respecting person. For instance, having a medical test done that involved the taking of and tinkering with one's bodily substances (e.g. presenting one's urine to the laboratory assistant or having blood drawn) was generally not a problem for young men. However, although elderly women and teenage girls were familiar with these biomedical procedures, some broke off their consultations with the Chinese practitioner at this point.

## *Hyper-Ironic Twists and Indirect 'Empotment'*

Difference and distance need not always result in hostility and violence, but can also awaken curiosity. No doubt there were patients who were drawn into Chinese medical clinics because they were curious about things Chinese. Most of them did not like the thought of being needled but had no objection to ingesting formula medicines, that is, pills, tablets and capsules.[8] Therefore, the majority of Chinese practitioners had only formula medicines on offer. But a few practitioners additionally engaged in more specialised skills. They said that this was in response to the clientele that sought them out. In what follows I discuss the specialist skills of wound dressing, gynaecological surgery and acupuncture. I argue that the Chinese practitioners deployed these not merely in response to a clientele that was keen on enhancing health through emplacement, but also in an effort to emplace themselves into the East African medical landscapes.

Dr Wu was trained as a biomedical doctor, and had several years of work experience, but after moving to Kenya in the late 1990s he could only hope to practise medicine by advertising himself as a Chinese medical practitioner, which put him in a grey zone legally. Kenya was in this respect no different from other countries that require biomedical professionals to be re-examined and approved by national medical authorities. Dr Wu felt he knew sufficient Chinese medicine because the usual biomedical training in the PRC included a minimum of two semesters of compulsory courses on acupuncture and moxibustion (*Zhenjiuxue* 针灸学) and the Chinese *materia medica* (*Zhongyaoxue* 中药学). The practice he opened in the early 2000s was located next to a Chinese textile shop in one of Nairobi's shopping malls on the outskirts of the city, catering to upper-middle-class clients who owned large cars and mansions. His consultation room looked more like an academic's office than a medical practice. All the surfaces were covered with magazines and books, the drawers were filled with medicines alongside electronic devices, and stacks and stacks of paper were everywhere. He had many friends who came to see him, most of whom were Chinese. Some of them needed medication, while others just enjoyed his conversation and company. By 2006, when I last visited him, Dr Wu had made so many friends that he had gradually glided into a second-hand car-selling business, given that there was great mobility among the Chinese expatriates and almost all really enjoyed driving.

In that very year, incidentally, on each of the few occasions that I dropped in on him, a different tall Somali man with gaping wounds on his legs or feet would be lying on one of several plank beds in the back room, while the doctor was handling cotton wool and disinfectant, tongs and scissors. The silence of concentration was protracted as he skilfully worked on the wounds, cleaning them, cutting off pieces of skin and finalising their dressing. The young, well-grown Somali refugees had no job prospects, but some pushed themselves very hard, training as athletes for long distance running (c. 20–40 km daily) in the hope of being selected by a sports team one day, and by an international trainer. They were not part of Kenyan civil society and had no access to Kenyan medical care, but Dr Wu had become known among the refugee community living in the open wastelands south of the southern suburbs of Nairobi for his hygiene and skill in dressing wounds. This involved re-enlivening aspects of his preferred repertoire, he said, having specialised in (Western medical) minor surgery (*Waikexue* 外科学) during his student years in China.

As a Chinese medical doctor, his practice involved 'pots' classified as biomedical, among them the highly specialised surgical knives, scissors and tongs that he imported directly from the PRC, but since he was treating marginalised non-Kenyans and did this with skill and care, he was not denounced. Regardless of the cultural distance between them in terms of language, religion and geographic provenance, the intercorporeal routines between practitioner and patients was facilitated by the practitioner's adept handling of the surgical tools, which assisted both parties in their different efforts towards making a living in a foreign country.

In this case, a dynamic interdependency of practitioner's body and tools affecting and being affected by the patient's body was the primary means for making possible and speeding up their different ambitions of emplacement or 'empotment' into different spatial textures. Their remarkable bodily skills, however different, elicited and enhanced intersubjective understanding and mutual respect. Their practices of place-making resided less in an anthropology of appropriating the substances of the land one aims to inhabit, but rather in the production of habits that involved dynamic intercorporeal interdependencies between the runner and the grounds they ran on. The Somali runners, aided by the Chinese practitioner, had the potential to reconfigure a space of apparent no-man's land as a place reanimated by sportive bodily cultivation, ambition and hope.

Another practitioner, Dr Wei, likewise engaged in minor surgery for people living at the margins of society, in this case sex workers who needed an abortion or suffered from STDs. Dr Wei was in her late fifties and had decades of clinical experience. Her practice was situated in a residential area, a stone's throw away from the hurly-burly of a central suburb's main street. She performed abortions as one does in the PRC, with only a local anaesthetic. The advantage of this procedure is that the risk of haemorrhage is greatly reduced compared to a fully anaesthetised abortion, but it can be excruciatingly painful. Once, when I dropped by, one could hear screaming from one of the back rooms of her practice, close to where she had her living quarters. The screaming was intense but not protracted. When Dr Wei opened the door about twenty minutes later, she still wore her rubber gloves, with bright red blood on them, and disappeared into an adjacent room containing a semi-mobile sterilisation unit that she had shown me on another occasion. She had arranged its importation from the hospital in Northeast China where she had worked before going into early retirement. In TCM, women's medicine, *fuke* 妇科, had always included Western medical procedures, with an overlap of around 90 per cent, she explained. This was because the traditional 'department of women', *fuke*, had been merged with the traditional 'department for birthing', *chanke* 产科. The latter's almost exclusive reliance on incantations and other superstitions (*mixin* 迷信), Dr Wei said, had been replaced by training students in biomedical birthing techniques. What Dr Wei said was indeed common knowledge among TCM professionals (see also Furth 1999). However, its historical accuracy may be slightly challenged, as only a cursory glimpse at *Fu ren da quan liang fang* 妇人大全良方 by Chen Ziming 陈自明 shows a good range of decoctions for managing not only pregnancy, but also birthing (including the changing of position of the foetus) and post-natal problems (Hsu et al. forthcoming), even if today their efficacy is queried. Although Dr Wei relied largely on biomedical skills, she insisted that she was a TCM professional, and one wall of her clinic was covered with photocopies of certificates to prove it.

Practitioners and medical anthropologists alike have described TCM as a Westernised, scientised and hybridised traditional Chinese and modern Western medicine (see introduction). Dr Wei insisted on calling it a modernised Chinese medicine (*xiandaihuade zhongyi* 现代化的中医). In other words, she was implicitly advocating TCM as an 'alternative modernity' (Gaonkar 1999; see Chapter 7). The fact that she made use of technology developed during the nineteenth and twentieth centuries in Western medical circles did not stop her from identifying herself as a Chinese medical doctor and an exponent of a long tradition of medical learning that had existed for at least two thousand years. In contrast to Dr Wu, who emphasised that he had to make a living in a foreign land and provide for his wife and daughter, and who claimed that there was no going back for him due to the rapid economic and scientific progress in reformist post-Dengist China, Dr Wei did not express the wish to stay in Nairobi. Her aim was to enrol her son at an American university, whereupon she would return to China and join her spouse. She was well known among the Chinese practitioners, and her clinic was considered one of the longest standing. In the seven years of my fieldwork it was one of the only clinics that remained in the same location throughout. It was in a lush, green and quiet neighbourhood that also attracted other clients.

Dr Wei was a foreign woman who engaged in work for marginalised members of the metropole's underworld that was polluting (Ngubane 1977). Handling female fluids, discarding unwanted life and keeping contagious STDs under control all involved hands-on skills, like those of Dr Wu. Yet where Dr Wu's surgery won wide recognition among medical professionals, males and females alike, Dr Wei's work, which was performed with an equal care for hygiene and which also involved a professional's careful navigation of technical and social know-how, was not spoken of. Dr Wei was unwilling to share the story of her life; it had no narrative plot resulting in an 'emplotment'. Rather, by means of her doings, she seemed to achieve an 'empotment' of her mostly female clientele as well as herself into this neighbourhood.

Finally, there was Dr Wang, who had stationed herself in yet another suburb and advertised herself as an acupuncturist. She was a young woman who had been a Western medical laboratory technician in the PRC. She had no training in Chinese herbal medicine but apparently attended evening classes in acupuncture while still in China. She came to Kenya as a refugee, fleeing from Burundi when the genocide started there. She too catered to people on the margins: white expatriate men and women. It is these expatriates who believe that Chinese medics cater primarily to the affluent middle classes in urban Africa, Europe and North America. They are right but, as shown above, only partially.

Dr Wang engaged in needling with fine needles according to the TCM teachings on acupuncture. She too paid great attention to hygiene by disinfecting the needles with alcohol and storing them separately, up to a dozen for each patient. These needles, which came in different sizes and lengths, she regularly imported from the PRC without going through the nuisance of customs. They were easy to transport in the suitcases of her many friends. Dr Wang was always very pleasantly dressed, very feminine, with long, shiny black hair that she swung from one side to the other from time to time. Her medical practice was in a bungalow, with a sloped red-tiled roof and a bed of roses in front of its windows, situated adjacent to her private lodgings; it was a view of a home that one might see on TV as the background to a rosy future thanks to life insurance. She had already spent several years in Nairobi at the time of my fieldwork, but she made clear that her dream was to move to Canada or the USA. For her, clearly, Nairobi was but a stepping stone. Interestingly, her toolkit – the fine acupuncture needles and the alcohol that could be purchased worldwide in any urban area – were those of a hyper-mobile practitioner. To make her living in the interim, she created through her skilled use of these needles an intercorporeal interdependency with Nairobi's mostly white expatriate employees, most of whom worked on temporary contracts.

## *Discussion*

The four ethnographic portraits above might be read as relegating the activities of Chinese medical practitioners to the margins of urban East Africa – catering to refugees with no means, to super-rich yet ephemeral expatriates, to the terminally ill and to the polluted and socially compromised. As a point of comparison, Das and Das's (2005) thorough research gives a rich and compelling account of similar 'local ecologies' where 'self medication' is practised in urban India:[9]

> [F]orms of belongingness in the urban context are fraught with tensions. An individual cannot be said to 'belong' to her kinship network, community or neighbourhood as, say, water belongs to the bottle or clothes belong to the wardrobe. The 'voices' of the community, the repeated quests for therapy for illnesses for which only temporary relief seems possible, and the constant need for brokers through which the outside world [of state medical care] can be accessed, all contribute to an individual's experience. A dependence on the medical system exists alongside a tremendous distrust of the services received. The 'self' in self-medication is a composite of these experiences – in which the real seems to constantly elude the hold the poor can establish over it. . . . These are the worlds of the poor – produced through complex configurations of policies and programmes, shaping medical realities that lie beyond the bedside of the patient. (Das and Das 2005: 81–82)

East Africa's urban textures in which Chinese medical practitioners worked were similarly diverse and entangled – multiply layered, cacophonous, criss-crossing, sometimes short-lived, sometimes not, and always marked by indeterminacy. The social profile of the patients was very varied as well. It differed between medical practices, but in general the suffering did not strike me as abject, as among the above 'worlds of the poor' in urban India. In general, there was a probing, yet positive and forward-looking feeling among those patients who ventured into Chinese medical practices.

## Reflections: Techniques of Transformation

This chapter went beyond the focus on the dyad of patient and practitioner that is usually in focus in studies of medical pluralism. Instead, it framed the medical encounter as a triadic configuration of patients, practitioners and pots.[10] The triad of patients, practitioners and the as-yet-to-be-more-closely-defined *pots* provides the blueprint for the entire monograph: Chapter 4 discusses the patients, Chapter 5 the practitioners, and from Chapter 6 onwards, in Chapters 7–9, the pots are discussed.

The *pots*, as part of the triadic relationship at the core of healing efforts, will be primarily defined through their relations to patient and practitioner. A focus on *pots* as part of a medical encounter therefore asks us to go beyond the epistemological concerns of most medical anthropological research on traditional medicines and medical pluralism. It requests us to reformulate epistemological concerns and turn them into questions regarding practice and craftsmanship, matter and materiality, and techniques and technology.

Insofar as in so-called 'traditional' medicines, and also in 'alternatively modern' Chinese formula medicines, ingredients are made of plant and animal parts (albeit in powder form), these might be seen to form part of a multispecies relationship with the human beings who are attracted to buy and ingest them. Since animals, plants and minerals form part of the Chinese *materia medica*, this instantly begs the question of how to think about minerals, which are classified as inanimate according to modern and Marxist materialism but are subject to a cycle of waxing and waning *qi*, and thus are considered animate and capable of being co-constitutive of a multispecies relationship in Chinese medical practice.[11] Questions of the kind that concern the sensory ascertaining of specific *pots* pertain to the 'new materialities' and 'new animism' (*qi* is tangible for Chinese medical practitioners as a sensed materiality), and are also discussed, to a limited extent, by some authors of the 'ontological turn' (Holbraad and Pedersen 2017, see Part III).

So instead of foregrounding questions of whether scholarly medical theories are rational or not, this monograph emphasises healing as a practice involving craftmanship. Healing is effected through judicious application of techniques that effect a transformation in the patient and the place that the patient aims to inhabit. We have already noted spatial textures, like a stuffy divination hut (in Chapter 1), and techniques, like phonemic misunderstandings (in Chapter 2), affect the temporality of healing procedures. In the above cases they contributed to generating moments of synchronicity and simultaneity. Evidently, different techniques become relevant at different stages of therapeutic procedures.

In this chapter, I attended to the physiognomy of the urban textures as I moved through them. With a view to an efficaciousness that makes whole and effects slow transformation, I pointed to Chinese practitioners who successfully secured the emplacement of their medical practice – and with it, often of their family – into different urban neighbourhoods by catering to a clientele as varied as travelling youths, refugees, sex workers and white expatriates. This involved the negotiation and handling of substances, practices, materialities and spaces that made each practitioner and patient part of the different habitats they inhabited, and thereby empowered them. Therefore, I spoke of an 'empotment' into these urban textures, a concept that complements, and even embraces, that of narrative 'emplotment' (Mattingly 2010).

## *Marcel Mauss on Technical Practice and Its Perfection*

The above brings into play Nathan Schlanger's collation of twelve texts by Marcel Mauss (2006b) on body techniques, practice and its perfection, craftmanship, and culture. In a triadic medical encounter, efforts of textured crafting are also texturing, and as Mauss already seemed to suggest, render cultural boundary-making insignificant.

For the gestalt psychology-inspired, techniques-oriented approach adopted here, there is no need to contrast the mind's disembodied theories, which are considered systematic, elegant and normative, with the 'messy' practice encountered in tangible 'real' life. Rather, our approach pays attention to the textured and texturing spatiality of practices as they present themselves to those involved in them (inclusive of the researcher). Anything crafted always shows variation, Mauss underlined.

> Nothing manifests more the difference between two social traditions than the difference, still enormous, even in our own days, between the implements and the crafts of two societies. The methods of handling and

the forms of implements which they imply, of two people as close as the French and the English, are still almost absurd. Each has their different spades and shovels, and *this difference requires differences in the mode of their use*, and vice versa. It is enough to make one doubt reason. (Mauss [1927] 2006b: 52, italics added)

Naturally, this passage can be read as highlighting cultural difference. However, Mauss also says: 'and this difference requires differences in the mode of their use'. This speaks to an embodied understanding of cultural difference. Body techniques as they are enacted and tools as they are skilfully applied each have their own rhythmicity. This comment on a craft, like shovelling, is not discussed in terms of there being a disembodied ideal and a 'messy' implementation in practice. Rather, to make sense of a neighbouring people's very distinctive differences, which border on the 'absurd' and 'make one doubt reason', it is important to remember an 'inherent quality to all social phenomena':

> be they the instrument best adapted to the best and most numerous ends, be they the most rational possible, the most human, *they are still arbitrary*'. (Mauss [1929/30] 2006b: 62)

There is a feature of arbitrariness to them, but this does not necessarily make them messy. When Sennett (2007: 20) says that craftsmen are 'dedicated to good work for its own sake', he expresses one central aspect of craftsmanship, which directly reflects Mauss's (2006b). To produce good work 'for its own sake' gives technological activity a texturing capacity – something that also interested Mauss – rather than seeing in it merely a function of a given texture. However, Sennett seems not to be interested in one issue of central concern to Mauss. This is the relationship between craft, that is, the activity of crafting, and *culture*.

Mauss notes that a craftsman's commitment to obtaining excellence, if not perfection, in the doing of a craft has an effect on how we think about 'culture'. Conceptualising people as craftsmen allows for the conception of culture as a craft that reconfigures elements from different provenances. Such crafting creates a new 'whole'.

> Like all social phenomena, then, techniques are on one side arbitrary and particular to the community which invents them. . . . At the same time, however, more than any other social phenomenon, the arts are apt

to cross the boundaries of societies. Techniques are eminently liable to borrowing. (Mauss [1927] 2006b: 52)

A preoccupation with craftsmanship dissolves clear cultural boundaries, as the craftsperson will borrow and probingly integrate into their craft whatever optimises their craft. Mauss accorded the techniques an 'extraordinary extrasocial position', and defined them as 'the means, this time physical, which society possesses to act on its milieu' (Mauss [1927] 2006b: 52). Mauss seemed to imply that hands-on, skilled practice in itself is patterned and generative, and even though it varies from person to person (or from culture to culture), it is not messy. In his study of techniques and technologies, Mauss highlighted movement and mutual borrowing, copying, improving, modifying and re-borrowing from each other as part of the craftperson's striving for perfection.

The topics of tool use (Leroi-Gourhan 1993), skill (Polanyi 1966), craftsmanship (Sennett 2007) and making (Ingold 2013) bring age-old archaeological themes into anthropology, sociology and philosophy. The above discussions will have made clear that among this set of authors belongs also Mauss (1936, 1973, 1979a, 2006a; 2006b).

For a medical anthropologist interested in how healing makes whole, Mauss also matters: the healer as craftsperson engaged in skilled practice – for its own sake – strives for perfection, irrespective of culturalising boundaries and stereotyping talk. This chapter proposed to conceive of the medical encounter as a triadic configuration that – through techniques of transformation that are probingly deployed – 'empots' patients and practitioners into the places that they aim to inhabit.

## Notes

1. The main hospital authorities granted me permission to purchase the ingredients of four Chinese medical formulas prepared for an anonymous patient, over four consecutive weeks. They are now exhibited in the permanent 'Living and Dying' exhibition at the British Museum, London.
2. This section elaborates on Elisabeth Hsu. 2017. 'Patients, Practitioners, and "Pots": Probing Chinese Medicine in East Africa', in Viola Hörbst, Pino Schirripa and René Gerrets (eds), 'Revisiting Medical Pluralism: An Old Concept Inspiring New Theoretical Horizons', special issue, *L'Uomo Società Tradizione e Sviluppo* 42(1): 27–47. Used with permission.

3. Trawick (1987) made this point most forcefully in a critique of Robin Horton's claim that traditional knowledge systems are closed systems, while modern science is an open one.
4. The microbe as *tertium quid* became the main causal agent for disease in so-called 'germ theory' (Latour 1988), which later was to become the prototype for biomedical theories of disease.
5. Furthermore, most network analyses assume a usually quantifiable uniformity of the elements considered, and actants tend to be reduced to a geometrical point, their complex interpersonal relationships made into straight lines between these points.
6. In Chinese this method is classified as an innovation in acupuncture and called *shuizhen* 水針 ('water/liquid injection'). See *Zhenjiuxue* (1985: 174–75). It usually involves the injection of a Chinese medical decoction into what biomedicine recognises as the interstitial fluids of the connective tissue.
7. Injections have been very popular for therapeutic and preventative purposes not just in Africa (Whyte et al. 2002: 104–16) but also in China (Hsu 1992; White 1998; Chen et al. 2020).
8. The hesitation vis-à-vis acupuncture is worth further study. It may have been motivated by public health campaigns against using razor blades and syringes to prevent the transmission of AIDS and other contagious diseases.
9. Das and Das (2005) however query this term as used in global health circles: 'The majority of analgesics and antibiotics used by the households are those *dispensed* by the practitioners in low-income neighbourhoods' (ibid.: 78) They conducted a combined study involving household interviews and practitioner surveys, and this medical anthropological gaze allowed them to see '*patterns of therapeutic strategies* where others have seen only self-medication' (ibid., italics added). By sharing the gaze of Das and Das (2005), what started as a study of Chinese medicine as a form of self medication (see Introduction, 'The Fieldwork'), has become an ethnography of emergent *textures* in urban East Africa's health fields.
10. We are reminded here that Latour (1988) famously pointed to the microbe as the *tertium quid* in the medical encounter, which led to a redefinition of the 'social' as a multispecies 'association': 'We cannot form society with the social alone. We have to add the action of the microbes. . . . millions of omnipresent, terribly effective, often dangerous and quite invisible microbes' (ibid.: 35, 38). The *pots* in this monograph are evidently part of a triadic medical encounter, but not a triangular one. Unlike microbes, they are defined through direct sense perception. Furthermore, the anthropologist in the field was also affected by the *pots*' spatialities and materialities.
11. Working with the concept of 'spatial textures' can bypass the artificially created problems of whether we are dealing with living kinds and biological species or whether we are discussing materials and matter.

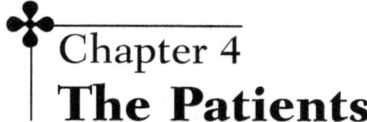

## Chapter 4
## The Patients

### Fieldwork: Semi-Structured Interviews

Refraining from asking any questions and just being with people and recording their mundane activities no doubt belongs among the most rewarding fieldwork methods. The multisited meshwork that I co-produced had me repeatedly return to a mid-range hotel in downtown Dar es Salaam, live in a local nurse's home on Pemba and stay with a TCM practitioner's family in Mombasa. It also reached into my interviewees' homes, and they were happy to let me get a glimpse of their daily lives, even if only for the length of an interview (one to two hours or more). In order to learn about the patients' perspectives on sickness, health and life more generally, and on why they consulted a Chinese medical doctor, I had to rely on interviews, however.

Harvey Russell Bernard's (1994) classic work on research methods discusses informal, unstructured and semi-structured interviewing in the same chapter (ibid.: 208–36), in contradistinction to structured interviewing, questionnaires and surveys. The semi-structured interview, he notes, is usually employed when one expects to see the interviewee only once. It is a favoured method among fieldworkers, I found, not only because it allows the fieldworker to conduct a conversation fairly unconstrainedly, but also because it will invariably produce 'data'. The sort of semi-structured interviewing that I undertook was more of an explorative kind rather than for producing reliable positive knowledge. It also proved valuable for gaining a sense of the variation in opinion and practice among a group of people, and of my re-search project's scale and complexity. Explorative semi-structured interviews give the researcher the possibility to test different facets of their research, since they are 'doable' fieldwork tasks that can easily be adjusted to the fieldwork situation. How are the results affected if one interviews only one gender, one age group, or at home rather than in the clinic?

In the context of immersive fieldwork, thirty semi-structured interviews is a common target. One gets a sense of the robustness of one's sample when answers start to become quite repetitive. This may be because of one's interviewing style; sometimes, when the interviewer gets tired, the answers become stereotypical. I found it important to stop interviewing when this happened. Incidentally, it was often when I had interviewed around thirty people. In some cases, it happened sooner, and in those cases the questions had to be reformulated or the study focus redesigned.[1] Oral historians have made interviewing a distinguished art for elucidating knowledge about little-known historical facts, but the approach that anthropologists take and the findings they obtain may or may not overlap with those of oral historians.

Patients were not always willing to be interviewed. Many thought I was doing marketing research. Some asked what I would pay for their participation. I explained that by conviction, I did not pay for interviews. For me, interviews were conversations that should enrich life on both sides and enhance insights and reflection into one's life history and doings. Other patients were vocally uncooperative and explained that they avoided situations that would recreate an asymmetrical social relation, as is characteristic of neocolonialism. Since I recruited them in Chinese clinics, they considered me an employee of the Chinese practitioners.

In order to get an impression of the range of disorders treated by Chinese practitioners, I attempted to obtain a random sample by asking every patient on a particular day to sign up (in one clinic on 19 December 2001, in another on 27 December). However interesting this sort of sampling may have been, it proved impractical, as the medical practices were sometimes extremely crowded such that it was impossible for me to practise equity and speak to everyone in the waiting room. I was less strict about sampling when recruiting patients into my research in Mombasa and on Pemba two years later.

*The Patients*

I planned to compare the first group of thirty interviewees in Dar es Salaam, Tanzania, with two other groups of thirty in two other field sites that were culturally similar; one was urban, but in another nation state, Kenya, with a different recent political and medical history, and the other was rural, on Pemba island, Zanzibar. This meant that I would have semi-structured interviews with about ninety clients of Chinese medical practitioners in total. For these conversations I memorised about ten standard questions that allowed for further developments. I found it important to make each of the thirty interviews to a unique event for both parties involved, and my standard questions were usually asked in a different sequence, and whenever possible in the patients' homes. The rapport with the twenty patients interviewed at home was so good that six months later, when I visited them again in their homes, I had no problems re-engaging in conversation. None of my interviewees had expected my visit, and many were visibly delighted to see me again.

I did not limit my visits to the patients' homes just to interviewing. The information elicited through my project of semi-structured interviewing was therefore of an entirely different quality than that derived from a formal interview or survey. After every interview, I asked to take a portrait photo, which usually was very welcome. I brought in person or sent by post a copy of these to each interviewee; it was my way of showing gratitude. The photos were also valuable as an aide-memoire. Combined with the notes, they helped me retain certain aspects of the spatiality and specificities of each interview situation (although not the information elicited itself).

Sometimes, I stayed for a while in the patient's house, seated on an all too comfortable sofa and watching TV with them while waiting for a downpour hammering against the corrugated roof to come to an end, or chatting with the women of the household who were taking a rest from their cleaning routines, which have been noted to be very extensive (cf. Obrist 2004). Or, while waiting for a patient, I would learn a culinary technique from their neighbour, such as how to make the *maandazi* (doughnuts) that would be sold on the street early in the morning the following day. This had the effect that on some days I did not manage to do more than two or three interviews.

The interview itself sometimes triggered extended discussion among the family and the household members present. It regularly also led to the handling of material culture, such as showing me the cartons and plastic boxes of medicines purchased in the clinic. Some thanked me for having gone to the trouble of finding them at home, often in suburbs of the city's outer periphery, and they seemed to appreciate that I took them and their ailments seriously.

## *Initial Findings*

The semi-structured interviews had the same format in the three locations in which they were conducted, in Dar es Salaam, in Mombasa and on Pemba island. They consisted of three sections: the first was on personal details, the second on the specific complaints and costs of the treatment and the third about issues of medical pluralism and treatment-seeking. Finally, in an attempt to get a sense of how the TCM practitioners' patients perceived the notions of 'modern' and 'traditional', I asked whether they thought their lifestyle was traditional (*maisha ya jadi/ya kiasili*) or modern (*maisha ya kisasa/ya kizungu*). Each interview ended with an opportunity to ask me any questions. The kinds of questions I was asked revealed that they considered me a health professional and a friend of the Chinese medical practitioner. This alerted me, in turn, to a bias likely inherent in all their responses.

Since the interviews lasted between one and two hours, it often happened that the persons interviewed started to contradict themselves. I took this as a sign of growing trust between us. What they initially told me was what they would tell a stranger. What they eventually revealed two hours later was more personal. The discrepancies were particularly marked regarding sociologically important information on their identities, specifically their marital status, ethnic prejudices, and attitudes to the 'traditional' African.

Only a few patients lived in neighbourhoods with streets and street numbers. Rather, they would indicate a neighbourhood to me, say, Tabata, and indicate landmark features, like derelict railway tracks or a parking lot, a named shop or bar. They then provided me with the name of a person in the neighbourhood whom everyone knew, say, Mama Zabiba. They were often known to these key figures by a different name, however – a nickname, as some later explained – yet this was rarely indicated to me on the sheet of paper onto which they wrote their 'address' and name, and which I treated like a consent form (ethical procedures at the time were just on the cusp of becoming administratively highly formalised). Finding patients in their homes was not an easy task. Not every home could be tracked down, and once located, not every patient was at home. I refrained from passing by their neighbourhoods more than twice or thrice. Nevertheless, interviewing patients at home was definitely worth the effort. Several lived in physiognomically strikingly similar newly constituted neighbourhoods. The physical appearance of these neighbourhoods typically included spacious grey cement brick houses, many of which were in the process of construction, loosely spread out in an area still generously interspersed with trees. When asked, the interviewees confirmed that the neighbourhoods were no older than five to ten years. The inhabitants of these neighbourhoods obviously did not live in well-established wards with tightly knit networks. Rather, these newly constituted informal settlements accommodated upwardly mobile citizens, many of them young men. In one clinic, the doctor allowed me to ask each patient separately for the consent to tape-record the medical encounter. This allowed me to confirm the information that the patients gave me in their homes regarding their symptoms, diagnosis, the medication and its costs. During the interviews with patients and their carers, I would often be shown the original Chinese packaging. Although most treatments consisted of several different medicines and were prescribed in different dosages, and hence were quite complicated, I found that most patients knew what they were supposed to do – for instance, '4 x 3' meant 'take four tablets three times a day'. As far as I could tell from my visits to their homes several days after seeing the patients in the clinic, they were compliant with the treatment prescribed. Most patients remembered clearly the instructions the doctor had given them, without however understanding what they were taking and what each of the different medicines was meant to treat. A patient commented: 'Chinese medical doctors know what they are doing, you follow their instruction and get a good performance.' No doubt, what might be called patient 'compliance' was enhanced by the fact that the medicines were ready-made. In only one case did I note a blatant discrepancy between the doctor's diagnosis and the patient's father's understanding. In this particular instance, the father spoke of a chest problem of his 1-year-old daughter and of bewitchment, while the Chinese doctor quite rightly had suspected malaria, and after having the child's blood tested in his clinic's lab, prescribed an antimalarial. As the father told me during my visit at their homestead ten days later, the medicines, which he said had been administered as prescribed, had led to an improvement, but he was not aware that the child had been treated for malaria. He also indicated that he did not consider the child well yet, and was already planning to consult another healer; he enumerated a long list of whom he had consulted, which amounted to very high expenditures (details given below). He was however the only person among my respondents whose understanding of the situation differed strongly from that of the practitioner.

## The Ethnographic Focus: Chinese Medicine Patients on the Swahili-Speaking Coast of East Africa

The semi-structured interviewing of c. 90 patients, and c. 20 of those twice, as well as another 30 (3 × 30 + 20, plus 1 × 30) constituted the first systematic inquiry that I undertook.[2] Those patients who had given me their address were generally interested in talking to me, and I – with admittedly very basic linguistic skills – asked about their positionality and socio-economic standing and how it related to their perceptions and understanding of Chinese medicine, which in Swahili was called *dawa ya Kichina*. I also raised the question with them of whether they thought that the healing effect through Chinese medicine worked on the basis of science, magic or witchcraft, in an attempt to explore what they associated with the terms 'traditional' and 'modern' (before, in a second step, exploring the health policy implications of these terms; see Chapter 7). Visiting the patients in their homes provided invaluable insights into my field site but also taught me about the limitations of my interviewing method. Many years later I noted veritable 'tactics' on the patients' part to make sense of the situation they had become part of (see Reflections).

## Chinese Medicine Patients in Dar es Salaam

In Tanzania, Chinese medical health care was provided by practitioners who were small-scale entrepreneurs, and the entrepreneurial aspect of their practice no doubt attracted many clients. Unlike clients in the USA, who sought complementary health care because they valued the extended personal time to talk and attend to matters of the heart, *xin* 心 (Barnes 1998, 2009), many Tanzanian clients praised the visit to the Chinese doctor for its brevity and the discretion with which they were met. Most patients did not know that Chinese medical diagnostics involved inspection of the complexion (*se* 色) and examination of the pulse (*mai* 脉), the two forms of diagnostics (*mai se* 脉色) that date to antiquity, nor had they heard of *yin-yang* or *qi*. Evidently, Chinese medicine in Tanzania was not primarily sought because clients were attracted to its 'holistic' philosophy of nature and life.

The interviews with patients produced some quite specific but nevertheless robust data. For instance, patients valued receiving a medical service without first having to pay consultation fees, which make little sense in traditional contexts of health care provision and are perceived simply as a 'loss of money'. Furthermore, visiting a Chinese medical practice on the high street in the course of doing one's errands in town was presented as a bonus, whereas the health bureaucracies of the state were a veritable 'loss of time'. Chinese practitioners employed African laboratory technicians and rented as a lab one of the many rooms that their practices had, which had the effect that patients only queued once to receive a diagnosis, a lab test and medication that was not generally out of stock. Contrary to the stereotype of 'African time' that implied that time management is of little concern to 'Africans', I found people to be very busy, often juggling three or more different jobs and their children and spouses, alongside observing the attendance of rituals of the extended family (e.g. funerals, which were very disruptive as they often involved long-distance travel) and engaging in regular prayer. Even those who had chronic and terminal conditions wished to get the nuisance of a visit to the doctor over with quickly. All these matters, which related to the entrepreneurial structure of health care provision, appeared to make Chinese medical clinics attractive to Tanzanians.

The interviews in the early 2000s showed that Tanzanian patients considered *dawa ya Kichina* to have 'rapid effects'.[3] It was 'rapidly effective' in at least three ways; these were, however, only tenuously (if at all) related to TCM theory and practice as historically practised in its country of origin. One concerned the organisation of Chinese medical businesses in Tanzania; the second, the ways in which Chinese pharmaceuticals were marketed and consumed; and the third, the reportedly 'rapid' therapeutic effects of skilfully administered treatment that combined Chinese and Western medicine. Relevant here is that what in Swahili is called *dawa ya Kichina* had many more shades of meaning than 'TCM' or 'Chinese medicine'.

## *Dawa ya Kichina*

The ambiguity of the term permitted several interpretations among ordinary local people. *Dawa ya Kichina* literally translated as 'China's medicine', which in some cases referred to 'medicine from China' – in the sense of 'Chinese medicine' – while in others, it related to the 'medicine of the Chinese', that is, medicine practised by Chinese physicians, which may well include 'biomedicine as practised by the Chinese'. In addition, it could designate 'medicines from China', which referred in some cases to 'Chinese medical pharmaceuticals', in others to 'Chinese-manufactured Western biomedical pharmaceuticals', and in yet others to both. In Tanzania, it was partly on the ambiguity of this term that the marketing of Chinese medicine thrived.

Faith in *dawa ya Kichina* is often attributed to the experience that Tanzanians had with the Chinese during the period of socialist orientation. A government employee explained: 'In Nyerere's times there were many Chinese doctors here, we trusted them more than our local doctors at that time.' A police officer said the same: 'We had faith in Chinese medicine. Historically, Mao Zedong was our friend. We had a Chinese dispensary in Moshi which was very good.' When in the 1970s 'the Chinese' came to build the railway (Monson 2013), 'They built it in only five years'. They completed a difficult task effectively, so effectively in fact that the idea of them being capable of witchcraft was widespread. Chinese teams that the Chinese government sent on short-term contracts to Tanzania were also involved in construction work, in military affairs and mining, and in the agricultural and textile industry. They were generally accompanied by a medical team (*yiliaodui* 医疗队) staffed by mostly biomedical doctors. As my interviewees told me, they apparently provided medical services for the local population on a regular basis too.

The trust in *dawa ya Kichina*, as I was told by a government-sent Chinese physician, derived primarily from the socialist project of sending medical teams to peoples in the developing world.[4] Over two hundred physicians were dispatched yearly by the government of Shandong province to work in medical teams in the major district hospitals of Tanzania. These Chinese, who were biomedical practitioners, built up an excellent reputation for 'the medicine practised by the Chinese', *dawa ya Kichina*, a reputation that paralleled that of the other efficient work performed by temporary contracted government-sent teams. After completion of their missions, they all returned to China.

There still were, in the early 2000s, a few teams of government-sent biomedical doctors who were serving on one- to two-year contracts within Tanzanian health services. The Chinese who practised medicine in entrepreneurial settings were also on short-term contracts, but renewable ones. These Chinese doctors were a different sort of people. They were private practitioners who, as one of them put it to me without any sense of shame, had come to Africa to 'do business'. Some told me that they had heard that it was easy to make money in Africa, particularly in Tanzania; people were so modest (*pusu* 朴素) and honest (*laoshi* 老实), one of them said. Thus, ironically, in one of the poorest countries in the world, the capitalist-oriented, entrepreneurial Chinese medical practitioners seemed to live off the good reputation that Chinese biomedical doctors of the period of socialist orientation had given *dawa ya Kichina*.

*Dawa ya Kichina* not only referred to 'medicine from China', but could also designate Chinese medicines, or rather, any drugs that came from China. In Tanzania, the Chinese *materia medica* (*zhongyao* 中药) that one simmered daily for half an hour over a small fire, and that required much time for preparation, were generally not available, and most Tanzanians did not even know of their existence. Instead, ready-made Chinese medical patent medicines (*zhongchengyao* 中成药) were on the market. They made possible speedy consumption and were, like biomedical drugs, easy to consume. They were often imbued with biomedical effectiveness, perhaps because they looked identical: they came in tablet, capsule or pill form in colourful cartons or plastic packages that were covered with Chinese script, illegible to the Swahili-speaking clientele. It is therefore not surprising that the term *dawa ya Kichina* referred not merely to Chinese medical drugs (*zhongyao*) or Chinese formula medicines (*zhongchengyao*) but to any medicines that came from China, including Chinese-manufactured Western medical drugs. To complicate the issue further, Chinese formula medicines sometimes (though rarely) contained chemically synthesised ingredients, such as vitamin C or aspirin (salicylic acid), which meant, strictly speaking, that they did not in all cases consist of ingredients extracted from living organisms (for more on their 'ethnochemistry', see Chapter 7). They were hybrids, often dispensed in 'alternatively modern' treatment procedures (see syphilis treatment in Chapter 3).

This brings us to the third reason that many patients associated *dawa ya Kichina* with rapid effects. Quite often, it was the formula medicines of integrated Chinese and biomedical treatments that patients reported as stunningly effective. This form of combined Chinese and biomedical treatment provided relief not only for complaints relating to the muscular and nervous systems, but also for certain infectious diseases and disorders of the digestive and endocrine systems. It had the potential to provide relief on a large scale in primary health care among the lower middle classes in Tanzania, where the system of medical services, once remarkably vigorous (Iliffe 1998: 204–6), had declined (ibid.: 212).

In the realm of traditional medical treatment, anecdotes abound that feature a culturally constructed component of 'miracles' that can effect 'real' improvement (Zhan 2001, 2009; see also below). What a patient reports is generally not imbued with great truth value. Biomedicine differentiates between subjectively felt 'symptoms' of the patient and professionally recognised, objective 'signs' that are meaningful to the physician. Medical anthropology, alongside narrative medicine, has revalidated patients' narratives (Kleinman 1988; Good 1994). Embedded in personal and historical circumstance, they account for the patients' lifeworlds and intentionalities. However, the question of whether a treatment is not only perceived to have rapid effects, but 'in fact' does have such effects – a question grounded in the 'realistic realist' approach (Latour 2000b) – does not usually fall within the scope of interpretive medical anthropology. Meanwhile, my fieldwork in Tanzania made evident, again, how important it is for anthropologists to reformulate this question, which regards the question of a medical intervention's efficaciousness. All experience is culturally tainted, but surely not all to the same degree and in the same way; there are specific immediate effects that are perceived as 'real', unmediated and practical, and that appear to be so intersubjectively and cross-culturally. There must be a way in which one can discuss these within an anthropological framework – perhaps by accounting for them in terms of hands-on techniques and non-verbalised tactics?

Furthermore, detailed recording is key, as it uncovers semantic nuance. When Tanzanian patients claimed that *dawa ya Kichina* had 'rapid effects', Chinese practitioners did not entirely disagree, as they said so of integrated Chinese and Western medical treatment (*zhongxiyi jiehe* 中西医结合). Most of them distinguished between integrated Chinese and Western medical treatments and Chinese medicine (*zhongyi* 中医) – the former worked rapidly, the latter not. However, most Tanzanians were not aware of this distinction and related to both as *dawa ya Kichina*.

In addition, practitioners delivering hybrid forms of care prescribed biomedical pharmaceuticals *tout court* that were known to have rapid effects, like aspirin or antibiotics. More importantly, however, 'the Chinese antimalarial' was known to have more rapid effects than all other antimalarials, and this observation certainly reinforced the view of Chinese medicine as having rapid effects. Evidently, as seen from linguistically informed participant observation, the ambiguities surrounding the term *dawa ya Kichina* and its rapid effects did not solely arise from a misunderstanding and misperception of what Chinese doctors were doing.

Meanwhile, the response by Tanzanian patients that Chinese medicines produced rapid relief was no doubt a very polite way of expressing their probing attitude, the main question being: will it work long-term? Among adults, cross-culturally, seeking rapid relief is considered immature – in Europe, China and Africa, it is the sort of thing adults teach children not to do. Meanwhile, some otherwise medically competent and caring Chinese practitioners, seemingly unaware of their racist formulation, would unabashedly say that 'Africans' (*Feizhou ren*) yearned for a treatment's instantaneous results. More educated Chinese were not as condemning of 'the Africans', although these same practitioners deplored their lack of education (*jiaoyu* 教育) and their abject 'poverty' (*tai pingqiongle* 太贫穷了), and implied that this was due to 'Africa' being 'backward' (*luohou* 落后). Meanwhile, several Chinese practitioners had not experienced higher education, or even the three final years of high school. Other practitioners seemed to imply that Africans were simple-minded, as was their language. Swahili, they claimed, was simple and 'undeveloped' (*bu fada* 不发达) as it had many Arab loanwords. Discussing these opinions with friends, they said that, indeed, their patients showed very little interest in complying with long-term treatment, not necessarily as a matter of mindset and lifestyle, but due to financial and other circumstantial hardship. Meanwhile, my research found evidence to the contrary in several cases of very long-term adherence to Chinese treatment regimes, some of whom had been n treatment over several years, This was the case particularly in Mombasa, where *dawa ya Kichina* had been on offer for over a decade.

In summary, the above has highlighted ambiguities surrounding the concept of *dawa ya Kichina*. One fairly predominant perception pertained to its ready-made, speedily consumed drugs, which like other interventions undertaken by the Chinese during the socialist-oriented period were considered highly effective. Finally, the attitude to *dawa ya Kichina* as a medicine with 'rapid effects' may also have been a polite way for members of the hosting countries to respond with civility to their uninvited guests. This will be further explored in what follows.

## *Upwardly Mobile*

Who were the patients who sought Chinese medical treatment? Their socio-economic standing depended on the location in which the medical practice was located. In what follows I compare two Chinese medical practices with a Tanzanian healer's practice.

The patients from the two Chinese clinics whom I interviewed were between 1 and 61 years old; twenty-one were male and nine were female; fourteen were married, twelve single, one a widower, one a divorcee and three children; eighteen were Christian and twelve Muslim. They were also ethnically extremely varied, from twenty different ethnic groups: My interviewees identified themselves as Arab Zanzibari (2), Indian African (1), Chagga (3), Diga (1), Ha (3), Hehe (1), Jita (2), Kuria (2), Luo (1), Mdengeleko (2), Mpimbwe (1), Musoma (1), Ngoni (1), Nyakyusa (1), Nyamwezi (3), Nyiha (1), Pare (1), Sukuma (1), Ugandan (1) and Zambian (1). They were from regions as disparate as Iringa, Kigoma, Kilimanjaro, Mara, Mbeya, Mwanza, Lindi, Pemba, Songea, Tabora, Tanga, Coast (Rufiji) and Rukwa. They lived in suburbs as varied as Buguruni, Kigogo, Kimara Baruti, Kinondoni, Kunduchi, Kurasini, Mbagala, Mbezi Beach, Mtoni, Pugu, Sinza, Tabata, Tandika, Tegeta, Temeke, Ukonga, Upanga and Vinginguti. Chinese medical doctors were only occasionally consulted by the kin of their Tanzanian collaborators, and very occasionally by Chinese contract workers.

In the two clinics, the patients differed however in educational background, profession and income. One clinic was situated near the Kariakoo market, in downtown Dar es Salaam, Ilala district, in a neighbourhood bustling with small businesses. It catered mostly to businesspeople trading shoes and clothes (second-hand, imported from Hong Kong, or batik), housewives and employees in the administration whose income varied between TZS 50,000 to several hundred thousand per month. The practice spread out over the first floor, which was considered safer than the ground floor. Many patients in this clinic considered it possible that 'witchcraft' may have affected their lives, although generally not in the problem that they presented to the Chinese doctor. Thus, a woman who suspected that witchcraft was responsible for her barrenness said that she consulted the Chinese clinic for treatment of typhoid.

Another Chinese clinic, also in central Ilala and also spread out over the first floor, catered to a more upmarket clientele. It included 'businessmen' who traded clothes or computers, government employees (two interviewees said that they had an income of over TZS 500,000) and housewives. This clinic offered acupuncture treatment, and several patients were treated for problems of muscular pain similar to those one would find in clinics of the northern hemisphere; the doctor in charge spoke of *bi* 痹 obstructions, and noted that they were worst not during winter, as in China, Europe and

North America, but during the days when the tropical heat peaked (Qiao n.d.). In this clinic, 'witchcraft' was not generally mentioned as an issue, neither during the interviews with the patients nor in informal conversation with the Chinese medical practitioner. This clinic also catered to some upper-middle-class clients interested solely in buying Chinese antimalarials (see next subsection).

The cost of treatment varied considerably with around TZS 5,000 in Kariakoo and around TZS 10,000 in central Dar es Salaam. These differences reflected the spending power of the respective customers rather than the costs of the medicines used. It is well-known throughout the African continent that monetary transactions accompanying health interventions represent an important communicative aspect of the social relation between the healer and their clients (van der Geest 1992), rather than being merely payments for medical services.

By comparison, in March 2002, I visited daily a Tanzanian healer who lived in Manzese, a district of Dar es Salaam known for its low-income population, crime and violence. This healer's patients, with few exceptions, had a 'Standard 7' education, and paid TZS 1,000 to 5,000 per treatment. The majority were 'businessmen' (or women) dealing with potatoes, onions, maize flower, bananas and petty commodities, or they were housewives; many were in their twenties. Income was not very regular, and certainly was less than TZS 50,000 /month. The patients consulted the healer for cases of 'confusion' (*kuchanganyikiwa*), 'epilepsy' (*kifafa*), physical and emotional distress of various kinds, 'sugar' (diabetes), fevers, malaria, stomach aches, headaches, chest pain, bad luck in business, protection for imminent travel, the search for a partner and marital problems. Some of these cases involved 'witchcraft' (*nguvu ya uchawi*), others decisively not.

The healer took on the role of a family doctor, and remuneration for his services was mostly, but not always, monetary; more than a third of the patients I interviewed said that they were relatives of his or one of his three wives. The healer was Muslim, yet Christians and Muslims alike consulted him; most were Tanzanian and lived in Dar es Salaam. While many interviewees who visited a Chinese clinic had secondary education (Form 4 or Form 6), the c. thirty patients of this healer in Manzese had elementary school education (Standard 7). This meant that they generally had less experience of talking to a foreigner and thus were what I interpreted as shy. Furthermore, they were not used to being asked to have an opinion. I had no choice but to exclusively rely on conversing in Swahili with them. In that situation, the interviews were undertaken as a routine in which I performed my work perfunctorily, with the help of a former patient who spoke a smattering of English. This interview situation instilled a certain trust from the healer and his entourage in me as an anthropologist, as they could watch me doing my work. As a result, several episodes that turned out to be ethnographically precious were communicated to me after the interviews. However, overall the information elicited from these thirty patients was too shallow to be systematically evaluated.

In summary, in the early 2000s, Chinese medical practitioners catered to all echelons of society in Dar es Salaam, though they seemed to be consulted mostly by patients who had had a secondary education. They were sought out by unrelated, enterprising individuals from throughout the city, and not only through kinship networks or neighbourhood relations. Most patients explained that they had followed the advice of a friend or relative, many of whom had been treated precisely for the complaint that they suffered, yet not necessarily in the same clinic. Only a few had responded to newspaper advertisements, which Chinese medical practitioners had been permitted to place in the mid-1990s, but no longer after the year 2000.

## *The Most Frequent Complaint, Malaria*

During the 'small' rains of December 2001 and January 2002, the most frequent complaint for which medicines were dispensed over the counter was malaria.[5] Clients who knew about the 'Chinese antimalarials' were unanimous in their opinion that malaria was best treated by them. Naturally, *homa ya malaria* ('fevers of malaria') can refer to many conditions, which need not always involve a fever (e.g. Winch et al. 1996; Hausmann Muela et al. 1998), and one of the reasons for visiting Chinese medical practices was precisely that their laboratories provided quick results for around TZS 300–500. Most patients knew that the Chinese had effective antimalarials, and some had been sent by Tanzanian biomedical doctors to the Chinese in order to prevent them from purchasing from other vendors; in the early 2000s, there were only very occasionally fake

Chinese antimalarials on the market (in contrast to Southeast Asia, see Newton et al. 2003).

Artemisinin had been a public health commodity for twenty-five years at the turn of the millennium. The Chinese doctors always asked their patients to take a blood test before they gave them a five-day treatment (at a time when the WHO recommended a seven-day regime; see Phillips-Howard 2002), after which patients were required to have another test that was meant to assure them of the efficacy of the treatment. Patients generally said that Chinese antimalarials had 'no side effects', an attribute usually given to 'natural' herbs, such as the traditional Chinese drugs (*zhongyao* 中药). Some patients knew that in contrast to other kinds of *dawa ya Kichina*, the Chinese antimalarials were truly 'scientific'. Artemisinin and artemisinin-derived biomedical drugs had long been proven to reduce malarial fevers within a few hours (95 per cent parasite clearance times of between six and forty hours, see Hien and White 1993: 605), and compared to all the other antimalarials, they did indeed have extremely rapid effects. It is ironic that, as a consequence, most patients consulted Chinese medical doctors for treatment with a purified chemical substance, artemisinin, that is a Western medical pharmaceutical, rather than for a 'natural' Chinese medical prescription. In some clinics, artemisinin-based antimalarials made up more than 50 per cent of the over-the-counter transactions.

The Tanzanian government listed the Chinese antimalarials on the Essential Drug List. 'There are two different classes of biomedical drugs; Class I drugs can be sold over the counter, but Class II drugs can only be sold by biomedically trained and licensed personnel', an official at the National Institute for Medical Research explained. The antimalarial chloroquine belonged to Class I while sulphadoxine-pyremethamine (Fansidar) and the Chinese antimalarials belonged to Class II. This newly endorsed classification meant that, in effect, all Chinese medical practitioners who sold the Chinese antimalarials with purified artemisinin and its derivations were doing unlawful business. Obviously, Chinese medical practitioners felt this discrimination to be arbitrary and unfair. They argued that artemisinin was the intellectual property of a highly idealised and essentialised notion of the 'Chinese people'.

However, the Tanzanian government endorsed the perspective of the biomedical professionals, that Class II drugs were to be sold by licensed pharmacists only. This led to the irony that a chemical substance extracted from a Chinese *materia medica* first described by ancient Chinese scientists, which was identified and purified by modern Chinese scientists, could not legally be sold by Chinese medical practitioners in Tanzania. As in other modern nation states, only licensed pharmacists could do so, and those were often of Indian descent. As any licensed pharmacist would do, they sold brands that were produced according to GMP standards or distributed by Western pharmaceutical companies, at a significantly higher price than the Chinese brands (see further discussion in Chapter 9).

## *Other Complaints and Treatment Outcomes*

Patients also presented a wide range of complaints other than malaria to Chinese medical practitioners: chest pain and asthma, *gesi* ('gas/bloating'), digestive problems, ulcers, lack of libido and 'impotence', pimples on the face, eczema and rashes, chronic tonsillitis, 'pressure' (hypertension), 'sugar' (diabetes), HIV/AIDS, hemiplegia, back pain, muscular problems, arthritis and many more. *Dawa ya Kichina* was considered highly effective in increasing the 'strength of men' (*nguvu ya kiume*) and several related complaints. Asthma and chest or lower back pain, symptomatic of this lack of strength, had to be recognised and diagnosed as necessary targets to be treated in a separate therapeutic cycle before the Chinese medication for treating the 'strength of men' could be dispensed (see Chapter 8, 'Technologies of Temporalities').

Some therapeutic effects bordered on the miraculous: 'After three days only, she could walk again, and join us dancing at Christmas!' (see also Zhan 2001; and below). In other cases, 'the problem recurred', as a patient who previously 'had been to the Chinese' told me when I encountered him in an African healer's practice in a northern suburb of Dar es Salaam. While some patients had not found relief anywhere, most expressed 'satisfaction' with the treatment they had received from Chinese medical doctors.

In this context, the data from the follow-up study are of particular interest. Of the twenty patients interviewed at home in December and January, three had changed residence and could not be found six months later. Of the seventeen that I could interview a second time, four had been treated with Chinese antimalarials, all four successfully. Two of the four lived in visibly better conditions than the other two (e.g. a flat on the first floor in central Dar), and they had not been ill with malaria since. Of the two who had experienced a reinfection, one continued to frequent the Chinese clinic, while the other had consulted it only on two further occasions. When this particular patient could not obtain the brand Cotecsin any more (on the different brands, see Chapter 9), he was not prepared to pay the same price for Artesunate (TZS 4,500); instead, he took Fansidar, which he found barely effective but which cost him only TZS 750 for the three tablets that, as he explained, constituted a full course of malaria treatment.

Among the thirteen remaining patients, the Chinese doctors had successfully treated six, three found improvement with other doctors, and four had no relief. Among the six successfully treated patients, three got better instantly (two had had acute stomach ulcers, while one experienced the above 'miracle' of being capable to walk and dance again, without relapse). Two patients had a chronic condition that was successfully controlled by regular treatment with integrated Chinese and Western medicine: one, who had a history of twenty years of stomach ulcers, very evidently looked much healthier and had gained weight, while the other was a diabetic whose condition had not deteriorated but neither improved. The sixth patient claimed instant improvement of her eczema (but this information, which was given over the phone, is not as valid as the other findings elicited in long face-to-face conversations).

All three patients who eventually were treated by other doctors had been seen by a very young, inexperienced doctor (the other Chinese medical doctor who worked in central Dar es Salaam had more than ten years of clinical experience). Two had been treated for facial eczema, with some but not satisfactory improvement. One then turned to biomedical treatment, the other to the well-known North Korean medical clinic in Megalomani, which he continued to frequent for other medical problems as well. The third patient continued to be treated for stomach ulcers for a further two months, without much improvement. She then turned to Muhimbili government hospital, where treatment apparently had effected change for the better.

Four patients did not return to the Chinese clinic because they had no relief. One young man, whom the Chinese practitioner had treated for unspecific chest problems, was diagnosed several weeks later with TB at a district hospital; he had been a soldier. One with arthritis and chronic 'fevers of malaria' was visibly worse; she was the second or third wife of an extremely wealthy police officer, and had spent a considerable amount on Chinese medication over a couple of years; the receipts she showed me from the past six months documented almost weekly visits to the dispensary in the neighbourhood. They amounted to many tens of thousands of TZS each month. There was little doubt that she had AIDS, but no one enunciated the word during the interview. Two others, young men with a considerable history of treatment-seeking, said that they now lived with their problems without seeking further medical care; one had been diagnosed with, and treated for, typhoid at the Chinese clinic, and later had another diagnosis done at the Aga Khan, a prestigious private biomedical hospital; again the condition was diagnosed as typhoid, yet again the treatment barely effected improvement, but cost him ten times as much as at the Chinese clinic (TZS 40,000 instead of TZS 4,000). The other, a government employee with a monthly salary of TZS 50,000, had a chronic stomach ulcer but could not afford the TZS 9,500 for the entire treatment that the Chinese doctor had prescribed in December, and admitted to taking painkillers, like Panadol, quite regularly instead; in the cases of malaria he had suffered since, he took no antimalarials any more of any kind because they were all very bitter and would affect his ulcer badly.

In summary, among the seventeen patients interviewed, several had life-threatening diseases, and yet the Chinese doctors seemed to have successfully treated ten. Nevertheless, this success rate was rather modest, which may partly have been due to the inexperience of one of the doctors (three out of the seven unsuccessful cases). The follow-up interviews also revealed how frequent malaria was, as I asked all patients whether they had experienced malaria in the six months between December/January and July/August 2002 (most rains fell in the period between March and May). Only five out of the seventeen I interviewed were adamant that they had not had malaria since December, and three of them were very wealthy. Among almost all of the others (ten patients), malarial plasmodia had been detected in their blood between once and four times or more in these six months. Of these ten patients, fewer than half had made use of Chinese antimalarials; several simply could not afford them.

## Choices of Care in the Patient's Perception

Available choices of health care were described to me in variant and sometimes even contradictory ways. Some patients said that they generally only went to dispensaries that offered services free of charge; others complained that doctors in government hospitals, particularly those at Muhimbili, had to be bribed, or that the medicines they prescribed would either not be available at the pharmacy or only at an exorbitant price, and they mentioned the problem of endless queuing. Doctors at private biomedical clinics were often perceived to be interested only in money; in some cases, it was explained, a bribe at a government hospital could be less costly than the cost for the same services at a private biomedical clinic (this applied to having an X-ray taken, for instance). Other patients claimed that private doctors really cared for their patients, and that one could be sure that the same doctor at the government hospital would not give one as much attention as at their own private hospital, which would be open after their work at the government hospital, say in the evening.

In this context, it is interesting to note that of the six patients who mentioned Indian doctors during the interviews, three were negative about them. A businessman, who himself was partly of Indian descent, remarked: 'There is more trust in Chinese people than in Indians, Indians are traders.' He evidently was unfamiliar with 'the Chinese' and unaware that they are well known as traders too. He continued: 'Also, the Chinese don't use consultation fees. I don't trust other Indian doctors, there are many of them, they want upper-class people, not middle-class people like myself.' A government employee of the Inland Revenue Bureau exclaimed: 'You ask whether we've consulted Indian doctors? We hate them, we know that Indian products are no good, generally. The Indians can make a profit out of your hat . . . Contrabandists have produced fake Cotecsin, so the importation of Cotecsin is now prohibited – only Indians could have done that.' Meanwhile, the expensive medicines from England and Germany, the countries of the former colonisers, were valued highly, but: 'Indian medicines are fake, at least most of them.' The pharmaceuticals produced in India were often generics, and hence much better value. With regard to 'Indian medicines' people usually distinguished between the biomedical and traditional ones, this in contrast with their situationally sensitive perception of *dawa ya Kichina*. The packages were labelled in English, and this is likely the reason that the Tanzanian clientele made these distinctions: 'I use Indian Fansidar, yes, and once I took an Indian traditional medicine, Maha Sudarshan Chuma, somehow it worked but nevertheless the malaria was still in me.' The husband of a woman who for fourteen years had suffered from what he called 'skin asthma' recounted: 'We went also to an Indian healer, private somewhere, who worked in the evening. He took no money. His herbal medicines were at first very effective but then the problem reverted.' This was the only time that a patient of a Chinese medical practitioner mentioned a doctor or healer who refused to take money, which underlines again that in the urban contexts of Dar es Salaam, medicine usually was business (Swantz 1990: 13), and very evidently not only for Indians.

With regard to 'traditional' African medicine, patients differentiated between consulting a *mganga* (traditional healer), buying herbs on the market and applying the knowledge they had learned from their father or mother in preparing certain 'leaves' or 'medicines from trees' (*miti*) for treating 'fevers of malaria' (*homa ya malaria*) or 'stomach problems' (*homa ya tumbo*), for instance. A Christian Chagga businessman, with 'Standard 7' education, who lived in a large house in a newly constituted neighbourhood, said that he had never been to the 'witchdoctor' – religion forbade him to do so. However, as became apparent later, he knew how to use the leaves of a bush in the garden for treating minor ailments, and yes, he had bought African herbs from the market, *ngetwa* and *ngoka* for instance.[6] His three children, whom he sent to elementary school in Kenya and who were therefore fluent in

English and acted as interpreters during the interview, were convinced that these two African medicines were indeed wonder drugs; the father did not contradict them. Several patients at the Chinese clinic in Kariakoo admitted to having sought *waganga* (eight of the nineteen recruited into the study on one day in December 2001). One couple said that they had been to five different *waganga* for the sake of their infant, and enumerated the following four: one in Mbagala whom they paid TZS 30,000, one in Kilawani for TZS 16,000, one in Vinginuti for TZS 18,000 and one in Gongolamboto for TZS 5,000. Patients travelled far, not only within the city of Dar. Thus, the above woman who suffered from infertility, after her husband's sperm had been tested at Muhimbili, had travelled to *waganga* as far as Moshi and Mbeya. By contrast, only one of the eleven patients interviewed at the Chinese clinic in central Dar es Salaam admitted to having been to a *mganga*; all of them had been exposed to more education than 'Standard 7'.

The above suggests that the clientele of Chinese medical practitioners considered the various health care choices in Dar es Salaam, whether offered by the state or in private biomedical, traditional African or Indian clinics, to all be fraught with deficiencies due to bribery, fraud or simply ignorance; only the North Korean medical establishments, of which there were two in Dar es Salaam, tended to be mentioned positively. The bias against South Asian professionals, and their wealth, was remarkable in the health field (see Chapter 8, 'Magic and The Efficaciousness of History', and Hsu 2002; see also Parkin 1968; Iliffe 1998: 63, 76, 121, 124 and 186). Meanwhile, the number of patients who were indiscriminately seeking help from diviners and traditional healers, referred to as *mganga*, seemed to correlate with their educational backgrounds.

## *Perceived Efficacies*

During my fieldwork in the PRC, people uniformly said that Chinese medicine (*zhongyi*) had no side effects, that its effects were gradual and that it was 'good' for treating chronic or recurrent conditions; acupuncture, for instance, was considered particularly effective in treating arthritis and muscular problems (fieldwork, 1988–89; Ots 1990a). However, in Tanzania in the early 2000s, people had not been exposed to this rhetoric that emphasised the complementarity of Chinese medical treatment to Western biomedical interventions. Only some patients, who for months and even years had stayed with a Chinese medical doctor, expressed the above ideas that are prevalent in the PRC. In this context the role of the 'grandfather' in family businesses, which some Chinese medical practices were, became obvious. While most patients barely spent more than five minutes with the doctor, they sat for between ten and twenty minutes in the waiting room. Several told me that the father of the doctor, who spent most of his time in the waiting room, had explained to them that Chinese medicines had no side effects, and that they worked slowly. Evidently, the grandfather's task was to teach the clients what to expect and how to evaluate their future bodily experiences with Chinese medicines, and thereby to strengthen their compliance.

With the exception of malaria, which was considered best treated by the artemisinin-based Chinese antimalarials, the Tanzanian patients I interviewed did not generally distinguish between conditions best treated by Chinese medicine and others best treated by biomedicine. Some knew that Chinese medicine was particularly effective for treating certain conditions (although the particular conditions mentioned varied considerably), yet the usual response was: 'It is good for everything.'

In this context, it is important to know that there were very few acupuncturists who opened shops along the Muslim Swahili-speaking coast of East Africa. In Nairobi and Kampala, with their sizeable expatriate and local Christian communities that had links to Europe or North America, acupuncture was mostly sought for *bi*-obstruction problems in the muscular and connective tissue. By contrast, the patients in the PRC considered themselves knowledgeable enough to be selective, and decided which problems to show the TCM practitioner: digestive problems and women's disorders were among the most frequent, as Ahern (1975) noted more than half a century ago in Hong Kong. This indicated a trend that one can observe also in other traditional medical settings. The stomach and the womb, sometimes referred to with the same word (the centre, *zhong* 中; *tumbo*), are often considered the innermost organs, which makes them both precious and vitally important (see Hsu 2010a: Cases 1, 128, and 5, 217–18). Thus, the observation that many reproductive problems were presented to Chinese medical practitioners may have to do with a perception coming into play of the TCM clinics' 'traditional medical' aspect (see Chapter 8), notwithstanding their claim to science and progress (see Chapter 7).

In the PRC between the 1950s and 1990s, TCM was presented as a science. So I asked patients on the Swahili-speaking East African coast whether they thought Chinese medicine was a science or whether they thought it worked through 'witchcraft'. This opposition of science and witchcraft surprised most of my respondents. Some patients were uncertain of whether or not the Chinese knew how to do witchcraft, but others explicitly associated 'doing witchcraft' with 'rapid effects', and the Chinese were generally known to produce effects rapidly, particularly 'in the domain of engineering'. Some patients even said that 'Chinese medicines have quicker effects than Western medicine.' This did indeed apply to the Chinese antimalarials. Simultaneously, it in all likelihood reflected a view dating to Tanzania's period of socialist orientation (1960s–80s), when the PRC was viewed as a more 'advanced' socialist nation than the capitalist ones.

An elementary school teacher who was fluent in English and had even enrolled in a long-distance correspondence course for an 'Advanced Diploma in Business English' from the Manchester Business School explained that, a year or two ago, he had seen an advert in a newspaper that apparently read: 'The Chinese doctor has come to liberate the Tanzanian patient.' He explained: 'I thought I was one who could be liberated.' His stomach ulcers had arisen while 'serving in the army' in his early twenties, 'due to the daily diet of beans'. He had initially treated an asthmatic condition for six months at the expense of *c.* TZS 10,000, which apparently effected only a 'relief of 40 per cent', before embarking on treatment with *dawa ya Kichina* for these chronic ulcers for another five months, at the same cost, effecting 'a relief of 70 per cent'. He showed me his medications. As was visible from the Chinese leaflets enclosed, this relief had been achieved through the combination of a Chinese-manufactured biomedical pharmaceutical and a Chinese herbal drug; yet since their packaging was alike, the patient was unaware that he was not merely on herbal treatment, but also on biomedical drugs.

In the same neighbourhood, another patient, who knew the primary school teacher by sight, without however knowing that they had both consulted the same Chinese medical clinic, expressed a similar view of Chinese medicine as being 'advanced'. 'Chinese medicine is based on observation', he said. 'The doctor used a stethoscope' (for examining the 'chest problems' of his brother – later diagnosed as suffering from TB – whom he had accompanied to the Chinese clinic). 'That's what other doctors do as well', I replied. 'Yes, but the Chinese stethoscope is more advanced.' 'Why?' 'You can just see it, from its make.' This 22-year-old high school attendant, who in Pugu, some thirty kilometres outside of Dar, studied at the same school as Tanzania's first president Julius Nyerere previously had, was certain that Chinese medicines were scientific: 'Their medicines have been researched in laboratories, they do not look like those of the *waganga* traditionalists [stored in recycled plastic bottles].'

As an 'advanced' medicine, Chinese medicine was attractive both to patients who said that they only used 'modern' medicine and to others who claimed only to use 'traditional' medicines. Thus, the primary school teacher, who said he was trying to live a modern lifestyle, remarked: 'I've never been to African doctors, I don't use African herbs, I just go to modern doctors, Chinese medicine is a modern medicine.' By contrast, the 34-year-old son of a Christian *mganga* from a village in the Tanzanian hinterland, who was trying to make a living in Dar es Salaam, said that he valued the traditional. He explained in English that he used Chinese medicine because it was traditional:

> I basically only take traditional medicines, for everything, for treating malaria, fevers in general, coughing, burning legs, for 'washing my kidneys' and 'men's sexual strength', and also against growing fat by 'flushing my body so that I keep a normal weight'. Traditional African medicines, too, have no side effects, bad effects arise only if you get an overdose ... I use traditional Chinese medicine only for treating malaria, it is an advanced traditional medicine. (Red notebook, 2001–2)

'Advanced' meant in his case that 'traditional Chinese medicines are well measured'. This statement indicated to me that he had struggled with getting the dosage of the 'African medicines' right, a well-known problem. 'Modern', another patient explained, meant 'to be open, to advertise and sell openly, and not to be secretive', and this, she thought, was what the Chinese were doing.

Ideas about the meanings of 'modern' and 'advanced' varied considerably, as became particularly evident in my probing of the patients as to whether they considered their lifestyles 'traditional' (*kiasili*) or 'modern' (*kisasa, kizungu*). In that context, 'modern' was often associated with having the money required to be modern, but interestingly, in the context of discussing traditional medicines with the patients of Chinese medical practitioners, the financial aspect of 'modern' versus 'traditional' medicines was not mentioned. Clearly, these patients who called themselves 'middle-class' were spread over a very wide range of socio-economic standing. For people at the grassroots who lived in informal settlements and, if employed, earned a salary of TZS 30,000 at most, even though they called themselves 'middle-class', Chinese medicines were not particularly cheap, if they were affordable at all.

## *Discussion: To What Extent Can We Speak of Patient Agency?*

Which expectations brought East African patients to Chinese medical practitioners? The above suggests that *dawa ya Kichina* was positively valued due to a) the history of socialist orientation in Tanzania and the PRC, b) the sociology of the upward mobility of patients who lived in fairly newly constituted informal settlements, yet considered themselves 'middle-class', c) their treatment-seeking strategies (ranging from curiosity to a lack of other health-care choices and last resort), and d) some stunning treatment effects. The study presented in this chapter was initially framed as one of 'glocalisation', with a view to stressing the commercial aspect of medicine and how commerce transformed TCM practices in Tanzania. The idea was that local consumers would shape the market, and that businesspeople would tailor articles of consumption to their expectations. Accordingly, the focus of this study was on patients. However, the concept of 'glocalisation' was less useful than originally assumed. Furthermore, I found that financial constraints were so important among the people I worked with that 'patient agency' had a ring of euphemism.

First, the concept of 'agency' as being located in individual actors has already been queried in the previous chapter. In Tanzania in the early 2000s, *dawa ya Kichina* tended to be viewed as an 'advanced' medicine with 'rapid effects', rather than as a 'traditional' medicine with 'slow' effects. This was in line with a turn towards an economy-driven, specifically Chinese form of globalisation (Pieke et al. 2004), and 'TCM' as practised in Tanzania was a prime example of this new 'mobility', which was mostly economically motivated (Hsu 2007a).

TCM practitioners who completed five years of higher education in TCM as 'regular students' (*benke sheng* 本科生) possessed both biomedical and 'traditional' knowledge. They would have had the education, the knowledge and the interest to make a significant contribution to Tanzania's primary health care. To ensure that this happened, however, it would have been imperative that the Tanzanian Ministry of Health set up regulations to ensure that the practitioners they licensed had adequate medical education. In the early 2000s, licenses for running a private clinic in the PRC were given to applicants who had five years of university training in TCM and a minimum of five years of work experience in medical practice (TCM practitioners in Kenya, Tanzania and Zanzibar, personal communications, 2001–5). But no such efforts were made in East Africa.

Clearly, there was a personal element to a medical consultation, particularly in an entrepreneurial setting, and in some very rare cases, there was even a sense of friendship between some patients and their doctors. However, partial knowledges, 'misperceptions', tensions, contradictions and 'incongruencies' were just as important. Thus, the generalising statements by TCM practitioners about 'Africans' and their perception (if not preconception) that 'Africans' wanted an instant fix 'after three visits max' were particularly detrimental to a long-term 'empotment' of Chinese medicine into East African health fields. This Chinese prejudice that Africans were simple-minded, I believe, could easily be changed through an educational effort, as many TCM practitioners were university trained and thus receptive to education, but not aware of how racist their preconceptions were, and that it distorted what some of their very polite and civilised clientele actually thought and did.

## Chinese Medicine Patients in Mombasa and on Rural Pemba

This research project initially aimed to complement the comparison of medical professionals in Tanzania and Kenya (and Uganda), as undertaken by John Iliffe (1998), with that of TM/CAM as practised in urban textures.[7] TCM as practised in Swahili-speaking Tanzania's Dar es Salaam was to be compared with TCM as practised in urban Kenya, specifically Swahili-speaking Mombasa. Both cities were economically defined by their ports on the Indian Ocean. Mombasa, due to its deeper waters, could host larger ships, was technologically much more established and had a much larger import-export volume. Both were serviced by a train line into the hinterland, namely the Ugandan railway to Kisumu on Lake Victoria, built between December 1895 and 1903 under British colonial rule by Indian labourers (Grillo 1973), and TAZARA leading to Lusaka, the capital of continental Zambia, and built in 1970–75 under Julius Nyerere's socialist-oriented government by Chinese workers (Monson 2009).[8] The Ugandan railway was famed for its anti-slavery impact at a time when in the harbour of Bagamoyo, 60 km north of Dar es Salaam, the slave trade was at its height. Yet one hundred years on, the corruption in Kilindini, Mombasa, was legendary, such that there was rumour of a Chinese BRI (belt-and-road initiative) plan to invest in Bagamoyo as the largest African port. In post-socialism-oriented Tanzania, as in post-socialist Russia (Lindquist 2005), there was an aggressive surge of late-liberal commerce, sometimes mixed with crime. Meanwhile, long-haul German mass tourism to Mombasa, which was economically considerable (e.g. Gess 1974: 22), countervailed the many violent ethnic eruptions of post-independence Kenya. Furthermore, there was an air of history and stability in the stone masonry of Mombasa, apparently already mentioned by the Arab geographer al-Idrisi in 1151 and visited by the Portuguese navigator Vasco da Gama in 1498, that Dar es Salaam, founded in 1891 by the German colonisers, did not have.

The comparison of urban and rural patient cohorts became a possibility due to good relations with a Chinese practitioner who had opened a practice in Chake Chake, the capital of Pemba island, between autumn 2002 and spring 2003. Pemba was, together with Unguja, one of the two main islands that made up the semi-independent state of Zanzibar. As we will see, the differences in the profiles of the patient cohorts in urban and rural textures pertained mostly to economic, educational and religious circumstances. The history of the nation state's health care certainly played a role in all three settings – in urban Dar es Salaam and Mombasa and on rural Pemba – but perhaps not as important a one as an anthropologist of TM/CAM might have expected. The urban–urban comparison of interviewing Tanzanian and Kenyan patients showed some place-specific differences, while the comparison with rural Pemba highlighted issues of a different order.

There is an extensive social anthropological literature on Zanzibar, an archipelago in the Indian Ocean that has been a Mecca for patients in search of traditional medical authorities and healers (e.g. Parkin 1995, 2000; see also Larsen et al. 2001; Larsen 2008, 2019); but times were changing, as for some, spirits were *upuuzi*, foolishness, e.g. Caplan 2004: 50). More recently, due to the predominant 'traditional' lifestyle, Pemba has become a target for public health interventions, in particular to promote family planning and women's health (e.g. Kielmann 1998; Young 2002; Beckmann 2015a, b).

Zanzibar was known for playing an important part in Indian Ocean trade routes.[9] Vestiges of the slave trade were very visible in the stonework of Stone Town, its architectonically stunning metropole on Unguja. The clove plantations dating to colonial times were in the early 2000s still a dominant aspect of rural Pemba. The ongoing ethnic conflicts were violent.[10] Since my research focus was on Chinese medicine, I could avoid any discussions to do with politics. However, it was impossible to evade them in interviews (see below) and in daily life routines (e.g. interviewing people living behind barbed wire).

In Mombasa and on Pemba island I again aimed to interview the patients in their homes. I could not rely on a taxi driver, however, as in Dar es Salaam and Nairobi. On Pemba I was guided by a local psychiatric nurse and we criss-crossed the entire island on his vespa to find the patients in their homes. In Mombasa I relied solely on public transport: the *matatu*, where pounding music, mixed with hot air draughts and dust, had me arrive nauseous at the patient's place. This effort of moving through textured spaces reminded me that according to Merleau-Ponty (1945), people throw themselves into the world with intentionality and accordingly get to know the world specific to the directionality of their intentionalities and social actions;

the body is the foundation through which people can project themselves into the world and get to know it. Acquiring any knowledge about the world is accordingly a bodily activity. This requires learning body techniques that engage with the materiality of the body's surroundings, be it a heavy pounding beat in a stuffy minibus or the mild scent of cloves in fresh air.

To compare the Tanzanian patients with urban Kenyan and rural Zanzibari patient cohorts, I held interviews during the small rains (December 2003–January 2004) with thirty-four patients of Dr Peng in Chake Chake, on Pemba island, and nineteen patients of Dr Ming in Mombasa, Kenya.[11] In Dar es Salaam in 2001 and 2002, the patients I recruited in Chinese medical clinics were generally curious and willing to be interviewed. In Mombasa in 2003 and 2004, however, many patients were reluctant. Some seemed jaded with being interviewed, regardless of the theme, having been asked to join focus group discussions or the like previously. Among those recruited, about one third had received higher education. This ratio may be misleading, however. My notes, based on sitting in the consultation room next to the Chinese practitioner throughout one day, showed a high ratio of young Swahili-speaking men who declined to participate in this study. Several were taxi drivers, accountants or shopkeepers, and they declined, perhaps, due to matters of entitlement, status and gender. In Chake Chake, by contrast, most patients who were adventurous enough to set foot into the Chinese medical practice would readily agree to be interviewed in their homes; they considered me part of the clinic's personnel, just as elsewhere, which clearly affected the answers they provided. On Pemba island, Chinese medicine was an entirely new phenomenon, the Chinese medical practice having been open for no longer than two months, and people were evidently curious about it.

As in Dar es Salaam, the semi-structured interviews in Mombasa and Chake Chake suggested that the TCM clinics' clientele consisted mostly of enterprising individuals. Their religion was not as diverse, however, being mainly Muslim on Pemba and Christian in Kenya, but there was great variety in their denominations. While in the urban areas of Dar es Salaam and Mombasa, the interview sample suggested that individuals were independently 'trying out', unrelated to each other, even if they lived in the same neighbourhoods, and presented with a wide range of different complaints, this was not the case on rural Pemba, where the news of a 'miracle' led to an entirely different patient profile visiting a pioneering medical practitioner.

In Mombasa, the nineteen patients recruited from Dr Ming's clinic, of whom nine were women and ten were men, fell into two easily identifiable age groups: one of ten patients between 19 and 38, the other nine patients between 48 and 71.[12] In both age groups there were two women who were housewives. Among the seniors, the remaining eight were all men, who, with few exceptions, had been schooled for seven years in elementary school and attained Form 4 or 6, followed by two or three years postgraduate training; five were teachers or school directors. Among the juniors, there were three women, alongside four men, who had been able to accomplish Form 4, and occupations ranged from teacher to security guard and from businesswoman to lab technician. The educational and social profile of the patients in Mombasa was not very different from those in Dar es Salaam, though perhaps slightly more elevated. The visits to their homes, however, revealed a much more pronounced inequality in living conditions. The houses of several patients in this sample had garages and even cars in them, whereas other patients lived in informal settlements,[13] say, a family of three cramped into a rented room in a dormitory.

In Mombasa, the sample comprising twenty-five patients (19 + 6) was predominantly Christian (seventeen in total): six identified themselves as Catholics; five said they were Anglican, some specifically CPK (Church Province of Kenya); five said they were Protestants, specifically one Lutheran, one AIC (African Inland Church), one belonging to the Ushindi Baptist Church and two Pentecostals; and one was an SDA (Seventh Day Adventist). Six were Muslim, three specifically Sunni; one identified as Hindu and one as Buddhist. Their ethnic backgrounds, as in the urban area of Dar es Salaam, were highly diverse, including Luo (5), Kamba (3), Luhya (3), Arab (3), Choni (2), Taita (2), Digo (1), Kisi (1), Kikuyu (1), Tareta (1), Chagga (1), one Indian and one Chinese (from Fujian province).

In Mombasa the complaints among the nine seniors were in the urogenital system (4), the chest (2), the legs (2) and in one case, typhoid or hypertension. Among the ten juniors, the complaints ranged from a knot in the breast, pimples on the face, a stomach ulcer, womb pain, diabetes and malaria to fungal infections, herpes and HIV. Evidently, both age groups presented with a wide range of conditions, many chronic and some terminal, which was much in line with the findings in Dar es Salaam.

## A Miracle Caused by Acupuncture Treatment

The clientele on Pemba identified itself as highly diverse ethnically, with a preponderance of Arabs (*Waraabu*). Twelve patients said that they were Arabs, of whom ten further specified themselves as: Siveri, Nophel, Hadharmy, Al-Rashidi, Al-Mashir, Al-Shardi, Rikesh, El-Habsy, and a Busaidi from Oman; furthermore, there was a Bajuki from Lamu and a Baluchy from Muscat; two were Mazrui; ten said they were Shirazi and one was a Mgunya; and four identified themselves as mainland Tanzanians: a Chagga, Nyamwezi, Sukuma and Makonde. All but one patient, who was Catholic, gave Islam as their religion; twenty-four said they were Sunni and nine called themselves Ibadhi.

Shortly after I arrived on Pemba (on 24 December 2003), news broke of a miracle effected by Dr Peng on that very day: a farmer who had been carried into the clinic could walk out of it herself after acupuncture treatment. This is not quite the miracle that I was told about by the male farmer himself, to whom I was directed a few days later. He had a stiff knee and could not walk: 'I have a problem with my knee, it is filled with water' (*ana matatizo ya goti, kujaa maji*), he explained when I visited him in the village of Ole-Muhogani on Saturday, 27 December. He had gone to the Chinese medical doctor on the previous Monday, he told me, received four different kinds of medicine, which cost him TZS 3,000 (*c.* GBP 3), and on the following day, that is, Tuesday, he could walk without crutches! He did not mention acupuncture treatment. I could not make sense of my findings, as the news of the miracle was that the doctor had worked it in a woman by means of needling. Perhaps this pioneering practitioner had effected two miracles in two different patients? In the following days and weeks the Chake Chake Chinese medical practice was crowded with peasants from nearby villages suffering from pain in the muscular-skeletal tissue. Dr Peng was one of the few Chinese medical doctors in East Africa who offered acupuncture treatment.

As would be expected, the 'miracle' skewed the profile of the clientele interviewed and the complaints presented: there were as many as seventeen whom I classified as 'seniors' (self-reporting to be aged between 50 and 80); six presented with leg pain, four with numbness, '*ganzi*', and one each with either gout or back pain. That is, in total, twelve of my interviewees presented with pain in the muscular-skeletal tissue. The other five patients had complaints of coughing and chest pain in four cases and a hernia in one case.

In the group of adults aged 17–45, comprising in total fourteen patients, by contrast, only one patient had a back pain problem. Otherwise, a more usual spectrum of complaints was presented, including chest pain (*pumo*, 1), asthma (1), headaches (*kichwa*, 1) and chronic flu (1) in the chest region; *gesi* ('gas'/bloating, 1), overweight (1) and malaria (1); and problems of the urogenital system and reproduction: urethral pain when urinating (2), erectile difficulties (1), heavy monthly bleeding (1), haemorrhoids (1) and a tear in the anus (1). Three were children aged 1–3.5 years, presenting with sickle cell anaemia and the more commonly seen cough and asthma.

The 'miracle' also skewed the occupation of the majority of the patients recruited into my study, of whom nine identified themselves as 'farmers' (*wakulima*, seven men and two women), in addition to the usual businesspeople (*watu wa biashara*, 4), housewives (*wake wa nyumbani/kinyumbani*, 4), accountants, secretaries and menial officers in the ministry (4), police and security officers (2), teachers (1) and students in engineering, computer sciences and at high school (3), and one driver, one builder, one tailor and one nurse.

Interestingly, all the farmers but one were above the age of 50, and most presented with what the Chinese doctor called arthritis in English (*fengshibing* 风湿病, literally a wind-damp disorder). Perhaps junior farmers had no pain or would not admit to having pain, or could not afford Chinese treatment? Back pain is an honourable complaint for a senior person among the Yap, as it testifies to the work and care done for the community (Throop 2011). Among the senior male farmers on Pemba, however, an overall sense of numbness, *ganzi* and pain in the legs, rather than back pain, seemed to prevail.[14] It is evident that a farmer's body would engage in taxing agricultural work on rural Pemba, and possibly the uniformity of complaints was therefore more pronounced than in the urban areas, and not merely due to the miracle.

## The Patients' Livelihoods: Traditional or Modern?
To identify the connotations of the traditional and the modern in general, and traditional medicine in particular, I asked all patients whether they lived a traditional or a modern lifestyle (*maisha ya kiasili* or *maisha ya kisasa*). In Mombasa, several said 'in-between' or 'a mixture'. Many of them were embarrassed and laughed: 'You tell me!' or 'What do you mean?' Some went into a reflective mode: 'Perhaps modern, because I don't stay in the village?' '*Maisha ya kiasili* is where you are born, but we came here to work.' 'We are staying in town, we are trying to live like townspeople, . . . *maisha ya kiasili* means you are not going to school, today we all have to keep learning.' Some specified: 'We used to have no electricity, freezer or cooker, . . . the environment changed due to education', 'literacy levels changed, we learned to adjust', and concluded: 'Our lifestyle is modern'.

On Pemba, as was to be expected, several said that their lifestyles were traditional, and that they were elders (*wazee*), living a lifestyle as is usual (*maisha ya kawaida*): 'We are not living in an advanced manner'. Yet others spoke of the lifestyle of the poor (*maisha ya maskini*) or of the lower classes (*ya chini*), emphasising that life was fraught with difficulties (*maisha magumu*). Others said that they lived a rural lifestyle (*maisha ya kijijini*). However, many Chinese medicine patients on Pemba also said that their lifestyles were modern. A tailor of thirty-two years commented: 'We are young, we follow the lifestyle we see;' a housewife of twenty-two said: 'This is not the way our parents used to live.' Some said: 'We are going with the times (*tunaenda kwa wakatiya*)' or 'we are following the religion (*kufuata dini*)'. Others explained: 'To live a modern lifestyle, you have to have money.' A housewife on Pemba said that her household's lifestyle was modern (*maisha ya kisasa*) and Arabic (*ya Kiarabu*), rather than Western (*maisha ya Kizungu*).

Some voices were very critical of modernity. The grandmother of the Chinese medical doctor's interpreter on Pemba was outspoken: 'A modern lifestyle is bad, it brings with it many problems' (*maisha ya kisasa mabaya, matatizo mengi*). Some were less condemning, particularly some respondents in Mombasa. A local government employee said:

> *Kisasa*, modern; this means you borrow the lifestyle from other countries, and fuse it together with theirs, and fuse it together, such that the chil-

dren can't understand their parents' language. That is happening here in town. I like *kiasili*, that is why Chinese medicine enticed me so much. It is succeeding where modern medicine is failing. (Notebook no. 3)

This Kenyan government employee, who had attended Form 6 and had several postgraduate diplomas, had many years of exposure to Chinese medicine. Indeed, TCM had been practised in Mombasa for about one decade longer than in Dar es Salaam, from the mid-1980s onwards. In Kenya, which never went through a post-independence period of socialist orientation, no one said that Chinese medicine was 'advanced'. A Mombasa-born, 48-year-old Luhya Western medicine doctor explained at some length:

> The first time I came here to this Chinese medical clinic it was for chronic typhoid. I tried Western medicine for a long time. Then, somebody told me about traditional medicines. I went to an Indian doctor, and got some herbal medicines; it did not work. One day a mother with a girl who had HIV got Mocrea for her; it was the aunt of my wife. So, I went to get some Mocrea from the Chinese clinic and asked Dr Ming about chronic typhoid. I took his medicines. I had first had my urine tested in a Petri dish, it was full; the second time it was spotwise; the third time only one colony was there; the fourth time none. Now I refer patients to him with chronic typhoid, chronic urinary infections, low libido and HIV/AIDS; excessive bleeding in women, fibroids in the uterus; and chronic diabetes. (Notebook no. 3)

'Western medicine can poison vital organs. When you look at traditional medicine, it is good because it does not do damage', he continued. Here he alluded to the Chinese medical saying that 'Chinese medicine has no side effects' (*zhongyi mei you fuzuoyong* 中医没有副作用), which, historically speaking, became popular in the PRC in the 1950s, while other attributes of Chinese medicine were celebrated in Republican times. Traditional African medicines, by contrast, were well known to be both poisons and medicines (Last and Chavunduka 1986); the dosages that resulted in recovery were very often not known to the healers' clientele. 'As for traditional [Chinese] medicine, you can take it for three months [i.e. a very long time]', the Luhya Western medicine doctor then explained. Although he knew that some are strong and poisonous too, his perception of Chinese medicines was of them being a slow medicine.

## From Science, Magic and Witchcraft to the 'Propensity of Things' (shi 势)

Interviews with patients on Pemba and in Mombasa suggested that Chinese medicine practitioners were not generally considered to practise witchcraft, in contrast to some interviews in Dar es Salaam. For one thing, I spent less time with patients in Mombasa, and even less in Pemba, where a nurse acted as interpreter. Furthermore, in Dar es Salaam, Chinese medical practitioners were clearly associated with 'the Chinese' who had built the TAZARA railway (a) at a great speed, (b) by working at night and (c) where others 'got stuck'. Although some patients said that Chinese medicine was 'just ordinary', for many its perception as traditional, natural or 'local', scientific, modern or (technologically) advanced expressed a certain mystification about its effectiveness (see Hsu 2002 for further detail). Chinese medicine was too new for people to have a firm opinion about it. There was an indeterminacy to it that is intrinsic to any process of perception.

If it was indeed a case of *uchawi* – no, *mazingira* – no, *sayansi* – no, what was it? In what follows, I will float the idea of the 'propensity of things' (*shi* 势) in order to explain the cascade of changes that a 'pot' (say, an acupuncture treatment) could trigger. *Shi* is a concept central to warfare (de Certeau 1984: xx; Jullien 1995) and the martial arts (Hsu 2018a; Hsu and Lim 2016, 2020). Here I transpose this concept from the martial into the medical field in an attempt to better understand the sort of transformations that a practitioner aimed to effect in the triadic constellation of a medical encounter through the patient's consumption of a *pot* perceived to have certain propensities.[15] I propose to use the word 'trigger' to highlight that doing one thing, for instance pressing on a trigger, can cause a cascade of interconnected transformations, depending on the given textures or the mechanics of the machinery just triggered. De Certeau, in the context of discussing the practice of everyday life, developed a concept called 'tactics' as a weapon of the weak. It was in this context that he compared tactics to *shi* 势, which Francois Jullien has theorised as the 'propensity of things'.

## Nine Farmers, Two with Tactics

It was striking how many respondents on Pemba referred to themselves as a *mkulima*, 'farmer' or 'peasant' – nine out of seventeen.

In the village in which the miracle happened, I interviewed three further farmers from the senior age group. One was a 50-year-old woman who was suffering from *ganzi*, 'numbness' (as the Chinese doctor explained to me in the clinic). Everywhere hurt, she said. She went to the Chinese clinic to get medicines, three different kinds, which cost in total TZS 4,500, plus an additional TZS 2,000. When I interviewed her a few days later, she was 'waiting to see' whether her condition would improve. Another was a 60-year-old man from the same village. He was suffering from 'lots, all over, heat' (*mwili ote unauma*); he had been to the clinic four times and spent TZS 12,500, to no effect. Nevertheless, based on what 'other people said' and the 'writing on the wall', he said that he thought he might get a cure from the Chinese. Finally, a 50-year-old woman said that she just wanted to try it out. Her main complaint was piercing chest pain, but she had a long history of health-seeking for a wide range of different ailments in private and state institutions. She spent TZS 11,000 for three different medicines and three injections. These three farmers had chronic pains 'all over', and the effects of the Chinese medicines that they had taken were not distinctive. The interviews, which took place in Swahili, soon reached their limits. However, on reflection, I doubt the lack of an interpreter at hand was the only reason for this. We will return to this issue after discussing the following five 'farmers' who, by contrast, spoke differently about their bodies and their perception of the Chinese medicines.

A 38-year-old man had been to the clinic thrice during the preceding two months, and had spent TZS 5,000 and twice TZS 3,000 – TZS 11,000 in total – which, considering that he had some relief, was 'not' very 'much money', he said. He had been suffering from chronic haemorrhoids for six years, among several other ailments. His health-seeking trajectory had him consult practitioners, initially in public and then in private clinics and hospitals, amounting to costs of over TZS 90,000. In the course of discussing the specifics of the Chinese medicines, he communicated perceptions of medical interest: when he took the drugs for the chest, they did not work only on his chest but more generally on his entire body. However, the medicines he got for the haemorrhoids worked only on those. He was an unusually committed, bodily aware and perceptive patient.

A 75-year-old *mzee* (gentleman) had a long list of complaints, from pain in the legs to numbness and dizziness, when I interviewed him. He said that he had spent TZS 7,000 on the one occasion that he had been to the Chinese clinic; he had not been told to return, and he also said that he had no means to do so. I had been present during his consultation in the clinic two days earlier and knew that he had asked for *Nanbao* (男宝), 'men's treasure', known to regenerate masculine strength (see Chapter 8); it was evident that he had scratched together for this one occasion the TZS 9,000 for which a box with two pills was usually sold. Meanwhile, the Chinese doctor checked his blood pressure, as required by his medical routine, and prescribed medication for treating hypertension, presumably for TZS 2,000. Two days later, naturally, the patient registered no effect. He was completely unaware that he could have gone to the nearby dispensary and got hypertension treatment for free. No doubt the idea of a miracle had driven him into the Chinese medical practice, but it had been a miracle of a different kind.

An 81-year-old self-identified *mkulima* had a hernia that reached halfway down to his knees. It started in 1978, he said. He had been to the clinic thrice for acupuncture treatment, every other day, which cost him TZS 3,000 each time. He said that he was a farmer, but he lived in an army camp and was wearing the uniform of a soldier. He had come to Pemba from Shinyanga in October that year. When I told him that Chake Chake hospital would surely offer surgery for free, he answered: 'I'm a foreigner'. Shinyanga was one of the regions of Tanzania where witchcraft assassinations had recently arisen, according to Mesaki (2009a, 2009b), not least due to mismanagement within the bureaucratic structures of the state. Perhaps this explained the army's decision to place this retired soldier on Pemba, in a comparatively safe place? The miracle happened on 24 December, and his first acupuncture treatment was on 26 December. He was due for the fourth treatment on the day of our interview, but he said that he could not afford the bus, nor, when I asked him, the fee for the treatment. It would appear that his 'trying out' lasted no longer than three times, which some Chinese medical doctors who had worked in East Africa for many years said was a magic number among their local clientele.

Another 80-year-old *mzee* (elder) had been to the clinic on the same day that I interviewed him in his homestead. The interview was brief. He said that he had lumbago and pain in the legs. The cost of the medication had been TZS 9,000, which was the price of the above medicine for boosting male strength, *nguvu ya kiume*. He, however, spoke of amidephrine, *diedawan* 跌打丸 and *furunbao* 福润宝, as though his visit to the clinic had been motivated otherwise. Although he said that he was a 'farmer' and lived in a rural area, his demeanour and dress were more like those of a recently retired government official; in the interview, he did indeed indicate that he was 'retired'. Perhaps my free movement on the island had caused some disquiet in his circles?

Finally, the grandmother of the Chinese medical doctor's interpreter, who was a high school graduate and could barely speak English, identified herself as a farmer. She complained about her eyesight, a cough and pain in her legs. She was given two kinds of medicines for TZS 7,000 in total. The interview with her was very brief as well, as she showed little interest in it. She was, however, one of the few who instantly took the routinely given opportunity to ask me a question. This concerned whether I was married.

## *Discussion*

The semi-structured interviews quite soon became utterly perfunctory among the *wakulima* on Pemba. While language barriers evidently existed, it appeared that semi-structured interviewing as a method perhaps also had its limitations. What was said could not be taken at face value but had to be considered in terms of linguistic pragmatics (e.g. Levinson 1983). We are reminded here of the term *dawa ya Kichina*'s wide spectrum of meanings. It could refer to drugs coming from China, regardless of whether they were Chinese formula medicines or Western medical pharmaceuticals, or it denoted medicine as practised by Chinese practitioners, regardless of whether it was traditional or modern. In a similar vein, five of the nine patients who self-identified as *mkulima* on Pemba, used the term in a very inclusive way, in the sense of 'just ordinary folks'. Likewise, the ages of 70, 80 and above meant simply 'very old'. Linguistic pragmatics are evidently central to the interpretation of any semi-structured interviews.

The semi-structured interviewing for this research was primarily intended for getting a feel of the scale of its complexity, although it actually yielded some very interesting 'data'. One of these positive findings was that the patients of Chinese medical practitioners in Dar es Salaam and Mombasa were ethnically very diverse, coming from different regions of the nation state and living in different neighbourhoods spread out over the city. They were similarly diverse by gender, age, education and profession, and presented with a wide range of different health problems. This suggests that in urban areas of the Swahili-speaking East African coast, TCM clinics attracted enterprising individualists, upwardly mobile men and women who were curious and willing to 'try out' something new.

Almost all identified as 'middle-class', a term that is not to be confused with how it is generally used in English. It expressed more, perhaps, their aspiration to be middle class, that is, modern and well off, as many lived in informal settlements. In Dar es Salaam these had a physiognomic aspect that, sitting next to the taxi driver on whom I depended to find the homes of my interviewees, I soon recognised as characteristic of the socio-economic status of Chinese medicine patients. These informal settlements often still had a rural feel to them, being lush and green, with trees and high grass overgrowing grey cement bricks stacked next to the skeletal structure of a house. By contrast, in Mombasa the 'middle class' patients who agreed to be interviewed belonged among the better educated (Form 4 or 6) and often owned houses in well-established neighbourhoods.

# Reflections: Tactics and the 'Propensity of Things' (*shi* 势)

Chapter 3, on the socio-substantial relatedness between patients, practitioners and pots, made very clear that there was no single 'authentic' way of practising Chinese medicine in East Africa: Drs Wei, Wu and Wang each foregrounded the use of different pots, with which they 'empotted' their clientele into East Africa's urban landscapes and thereby indirectly achieved an 'empotment' for themselves and their kin as well. This process of 'empotment', I argue, reconfigured the triad of patients, practitioners and pots.

This chapter has focused on the patients. Given that I relied largely on semi-structured interviews, it was difficult to ascertain whether, and to what degree, an 'empotment' would reconfigure wholeness between them and their entourage. This was not least due to what I call 'hyper-ironic twists', by which 'traditional' knowledge and practice are transformed in the course of their transposition into contemporary urban textures. Patients could not quite make out how the Chinese formula medicines worked. I was asking was it due to science or magic or witchcraft? But they approached the situation differently, and some astutely turned the tables by resorting to 'tactics', what de Certeau (1984) called the weapon of the weak, to investigate the interviewer's motives. The following year I learned that the TCM practitioner in Chake Chake, who during my two-to-three-week stay was famed for the miracle(s) he had effected through acupuncture, had closed the clinic a few months later.

## Tactics

On Pemba, it was intriguing that the retired government official who said that he was a farmer and the grandmother of the TCM practitioner's interpreter were transforming the interview situation into a different social encounter. Perhaps they mobilised the 'tactics' of 'the weak' in de Certeau's (1984: xix) sense when they showed willingness to be researched, but ultimately were more interested in researching the researcher? De Certeau specifically speaks of non-verbalised tactics (in contradistinction to verbalised strategies):[16]

> A tactic depends on time – it is always on the lookout for opportunities that must be seized . . . It must constantly manipulate events in order to turn them into 'opportunities'. The weak must continually turn to their own ends forces alien to them. This is achieved in the propitious moments when they are able to combine heterogeneous elements . . . (De Certeau 1984: xix)

De Certeau (1984: xix–xx) speaks of 'ways of operating' and invokes the Greek *metis*: '[C]lever tricks, knowing how to get away with things, "hunter's cunning", manoeuvres, polymorphic simulations, joyful discoveries, poetic as well as warlike.' He locates these ways of operating in a non-space, namely in time, in being 'on the wing'. He discusses the art of practice, spatial practices and the pragmatics of language, and he attributes tactics to persons, but he does not dwell on body techniques. He speaks of 'propitious moments in time', but in a disembodied way. It is worth noting that when he discusses 'opportunities' and 'propitious moments', he furthermore refers to the Chinese art of war, and to the insights, grounded in *shi*, namely the 'propensity of things' that the legendary military strategist Sunzi 孙子 expressed in that context. Chinese philosophers and military strategists located opportunity in material stuff, in the situation, in the configuration and in their propensities.

We will reflect on skills and the 'propensities of things' intrinsic to configurations like the triadic medical encounter in what follows. Rather than theorising (patient) 'agency' in contradistinction to 'structure', let us think of figurations, configurations and reconfigurations specific to a situation.

## The 'Propensity of Things'

Patients and practitioners had a probing attitude to *dawa ya Kichina*. Where earlier I had emphasised the 'patient's perceptions', more recently, the specific techniques with which patients and practitioners jointly implicated the Chinese medicine pots in a process geared towards reconfiguring sorts of wholeness in the patient and the social association, of which the patient was part, have attracted my attention. Where the word 'perception' clearly locates agency in the perceiver, and thereby in a person, it is interesting to note that other concepts do not attribute agency to specific agents, such as Lefebvre's spatial textures.[17]

Two Chinese concepts, the *li* 理-pattern and the *shi*-propensity, allow us to conceptualise change as happening due to spatially and materially given textures that have a texturing effect on the transformation. The latter concept, *shi*, is particularly interesting because it involves change that is triggered. The 'propensity of things' can work like a trigger that causes a cascade of different, but inherently interrelated changes.

Jullien (1995) traced the texts on *shi* from antiquity to the seventeenth century, when such texts proliferated, and he attributed, as legend does, the coinage of the concept to the warfare strategist Sunzi. The concept of *shi*-propensity, unlike that of *li*-pattern, involves a triggering of change. Once a process of change has been triggered, it takes its own course in accordance with the texturing textures contained in the situation. A strategist – be it Sunzi or a martial artist – will be particularly interested in triggers that remain unchanged, leaving them unaffected by the changes they cause.

Following Jullien (1995), I understand movements that take account of the propensity of things as achieving efficacious interventions. Accordingly, a certain spatial texture, such as the configuration of patients, practitioners and pots in a Chinese medical practice,

*The Patients*

would contain within it texturing devices that, once triggered, texture a new whole. Agency is accordingly not to be located solely in the person (free will and free choice) or solely in the (natural/social) environment (requiring 'adaptation' to given structures).[18] Rather, it is the situational constellation, with its inherent tensions and tonus that give it momentum.

In summary, to understand a patient's movements we need to consider not merely their perception of the practitioners and their 'medicine pots', but also their engagement with the situation as a whole. By studying primarily those practitioners who are intent on perfecting their craft,[19] rather than those mainly interested in maximising business profits, we might identify the skills with which people, even those from different provenances, achieve a spatial practice leading to a new sense of wholeness through attending to the 'propensity of the things'.

# Notes

1. Bernard (1994: 221) advises interviewing a minimum of forty to sixty respondents; he too warns against letting these interviews become mechanistic.
2. This section elaborates on select parts of Elisabeth Hsu. 2002. '"The Medicine from China has Rapid Effects": Chinese Medicine Patients in Tanzania', in Elisabeth Hsu and Erling Høg (eds), 'Countervailing Creativity: Patient Agency in the Globalisation of Asian Medicines', special issue, *Anthropology & Medicine* 9(3): 291–314, a publication based on twice thirty interviews, with twenty follow ups six months later.
3. This was surprising considering the reputation of TCM in the PRC and the West, which is that it works slowly (Karchmer 2015).
4. On medical teams, see Li Anshan (2006, 2009, 2011, 2021 and many more). Shandong province was in charge of Tanganyika/Tanzania, Jiangsu province of Zanzibar, and Yunnan province of Uganda. Kenya was a stronghold of the Allies after the Second World War, and no medical teams were dispatched there.
5. By contrast, most consultations concerned STDs and other problems of the reproductive system (Qiao n.d.). See Chapters 3 and 8.
6. See, for instance, *The Guardian*, 19 December 2001, 8.
7. DelVecchio Good et al. (1999) discussed the clinical realities and moral worlds common to institutionalised medicine in Tanzania and Kenya without foregrounding differences between them.
8. Participant observation included a journey on TAZARA to Mbeya in 2002 and another one on the old Nairobi–Mombasa line in 2005 (this was before the Chinese built the current standard-gauge railway line, opened in 2017). My field notes remark on the integration of the railway into lo-

cal markets in southern Tanzania; petty enterprise with fresh agricultural goods thrived. Meanwhile, the Kenyan route was deserted and used mostly by foreign tourists.

9. The historical and anthropological literature on Indian Ocean trade is too diverse to be referenced here. I (Hsu 2007a) have pointed out that the Chinese noodle-makers on Zanzibar trace their genealogy to fishers who settled on its shores between the world wars in order to provide shark floss and sea cucumbers as delicacies to the Chinese food industry, thereby highlighting trading connections beyond the Indian Ocean and Singapore to the South China Sea.

10. Young (2002), based on a master's thesis, provides rich detail on both the history and ethnic conflicts of Pemba, and Zanzibar more widely.

11. For the systematic review presented here, I rely on notebooks nos. 2 and 3; they were tidy, with corresponding page numbers in the index, waiting to be analysed fifteen years later. Notebook no. 1 of April 2003 contained another six interviews with patients of another doctor in Mombasa, Dr Meng, but their profile was too different to be included in this analysis; several patients were in longterm treatment.

12. If we include in the sample reported on in the main text the six patients interviewed in April 2003, the statistics would be quite similar: the twenty-five patients, of whom eleven were women and fourteen men, fell into two easily identifiable age groups, one of twelve patients between 19 and 39, the other of thirteen patients between 48 and 71. In what follows, I will only focus on the nineteen patients interviewed in Mombasa in January 2004.

13. On the precarious living conditions in these informal settlements, see Gilbertson (2013, 2015).

14. Legs are considered erotic and sexually attractive, and women must cover them. It would be interesting to know whether *ganzi* in the legs was an honourable complaint, like back pain among the Yap (Throop 2010). A 'TCM' practitioner comes to mind (see Chapter 7) who according to Jennings (2005: 462–64) claimed to treat 'arthritis and joint problems', but the patients' records in his Chinese handwriting revealed that most were being prescribed sulfonamides (the usual Western biomedical treatment for STDs). Relevant to the discussion here is that the patients said they suffered 'problems in their "legs"' (ibid. 463).

15. Law and Lin's (2016) provincialising project parallels the decolonising one here, but their interpretation of *shi* as a 'strategy' (marked by flexibility, fluidity and subtlety) is directly opposed to de Certeau's (1984) definition of strategy. They then attempt to interpret *shi* was an aspect of *xingshi* 形勢, 'tidescapes', a creative interpretation, which is not given in Chinese texts however.

16. 'I call a "strategy" the calculus . . . which becomes possible when a subject of will and power . . . can be isolated from the environment' (De Certeau 1984: xix; see also 34–39).

17. Concepts like 'automorphic' symmetry, as proposed by Weyl (1952), or arguably 'autopoiesis', as first posited by the Gaia hypothesis (summarised in Margulis 1997), suggest that change, regardless of scale, is always already textured, and that these textures, which are proportionate to the self, affect the outcome of the transformation.
18. Hallowell (2017: 89) also made this point when he spoke of the 'outlook of the self in its behavioral environment'. It is basic to the phenomenology of the body.
19. In the martial arts, the term *shi* specifically refers to embodied skills that are learned through perfected responsiveness (Hsu 2018a; Hsu and Lim 2016, 2020).

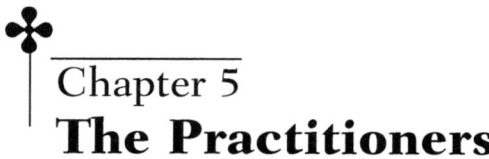

# Chapter 5
# The Practitioners

## Fieldwork: Working with Narrative

In Dar es Salaam, Chinese medical practitioners were generally hesitant to speak to me, let alone to give an interview. At the turn of the millennium, TCM clinics and their 'mushrooming' had become a media item. Viceversa, in the PRC the Chinese spoke of an 'emigration fever' (*chuguo re* 出国热); businesspeople, mostly from northeast China (Dongbei 东北), streamed into Dar es Salaam.[1] When a field site is polarised by the media, it is always difficult for anthropologists to do research. For one thing, interviewees should not be invited to make statements that render them vulnerable or invite further antagonisms. Furthermore, it is difficult to obtain information that is not tainted by the antagonisms of the situation. Therefore, I refrained from systematically eliciting life histories from the Chinese practitioners in Dar es Salaam.

In Kenya, the situation was different. Firstly, the health services in independent Kenya had not seen violent disruptions as in Uganda, nor had they been subject to socialist-oriented 'detours', as some Tanzanians put it. However, Kenyan health professionals were marked by 'burnout' and constant crises, not least due to the ongoing problems of HIV/AIDS (Good et al. 1999; Raviola et al. 2002). Furthermore, late liberalism in Kenya, as elsewhere, saw the promotion of vertical programmes, again not least due to HIV/AIDS (Booth 2004), which led to a fragmentation of holistic health as originally envisaged by the WHO. Into this fragmented urban landscape, dotted with uncoordinated vertical programmes, Chinese medical entrepreneurs found ready entry, particularly in the informal sector. In Kenya, the first practitioners immigrated in the late 1980s, about one decade earlier than in Tanzania. As seen in Chapter 3, they 'empotted' their patients and themselves into specific niches in the Kenyan health field. One of the first practitioners to set up a practice, for instance, was a Chinese *tuina* 推拿, 'masseur'.

Second, the migration pattern of Chinese medical practitioners into Kenya differed from that of Tanzania and Uganda. Most had come to Kenya with the assistance of a Chinese medical doctor who had emigrated in the late 1980s and become a so-called 'gatekeeper' (see Introduction, 'Kenya'). This pattern of migratory flows between defined areas of origin and destination is well known in migration studies.[2] The gatekeeper was respected and well known to the relevant Kenyan authorities, and he invited a series of colleagues and juniors to work with him on his Kenyan premises. However, due to conflicts, most of these individuals soon went elsewhere in the country after an initial period of working with or for him. Thus, most of my Kenyan interviewees had work experience with the gatekeeper and were vaguely aware of each other. The media reported on Chinese medicine in Kenya as well, but instead of ridiculing and demonising Chinese medicine, it at the time reported on what was presented as a prestigious research project financed by the Ford Foundation in collaboration with said gatekeeper (see below).

I interviewed the Chinese medical practitioners in Kenya twice, once in December 2001 and once in April 2003. My main method was life history elicitation. Furthermore, I drew heavily on participant observation of interactions taking place in and around the medical practice before and after the interview. In December 2001, a Kenyan social anthropologist interested in 'popular culture' was interested in a collaboration. He had located eleven TCM clinics, which were stationed mostly in wealthy suburban supermarket complexes, and he drove us there in his Land Rover. He had carried out a preliminary survey in English one month before I arrived, but made it no secret that he was frustrated about the dearth of information elicited. The Chinese evidently considered him a Kenyan government representative, and like other migrants, most had a considerable history of dealing with state bureaucracies that had made them weary. Furthermore, the language barriers between them were obvious. His and my collaboration was most fruitful when he started to informally speak with the receptionists in the front room, while I spoke in Chinese with the Chinese medical practitioners in the consultation room.

This elicited invaluable information about the clientele, the Chinese medical practitioners, and their collaborators and employees that no local would tell a foreigner, and certainly not upon first encounter. However, our styles of doing fieldwork differed, and he generously withdrew and, without further interference, let me get on.

When visiting medical practices in Nairobi, I introduced myself first in English, and instantly thereafter in Chinese, as a student of TCM who had learned the language and studied in the PRC. I also explained that my research and teaching fell into the field of medical anthropology (*yiliao renleixue* 医疗人类学), well aware at the time that this was a term that no one had ever heard. So I explained my research topic as being about cultural exchanges (*wenhua jiaoliu* 文化交流) in the medical field, and asked for permission to take handwritten notes. I started with the usual questions of a semi-structured interview regarding sociological data, which I introduced in a formal voice and register. These were questions that my respondents expected me to ask, and with which I could demonstrate that I was professional by doing what they expected a social scientist to do. Thereafter, I asked a few general questions about their clientele and the treatments they delivered, as well as about the perceived outcome of their treatments.

I turned to working on narrative, not least because one routine question from the semi-structured interview turned into an independent piece of research. This was when I asked the practitioners to tell me their life histories, and how and why they set foot in urban East Africa. Their life experiences were multiple and varied, and the numerous hardships encountered remarkable; they had all dealt with the existential questions of life. Our conversation almost always took place in Chinese, and some encounters turned into emotionally highly laden events, eliciting on one occasion a flood of tears and once a bout of anger. Evidently, the interview situation generated an unusual kind of closeness, even a sort of intimacy, even though I was a complete stranger to my respondents and surprised them with my visits. Talking in their mother tongue about their personal life history was compounded by the situation of living a sometimes rather isolated life in a foreign place. I was neither completely ignorant of nor entirely unaffected by the historical events in my own family's country. Each life story was very different; some were complicated and complex, interweaving several storylines; some had tragic and others ironic moments; most were very moving. It is impossible to report on all their many facets here. It is furthermore clear that in these intense moments, which barely exceeded an hour, not all had been said, or indeed could have been said.

In March and April 2003 I arranged formal visits to the same doctors again, this time on my own but with a tape recorder in hand, specifically for recording life histories. In the meantime, I had identified through the snowball method a total of twenty-four Chinese medical practitioners who at the time were active in urban Kenya; most worked in Nairobi, three in Mombasa and, according to hearsay, three elsewhere. I interviewed all practitioners in Nairobi and Mombasa, of whom more than half were new acquaintances. Most of those whom I interviewed the second time were much more welcoming than they had been the first time. I had dropped in on some several times in the meantime, such that I had become, if not a friend, an acquaintance with whom they felt at ease. Some did not quite understand why I needed to hear their life story again, but I explained that my notes had in places been unclear and that I needed more reliable information. I was also curious to test the anthropological method. Would I elicit very different information depending on whether respondents spoke freely or were tape-recorded, where the latter is a widely accepted ethnographic method?

Overall, the second visits, during which I elicited the tape-recorded life histories, were less eventful and significantly less emotionally charged than the first ones had been. I had hoped that in meeting for a second time we would go into previously unexplored territory, but this did not actually happen; the interviews were held with an air of professionalism on both sides. In a few cases, the sequencing of life events was not as accurate as during the first interview. I interpreted this as arising from a lack of effort to remember details precisely due to our increased familiarity, rather than due to wilful misinformation. Overall, I was pleasantly surprised to find that the information in the notebooks from the first visits and on the tape from the second ones (complemented by notes in my notebooks) was surprisingly similar in content. There were two exceptions. This was an interesting finding in itself. The two exceptions were two respondents who in that year had converted to Christianity. The life stories they now told as Christian converts were radically transformed.

Another incident made clear that eliciting life histories has therapeutic potential, but might adversely affect the interviewee if not handled well. On one occasion, I noted half an hour into the interview that the tape recorder's batteries were exhausted, and interrupted our interview. My respondent instantly understood and volunteered to retell her life's story again. She did so word for word, almost verbatim, for over half an hour. This raised questions. Had she retold her life story so many times that she had a routine version to present? Her narrative referred to several events that were harrowing, as she had come to Kenya as a refugee from Burundi at the height of the Rwandan genocide in the mid-1990s. She likely was suffering from what might have been diagnosed as post-traumatic stress disorder (cf. Loizos and Constantinou 2007). Would the elicitation of a life history have therapeutic effects for narrators like her? One is reminded that narrative emplotment has the potential to be therapeutic (Mattingly 1998). She could see that I was strongly affected by what she said. However, rather than wishing to talk about her memories in a conversation, which involves listening, turn-taking and waiting in suspense for a response, she appeared to take comfort in telling, retelling and re-retelling her narrative, with the same sequence of events in one long uninterrupted flow. On later occasions, when I visited her to briefly touch base, she was extremely nice to me, and although I was her senior, she treated me like a younger sister; she was much taller than me and would take me by the arm or pat my shoulder. Neither of us touched on any of the issues that she had related to me when tape-recorded. This information was locked off, tightly bundled, it seemed, in a sealed memory box.

In summary, as indicated in the previous chapter, semi-structured interviews did produce 'data'. However, for several reasons – among them bias in sampling and statistical validity – the reading of this 'data' has to be undertaken with great circumspection. I knew that the life histories I elicited were specific to the situation in which my interviewees found themselves at the time. We knew that we each were part of different meshworks, and that our meetings were but fleeting moments; a lot was not said. This gave the conversations themselves a pricelessness and intensity, creating enduring memories; in these instances the research method itself generated synchronicity, and moments of relatedness emerged that transgressed racial boundaries and preconceptions. These practitioners' narratives have an undeniable explorative value, and their variability inhibits any generalising statement.

Did these life histories affect the way in which the Chinese medical practitioners and their patients engaged in healing techniques? After all, our aim is ultimately to explore the extent to which the triadic medical encounter consists of body techniques, skills and tactics that are part of a craft oriented towards generating a reconfigured wholeness. How is a practitioner's self implicated into the medical treatment delivered (Hallowell [1954] 2017: 89)?

## The Ethnographic Focus: Chinese Medicine Practitioners in Kenya

From the late 1980s, Kenya saw a constant coming and going of Chinese medical practitioners (the first arrived in Nairobi in 1988). These travelling medical experts were not excessively numerous and ranged between only twenty to forty persons in the Kenyan, Tanzanian and Ugandan nation states respectively.[3] They were not primarily a public health phenomenon but a cultural one, as their presence was noted.[4] One question that the patients in the Chinese clinic, the health personnel in other medical institutions, acquaintances on the bus or colleagues at the university asked was as follows:

### Who Are These Doctors and Why Have They Come to Us?

The question was straightforward, and the stories it elicited are moving and stand for themselves. Yet this question, which came from the grassroots, pointed to issues that are still today fairly sparsely explored in the medical anthropological literature. First, while medical anthropology has made a difference in the health field with its research on patients' perspectives through illness narratives (e.g. Kleinman 1988; Good 1994; Mattingly 1998, 2010; for Africa, see e.g. Davis 2000; Geissler and Prince 2010a; Livingstone 2012), monographs on doctors' stories are still few and far between today (Hunter 1993 is an early exception, from an English Literature vantagepoint). Healers' narratives abound, which highlight the personal aspects of their lives, inclusive of their vulnerabilities. However, the study of the life histories of health professionals who work in health bureaucracies has been downplayed.[5]

It is as though medical anthropologists have been blinded by the ideology of professionalism of the health professionals. Rather than appreciating the personal life experiences of health professionals when discussing the personal element, there has been a tendency to highlight malpractice and insensitivity, and even opportunism (Katz 1985) – in opposition to the trustworthy but bygone 'family doctor' (Lupton 1997) – and to idealise the effectiveness of robots and AI (artificial intelligence). And yet the personality of health professionals, and even their physical stature, have been found to affect the efficaciousness of biomedical treatment (Moerman 2002: Chapter 5). Finally, these health care providers were also businesspeople benefiting from a 'mixed embeddedness' like other 'cosmopolitan' migrants (e.g. Glick Schiller and Çağlar 2013, 2015). Since many were in early retirement, they had faced the dilemmas and made the choices currently discussed through the interpretive lens of lifestyle migration (e.g. Hoey 2005, 2014; Benson and O'Reilly 2015).[6]

Interestingly, a simple question from the grassroots on a curious phenomenon in contemporary health care – Chinese medicine in Africa – highlighted, apart from this bias concerning narrative, a dearth of medical anthropological research on some further pressing social and cultural themes of health care (spelled out in Hsu 2012a): specifically, the doctor's attitude, lifeworld and narrative (as opposed to the patient's illness narrative); CAM in the Global South (as opposed to CAM in the industrialised North); and mobile medical experts (as opposed to mobile clients of reproductive health, transplant, enhancement and wellness businesses). Within the domain of mobility for medical purposes, there was a blatant sparsity of research on South–South mobility, and in the early 2000s, regarding general Chinese migration, on north-eastern rather than south-eastern migration flows out of China.

Does this make the research presented here marginal, exotic and insignificant? Or has medical anthropology become too biomedicalised, following research agendas determined by public health and developments in bioscientific technology, rather than problems that the person at the grassroots is confronted with in the Global South? Of the above short-comings in medical anthropological research agendas that the grassroots question 'who are these doctors and why have they come to us?' highlighted, this chapter will discuss: (a) narratives of health professionals, (b) CAM in the Global South and

(c) the East–South or South–South connectivity in the health field, and in this context also 'lifestyle migration' (detailed below). Our underlying question is: How were these mobile medical experts, with their new, strange and foreign medicine pots, aiming to emplace themselves into a new locality, urban East Africa? To what extent did their care contribute to healing and making whole specific aspects of East Africa's urban fabric?

## A Portrait of the Practitioners: Their Social Profile and Education

In the mid-2000s, the Chinese medical doctors in Kenya were Chinese-speaking Chinese nationals from the PRC who advertised themselves as such and who made a livelihood of it. They were mostly petty entrepreneurs, like many other Chinese in Kenya, and Africa more generally (Large 2008; Dobler 2008, 2017; Chatelard 2018). They furthermore had in common that they had all moved to Kenya since the late 1980s and 1990s. They were mostly men, but also women, who came on their own (single, married or divorced) or with a partner or family. Some were in their late twenties, but most were in their forties and fifties, and several had left China after going into early retirement. In April 2003, they numbered around eighteen in Nairobi (five were women) and three in Mombasa (one a woman). I interviewed them all. Furthermore, I heard of one doctor stationed in Kisumu, one in Eldoret and one in Nakuru, none of whom I visited.

The Chinese medical doctors in Kenya, and Africa at large, were generally not held in high esteem in the PRC; they were not considered 'real' or precious (*zhengui* 珍贵) Chinese medical doctors whose insight into Chinese medicine was 'deep' (*shen'ao* 深奥). Indeed, if one inquired into their formal training, one could find reasons for which Chinese medical practitioners in their homeland generally disapproved of them. Their educational levels varied. Nevertheless, all, even those who had had exposure to Chinese medicine within a family tradition, claimed to have undergone training in Traditional Chinese Medicine (TCM), which is the standardised form of Chinese medicine taught at government institutions in the PRC (Taylor 2005; Hsu 2022).

In the sample of twenty-one practitioners interviewed, five had been regular students (*benkesheng*) at a TCM university and had five years of training in both Chinese and Western medicine. These five were fully trained TCM physicians (*zhongyishi* 中医师), but they constituted a minority; one of them enrolled thereafter for another three years in a postgraduate degree (*shuoshi* 硕士). Two had three years of vocational training in acumoxa (acupuncture and moxibustion), which also involves being taught Western medicine; they qualified as vocational acumoxa practitioners (*zhenjiushi* 针灸士). Two had attended, as full-time students, special classes in either acupuncture or 'integrated Chinese and Western medicine' (*zhongxiyi jiehe* 中西医结合) for four years. Both had learned Chinese medicine through the family (*jia chuan* 家传) and attended additional formal training. Of the remaining twelve, several had only attended evening classes at a TCM university, for between one and four years. Among the latter were biomedically trained physicians, biomedically trained health workers and members of non-medical professions. Some had many years of work experience, some none.

Put another way, of the twenty-one medical practitioners interviewed, about ten (i.e. c. 50 per cent) had received higher education – that is, they had been regular university students – of whom five had regular university training in TCM and five in Western medicine. Overall, nine had been thoroughly trained in Chinese medicine (five at university, two vocationally and two in the family). Of the remaining twelve, several had formal training as Western medical health professionals and knew Chinese medicine only through evening classes or otherwise. In summary, levels of education varied and work experiences were very diverse. Meanwhile, it needs to be borne in mind that learning after graduation is also crucial for good medical practice.

Regardless of their education, they all advertised themselves as competent in 'Chinese medicine' or 'Traditional Chinese Medicine', often in blue script on white panels, but the various forms of medicine that they delivered are probably more accurately described as highly diverse and partly idiosyncratic interpretations of 'Chinese medicine and pharmacotherapy' (*zhongyiyao* 中医药) (Hsu 2008b).

Apart from the above, a core question concerned the 'thickness' of the Chinese practitioners' sociality: the degree of separation from their homeland, the motivations that instigated their mobility, the difficulties encountered on the move, the cultural differences perceived between sending and recipient countries, and their aspirations for the future. According to Charles Stafford (2000), publishing in the year before my fieldwork started, 'separation and reunion' were dominant, if perhaps not uniquely Chinese themes, and the Chinese medical practitioners I interviewed played on these in interesting ways: their life stories and self-presentation emphasised a simultaneous 'mobility and connectedness', thereby collapsing the distinctive episodes of separation and reunion into a single, all-encompassing mood of – tactically – 'being on the wing'.

This ambiguous state in which they perceived themselves to live became particularly evident from the question I asked at the end of the interview, which was whether they thought of moving back to China in the future. It put their voluntary movements into perspective: almost none considered spending their old age in Kenya. One of my respondents commented: 'None of us doctors has bought property here.' She herself was using Kenya as a stepping stone to get to Canada. This observation is in line with others that Chinese migratory processes since the 1990s have not only been driven by an unusually overt economic zest but also by heightened mobility (Pieke et al. 2004). The contacts in the home country are not given up, but cultivated, not least for business. Although all practitioners in Kenya had learned to speak English, and some had emplaced themselves very strategically into Kenya's urban textures, few took part in more formal activities of 'integration' in the receiving country. One would hesitate to speak of these mobile Chinese medical experts as 'settlers'.

Having just stressed their constant state of being on the hoof, three of the twenty-one Chinese medical practitioners interviewed did actually speak of settling in Kenya. One was Cantonese, a biomedical doctor by training who had married a Kenyan whom she had met in medical school in Guangdong and with whom she founded a family in Nairobi. The other was also a biomedical doctor, one who made his first visit back home to Shandong after living for seven years in Kenya. He realised on that occasion that it was most unlikely for him to settle ever again in China. In the era of the economic reforms, his colleagues had acquired biomedical knowledge and skills at a speed that was prohibitive and robbed him of any chance of catching up again. The third was one of the first Chinese medical practitioners to emigrate to Kenya, in the late eighties. He hoped to accumulate enough money in Nairobi to be a pensioner in China. However, he was well aware that life among the middle classes was in the meantime more modernised and more expensive in China than it was in Kenya, and that the Chinese economy was rising, while the Kenyan one was declining: 'If I am constrained to stay here long-term, I can do it, but I can't eat African food 如果我被迫长期留在这，我能做到，但我不能吃非洲食物' he said. The separation from China was in his and other cases geographical but, as far as culinary practices were concerned, hardly cultural.

Chinese grocers provided the basics for Chinese cooking to the Chinese communities in Nairobi, and some Chinese only ate rice that was imported (cf. Ohnuki-Tierney 1993). 'This rice is white' (*zhe fan shi baide* 这饭是白的), one said; he seemed to allude to hygiene, primarily, in the sense of it being clean (*ganjing* 干净). The white, like the transparent (as in *bai shui* 白水), implies clarity and purity. White rice, like white bone, is the enduring substance (after the flesh has decayed) in the place of one's ancestors (Seaman 1992). This was not said, nor do I suppose it was a consciously implied subtext. However, it is a semantic aspect of the Chinese word *bai* 白 (white), which can easily become textured into the above comment.

In summary, Chinese medical practitioners in Kenya were petty entrepreneurs, who lived in an ambiguous state of connectedness to China and elsewhere, and who regularly engaged in mobility in and out of Kenya. It is difficult to make generalisations. Demographically, some came with family, while others were on their own; economically, some sent remittances to China, others received household monies from the PRC; socially, a few had already stayed in Kenya for over a decade and were on the cusp of becoming settlers, and others were new or had moved from elsewhere in Africa to Kenya; some were very visibly committed to their clientele; all were on a learning curve and committed to a project of actively shaping their future.

As we will see, one rather specific way to make sense of the Chinese medical practitioners' movements is by highlighting two ancient Chinese concepts that, as argued here, aptly capture their dispositions, *ling* 灵 (being agile and flexible) and *tong* 通 (being connected). Although the Chinese medical practitioners I interviewed mentioned neither *ling* nor *tong*, their narratives conveyed a sense of being alive through *ling* and *tong*. Agility and flexibility (*ling*) is a cherished quality in China and Taiwan, particularly in religious contexts (Sangren 1987), but also in medical ones (Farquhar 1994 renders *ling* as 'virtuosity'). Connectedness, *tong*, is a quality that the ancient sages sought: they aimed to be connected with the universe (Sivin 1991 renders *tong* as 'continuity'; Hsu 1994 as 'to connect'). There is a saying that if there is connectedness, then there is no pain: *tong bu tong* 通不痛 (Zhang 2007: 44), which acupuncturists today often mention, but which in fact expresses a general disposition to being alive.

## *Patterns of Mobility*

The mobility of the Chinese medical practitioners was rather remarkable in the years between 2001 and 2003, but it decreased in the period between 2003 and 2006 (the Kenyan arm of this study ended in 2006). The mobility was sometimes pendular, involving a back and forth between the PRC and Kenya, while sometimes it had weblike nodes of intersection spread out all over the globe. Finally, it was also marked by a 'shifting', involving micro-movements within or across different cities while maintaining Kenyan residence. These three patterns of mobility, which put the lifeworlds of the individual centre-stage, are presented in what follows.

## *Starlike Patterns of Mobility*

Dr Mou, after working seventeen years at the Railway Central Hospital in Harbin, took advantage of an early retirement scheme in 1992. In the late 1980s and early 1990s, such early retirement schemes made it possible for work units (*danwei* 单位) to free up positions held by victims of the Cultural Revolution, whose education was not as reliable as that of young professionals trained in the 1980s, after the Dengist reforms. Dr Mou emphasised that he had passed the entrance examinations to medical school – in 1965. Although he did not mention it, it is clear that anyone at university in 1966–69 would not have received much formal training, because during those years universities were closed and academics were persecuted. In the early 1990s, many work unit members undertook entrepreneurial activities (*xiahaile* 下海了); there was a fashion (*re* 热) in Northeast China to emigrate to post-Gorbachev Russia. Mou had work experience as a Western medical doctor, but then worked as an acupuncturist at a Lada car factory in Russia. He said that he liked the Russians – they were honest (*laoshi* 老实). He thereupon returned to China to divorce his Chinese wife in order to marry a Russian woman, whom he divorced only a few years later when he returned to China, in 1998. He said this with a laugh (which sounded sad to me). While it is often the case that Chinese Western-trained doctors offer their services as Chinese doctors and acupuncturists outside their home country, usually after taking one to four years of evening classes, only a few get married to locals. Dr Mou said that it was a 'young and beautiful girl' who wanted to marry him, and that this in turn enabled him to get a residence permit. Romantic feeling was thus coupled with overcoming the bureaucratic problems of the migrant. Dr Mou did not explain why he returned to China in 1998. Given that his first wife was the daughter of a high military commander, he said that he now encountered increased difficulties in his home province. He bought property in Dalian, a sought-after resort on the shores of Bohai, but soon became bored as a pensioner of only 52. So, he emigrated to Ghana.

Dr Mou explained that he had worked for two years as a member of a 'Chinese medical team' for TAZARA in 1977–79.[7] In the 1970s, he had become quite fond of Africans – they too were honest. However, times had now changed. 'African people today', he said in broken English, 'they give you many traps, they are very tricky, I was cheated many times.' In the late 1990s, there were, according to Dr Mou, about four or five Chinese doctors in Accra, among them himself as an acupuncturist. As an explanation for his return from Ghana to China after only two years, he said that four Chinese nationals had died of malaria (he said 'cerebral malaria') within only six months. He bought another house in China, this time in a popular resort in the south, on Hainan island. However, at 54 years of age, he felt that he was 'not yet so old' and could still 'make money', although he quickly added: 'I have not come here only to make money.' He now moved to East instead of West Africa. He first visited Tanzania, but Tanzania was too poor, he said, not a suitable place for making money. A chance encounter with a native (laoxiang 老乡) of Northeast China brought him to Nairobi. However, within a few weeks of living there, he was robbed at 7 a.m. one day,[8] and anyway, 'Nairobi was too crowded'. He moved to a town on the periphery of Kenya.

Dr Mou's narrative portrays a pendulum of inward and outward movement, to and from China. It is not exactly an oscillating mobility, in that Dr Mou did not shuttle, like an 'astronaut' (Ong 1999), back and forth on one trajectory, but he moved to very different places inside and outside China. If one takes the PRC as the centre, it was a starlike movement, with Russia, then West Africa, then East Africa as destinations of outward movement. Although Dr Mou had residences in different places, namely China's far north and far south, he referred to 'China' as one place, and as the epicentre of his movements. Naturally, while resident in Kenya, he was physically 'separated' from his homeland, but in his narrative his sense of being simultaneously 'mobile' and 'connected' was more pronounced.

One could also say that Dr Mou's narrative testified to the fate of the 'lost generation': his marriages failed and his entrepreneurial achievements were only temporary. His mobility could be viewed as the response to such failure. The seed of his failures, one could say, was the fate of being enrolled in medical school during the Cultural Revolution. On the other hand, Dr Mou was also an agile navigator of adverse situations: he had married the daughter of a high military commander, and although he only mentioned the disadvantages of the divorce, there must have been advantages in professional life and general livelihood during the marriage; he experienced love in Russia, and once he put his mind to 'making money' was able to buy two houses in highly desirable Chinese resorts. In the PRC, those who migrate to Africa are likely to be viewed as losers, due to stereotypes about Africa and a general bias that views the foreign as barbaric. But even if to a certain extent, he was a 'loser', since he did not compete to stay in the PRC, his mobility was that of a skilful entrepreneur who lived life with a tint of adventure.

## *Weblike Patterns of Mobility*

There was another pattern of mobility that did not have one single centre like the starlike pattern of inward and outward movement from and to China, the way that Dr Mou experienced his life. Rather, it was weblike, in that it connected a variety of destinations on the globe to each other. It may not be a coincidence that several Chinese medical practitioners who lived this pattern of mobility were a generation younger than the Cultural Revolution cohort to which Dr Mou belonged. Nevertheless, like most life histories of Chinese citizens, those of these young Chinese medical practitioners revealed that they too had been affected by political circumstance. Dr Ming explained that he had been among the active student demonstrators in 1989 and that he had a file with the police. Neither Dr Mou nor Dr Ming presented themselves as victims of political movements, however, and they did not consider themselves political refugees. They spoke in a matter-of-fact manner about political movements, as though these were part of the geographic landscape into which they were born. Dr Ming was studying English at the time at an inferior university (he had failed the entrance exams to study history at a prestigious university), and already before the movement of 1989 he had the desire to go abroad. He worked as a tour guide in Tibet, set out to learn the art of Chinese cuisine from an acquaintance who was a cook and enrolled in evening classes on Chinese medicine. When suddenly, in 1994, the opportunity arose to go abroad, he seized it. It was to work as an interpreter for a firm operating for the provincial administration that was involved in a project at the electric power station of Owen Falls in Uganda.

Generally, Dr Ming was vague about his past movements in China and Africa; I pieced the above information together from different conversations with him and his wife, and also from comments that other doctors made about him in passing. However, he was articulate about future movements. He had a girlfriend from the times before he emigrated whom he had married in Mombasa, but shortly after their wedding she moved to Chile, because, as he explained, a friend working at the Chilean Chinese embassy had told them that Chilean citizenship could be easily acquired once one had been resident there.[9] So, for several years, the couple moved between China, South America and Africa, and before long his wife became pregnant. In December 2001 the future father explained that the child should not become a 'banana' (*xiangjiao* 香蕉), yellow outside and white inside – with the yellow skin colour of a Chinese person but with a Westernised heart and mind. He wanted his wife to give birth in China, but eventually, their daughter was born in Mombasa. 'The Indian doctor we had was so competent', Dr Ming's wife explained.

During my subsequent visit in spring 2003, father, mother and baby were enjoying the dream of the nuclear family, living in a one-family house in a chic suburb, with an African nanny, a quality car (air-conditioned) and special access to a Mombasa beach resort. They were adamant that they intended to make 'big money', and this, according to them, was possible only in Third World countries, not in the First World with its tight tax regulations. They spoke of moving on, not to the USA, nor to Europe, but to Chile and, perhaps eventually, to Canada. Their minimally furnished house was tangible testimony to their commitment to mobility.[10] Unlike the pendular movement to and from a centre, this couple engaged in a pattern of mobility that appeared more like a web, spread out over the globe, with various points of contact.

## *Shifting, but Staying Put*

Most Chinese medical practitioners in Kenya, and East Africa more generally, did not work in the same medical practice in which they had originally started to work. Most moved around the suburbs of Nairobi, opening and closing their different clinics at a fairly high speed. Of the eleven clinics visited in December 2001, two moved within the same suburb, two had closed and three had opened or reopened in a new place by April 2003; some practitioners left Kenya before I had a chance to interview them. Ever since 1988, when the first practice opened in Nairobi, there had been a constant toing and froing of Chinese medical doctors. However, as my final field trip to Kenya in 2006 revealed, the Chinese practitioners in Kenya were 'shifting' more frequently in the early 2000s than thereafter, regardless of whether the movements were intra- or inter-urban.

Regardless of how often practitioners shifted within Nairobi or Kenya initially, once they had come to terms with making their livelihoods in Kenya, at least for the foreseeable future, they stayed put. This did not usually diminish their close connection to China, which was easy to maintain electronically through the internet, email and Skype, while the mobile phone was used mostly for local communication. Furthermore, the Chinese practitioners also maintained their connectedness to the PRC physically: one commuted for business purposes on a fortnightly schedule, others at longer, regular and irregular, intervals – some because their spouses, their children, both, or their parents required their care. Some returned for Chinese New Year, but not necessarily every year, nor would everyone buy airplane tickets when they were widely desired and expensive.

## *Patterns of Mobility: Summary*

The above patterns of mobility arose from speaking to individuals about their lifeworlds and the horizons of their livelihoods. Most were oriented towards the PRC, and their starlike movements were perceived to be like the limbs of a starfish, moving in all kinds of different directions out of China. However, particularly among the younger generation, life was less centred on the PRC as an alma mater. This generation of Chinese saw themselves not exactly as citizens of the world, but nevertheless as more detached from China than they perhaps were. They presented themselves in weblike movements, hopping from one node of interconnectedness to another, each offering a multidirectional bouquet of new opportunities.

Finally, the practitioners who moved in and out of different neighbourhoods in Nairobi spoke of these movements as 'shifting', as though their 'shifting' entailed micro-adjustments in the course of their emplacement into urban Kenya, not unlike the rustling before an animal goes to sleep or a person settles comfortably into a chair. Some life stories also contained references to similar micro-adjustments in preparation for their emigration from China. Among these were taking evening classes in cooking on the one hand and in acupuncture on the other, as these were exotic skills that foreigners were perceived to appreciate; working first for this and then for that tourist agency; and being sent out on a short-term contract, once as an accountant for an import-export company, then as an interpreter. They were shifting about, making micro-adjustments before the opportunity presented itself to make the leap out of the PRC. Naturally, all of these movements had a strategic edge, but the shifting movements came closer to 'tactics' than to calculated 'strategies' (de Certeau 1984).

## *Motives for Mobility*

What motivated the different Chinese medical practitioners to come to Kenya? This was a question from the grassroots that rang in my ears over many years. Was it the wish to get out of China, to navigate the world; was it adventure or curiosity; was there a social, economic or other constraint? Or were people driven out of China when things went wrong back home, was it a matter of competitiveness, greed, failure, desperation? Was there a wish, from the beginning, to become substantially entangled with African soil and people? Or was Africa merely a stepping stone?

## *The Gatekeeper*

In many cases, the name of one individual, Dr Lai, was mentioned; he acted as what in migration studies is called a 'gatekeeper' (e.g.

Levitt and Glick-Schiller 2004: 1009). He had been a member of the prestigious medical teams from Shandong province that were sent to Tanzania in the 1970s. He had treated Julius Nyerere, the then president of Tanzania, in person, as large photos in the spacious waiting room of his practice showed. He had become involved in local politics, other doctors told me; was sent back to Shandong; and then emigrated from there to Nairobi in the late 1980s. He was not the first doctor from the PRC to emigrate to Nairobi, but he was well received in the city's expatriate community. Between 2001 and 2003, he was involved with a research project funded by the Ford Foundation to evaluate the efficacy of his brand of herbal tea, with which he treated HIV/AIDS patients.

When I asked Dr Lai why he had moved to Kenya, he said one word: 'Freedom (*ziyou* 自由)'. It implied that he knew that people in Kenya considered democratic states to have more freedom than socialist ones. In response I mentioned to him that other Chinese medical practitioners, in particular those from Northeast China, had mentioned 'medicine as business'. 'Not only', he said, meaning that this was not the whole story of why he emigrated to Kenya. Meanwhile, he could not deny that he was a good businessman. In March 2003, he was the director of a very successful Chinese medical clinic and a 'factory' for making herbal pills, tablets, capsules and gels, and he said that he employed over thirty staff. His intentions of expansion had brought several other Chinese medical doctors from Shandong province to Kenya. He had invited them to work in his clinic, and several of them later set up their own clinics. One practitioner had worked in Burundi for eighteen months, another had collaborated towards the setting up of a hospital in Sudan for four months; both had moved to Nairobi, and despite being without means, were well received by Dr Lai, and also briefly worked for him thereafter. Dr Lai's practice thus represented the gateway to Kenya for the majority of the Chinese medical practitioners who worked in Nairobi and told me their life histories. The reason that many Chinese doctors in Kenya were from Shandong was that this was the province in charge of neighbouring Tanzania, just as Yunnan was of Uganda or Sichuan of Zambia, while Kenya, a stronghold of the British Commonwealth, never had such close political relations with the PRC. A doctor who had fallen into disgrace with a socialist regime was no doubt welcome to set foot in Nairobi.[11]

Whereas Dr Lai's move to Kenya may have been motivated by political rather than economic circumstances, the medical practitioners he attracted seemed more economically than politically motivated. Chinese medical doctors would state that they were doing business – often with a disarming candour – as though they had no sense that medicine is generally considered an altruistic service to humanity. It appeared that they had learned in reformist China that 'doing business' was a laudable activity, much approved by the government, that required no further explanation. However, other motivations also surfaced in the course of our conversations; they were political, ideological, idealistic and, in particular, educational.

## *Lifestyle Motivations, with Political Overtones*

Politics shaped the fates of all three doctors discussed so far, Drs Mou, Ming and Lai. Several other Chinese medical doctors in Kenya could be considered 'victims' of the Cultural Revolution insofar as their knowledge and skills were considered insufficient in the era of the economic reforms that set in after Mao Zedong's death in 1976. As university graduates who had passed the highly competitive nationwide exams of 1978 became employable in the mid-1980s, less well-educated and older cadres were made to free up their positions for younger staff. To be sure, not a single interviewee said so. Some said that they were offered early retirement packages, others were eased out in other ways. One practitioner once said, completely out of context, that he did not like the Chinese Communist Party, but it would be wrong to describe him as a dissident. He was not a political activist but had evaded a certain lifestyle. As he put it:

> There are advantages and there are disadvantages to making your living here (*you de you shi* 有得有失). In our country you always have the feeling that people are in charge of what you are doing, you cannot progress, you can't develop, ... although you [EH] just mentioned the dependence on connections (*guanxi* 关系), these are, in fact, not as important as generally assumed.... it's just that so many things restrain you. Here it's different. Life is not that complicated, we mutually understand each other, there is not this sense of constant reservation towards the other, and if our livelihoods are unequal, it's not an issue; if you are happy, fine, if you are not happy, then you yourself look after yourself, you don't have to pretend you're happy. (Notebook no. 3)

Many doctors also complained of the enormous competitiveness in Chinese society, and the arbitrary ways in which control was exerted: 'Today they let you do this, but tomorrow the rules will have changed.' One confided in me that she came on her own to Nairobi for one year but got so homesick that she returned to her previous workplace – but then: 'At work, I could not get used to it' (*shang ban'r bu tai shiyingle* 上班儿不太适应了): getting up early in the morning, taking on night shifts and so on. So, she and her husband emigrated together, first with their daughter, who did not like it in Kenya and returned to finish her high school in China (in the custody of her grand-parents). There is no doubt that the sociopolitical climate of everyday life in China, rather than specific political events, brought some doctors to Africa, and Kenya in particular. For them, Nairobi was not only Africa's most affluent, prestigious and climatically pleasant city, but also a stronghold of capitalism (which nobody explicitly said) and of democracy (which was also only indirectly said).

The only practitioner who admitted to having been politically active during high-school had mellowed in the meantime:

> I once demonstrated for democracy but now I see its disadvantages as well. For instance, in democratic countries there is endless discussion without decisions being made. Sometimes it is better [that] a good leader just takes the responsibility and does what needs to be done. (Notebook no. 2)

We were driving at high speed on a double-track road into a junction with dense traffic when he started blinking his headlights and accelerated instead of slowing down so that the other cars would let him go first; he obviously did not suffer from an imperialist history, which prevents some Europeans from demonstrating superiority with the brute force of driving aggressively. 'Look at all this rubbish', he continued, seemingly unaware of what I was thinking, 'all these plastic bags by the roadside, all the degradation of nature that capitalism has brought to democratic countries.'

Another practitioner, who was promoted during the Cultural Revolution but later made redundant, revelled in the education they had received in the early 1970s:

> I consider the people who graduated from the worker-peasant-soldier (*gong nong bing* 工农兵) universities very good. At the time, the [mor-

ally] best people were selected [and sent to university]. The quality of their thinking (*sixiang suzhi* 思想素质) was exceptionally good, perhaps their culture was not the best, but their morals were exceptionally good. (Notebook no. 3)

He lamented over the changing morals in Dengist China. He had left his hometown in the late 1980s and his wife had divorced him in the mid-1990s, he said, because his business had not been successful. 'This person's morals had already changed . . . she [his wife] said: "You were so long in Kenya, and you made no money. Compare yourself with those from Shanghai and from the north-east, they all made lots of money."' He praised Mao Zedong (or rather, Chairman Mao, as he is tape-recorded to have corrected himself) and Mao's emphasis on a person's internal integrity, while now everyone in China was only interested in money. 'When I came to Kenya', he explained in Chinese, 'it was the opposite of how it was then in China, but now it is in China as it was then in Kenya. In Kenya, what one then used to talk about was economics, in their brains everything was about economics, whoever was rich, whoever had money, he was morally good. Now, in China, they ask me: "Have you made money in Kenya, and when I say no, they are not interested [in speaking to me]."' This practitioner resented the economic reforms that resulted in the rich being morally righteous.

Clearly, these mobile experts were not political dissidents. They were evading a lifestyle. Many were retired, and like other retired people who fell into the category of lifestyle migration, they were fairly well off, but they had evidently experienced precarity and vulnerability to a degree that blurred the boundaries between them and economic migrants (Green 2014). They presented themselves as people aiming to live an undisturbed, quiet, yet personally meaningful life; they were not necessarily after 'the good life', as were Hoey's (2005) interviewees in the USA, but a life that allowed them to be and do 'good' as their socialist education had taught them in their childhood (*wei renmin fuwu* 为人民服务). They had 'moral narratives of self' not unrelated to the terrain into which they had placed themselves.

> The people here are not as wild as they are depicted in China, in fact, they are extremely cultured, very polite, and towards us Chinese they are especially accommodating (*bu shi guonei shuode name yeman, hen wen-*

*mingde, hen limao, dui Zhongguoren you qi youhao* 不是国内说得那么野蛮，很文明的，很礼貌，对中国人尤其友好). (Notebook no. 3)

The drawback was that 'the livelihood here is rather restricted' (*shenghuo jiu hen you xian* 生活就很有限); yet the people and their demeanour were so very good-natured (*piqi hen rouhe* 脾气很柔和). Another practitioner commented on the climate at work: in China, there was so much backbiting, but here, people admired you when you did good; you did not need to engage in fake advertising, they could see it themselves; and once they recognised in you a moral person, they would bring you more business by informing their kin.

## *Education*

The most openly avowed motivating factor was education, while discomfort with the sociopolitical climate was played down. It would be wrong to say that Kenya attracted the losers of the Dengist reforms, just as it cannot be said that it attracted dissidents. Naturally, the two are linked in that access to good education depends on one's sociopolitical situation.

Several Chinese doctors had teenage children whom they aspired to give a better education than they themselves had received. One couple of the Cultural Revolution cohort had emigrated in the early 1990s, first to Nairobi, then, due to a iatrogenic death (as insinuated by other practitioners), from there to the periphery of the country, where they set up a very successful acupuncture, moxibustion, massage and rehabilitation clinic. They saved enough money to pay the high fees of the American university where their two sons were enrolled as students at the time of the interview. Interestingly, this sort of strategic movement, which spread the move from the PRC into the USA over two generations, is not prominently discussed in the literature on lifestyle migration. Evidently, the Chinese interviewees worked with a concept of self that spanned a movement out of 'backward' contexts over several generations when it came to education.

Two Chinese medical physicians were mothers whose husbands ran more lucrative businesses in the PRC. They had moved to Kenya with their teenage daughter and son respectively, intent on giving their offspring the necessary knowledge to pass the entrance examinations into an American university. They ran their Chinese medical businesses part-time, as their *raison d'être* in Nairobi was childcare.

One was very vocal in expressing her wish to spare her child the stifling competitiveness of Chinese high schools, and her Chinese medical business was more of a pastime. Her daughter made an appearance once during my brief visit. Her English was American, her straight hair finely braided. She embodied her family's mobility and connectedness. The other TCM practitioner had a hardworking teenage boy who wore thick glasses and had indeed endured competitive schooling, but he was going to sit the US university entrance exams again in Nairobi rather than in China.

The education of children figured in many life stories, and there is little doubt that this was one of the prime motives for moving out of the PRC to Nairobi, where work permits were easier to obtain than in the USA, and where high school education at private schools was more affordable. Obviously, the individualistic concept of self that figures centrally in many lifestyle migration studies would need to be modified were it to include care for offspring and educational strategising within the family, and along generational lineage relations, as relevant to the self.

## *Reinforcing the We-Relation*

Most practitioners with whom I was allowed to stay and watch them practising medicine did so with responsibility and interpersonal care. Some were verbally explicit about their altruistic and humanitarian concerns. One was an openly declared Chinese Communist Party member who framed his medical activities within the ideology of the party. Another one, who had sought legitimation of his Chinese herbal medicines through the FDA in the USA, came across as an idealist, driven by the thought of saving humanity.

The senior doctor Dr Cheng said that he had come to Kenya for world socialist reasons, namely 'for developing Chinese medicine in Africa' (*fazhan zhongyi zai Feizhou* 发展中医在非洲). In Africa, Chinese medicine had a great future. There were so many different diseases. Western medicine could not treat them all and Chinese medicine had the means to do so. He further explained, much in line with what leading TCM officials say, that the 'integrated treatment of Chinese and Western medicine' (*zhongxiyi jiehe*) was particularly suited to African health care. Unfortunately, African governments did not understand this. Dr Cheng insisted that Chinese medicine in its most progressive form made use of Western medical knowledge and practice in an integrative way. African governments, however, misunderstood the situation. It was not a matter of traditional medicine as a placebo that was effective due to the added ingredients of 'Western medicine'. Rather, 'integrated Chinese and Western medicine' was an up-to-date and efficacious medical system, combining the best from both sides. The African governments were short-sighted to forbid Chinese doctors from using any Western forms of treatment and medication,[12] when TCM practitioners in fact had the know-how to assist Africa in its fight against diseases, with adequate means. What Dr Cheng said reflected an intricate knowledge of ongoing debates in policymaking circles. It could not be dismissed as empty ideological rhetoric. The points he made clearly spoke to ongoing debates in the Kenyan medical profession, and represented very well the official TCM perspective in a language that everyone in the room could understand.

Dr Cheng was a senior party member, the son of a peasant who had worked his way up to leadership positions in the hospital administration and acquired governmental recognition as a 'renowned senior doctor' (*ming laozhongyi* 名老中医). He and his junior female colleague – his former student – produced ample evidence in the form of certificates and honorary degrees upon my first visit. He clearly had achieved the highest of medical orders (although other doctors, somewhat viciously, claimed that they were not fake, but bogus). The busy practice of teacher and former student, protected by a soldier in a watchtower, was located in a quiet neighbourhood. Dr Cheng explained that he had come to Kenya because Dr Lai had invited him to set up a medical hospital in Nairobi, but the two fell out with each other. Evidently, they both had leadership qualities. Since Dr Cheng had already asked for special leave from his work unit, and from an administrative leadership position in it, he found it difficult to return. He thereupon retired from his post in the PRC prematurely.

Instead of becoming a hospital director, as initially planned, Dr Cheng opened a small Chinese medical practice, as his junior colleague explained. It was evident that she felt both compassion for his plight and an obligation to save face on behalf of her teacher. Meanwhile, her husband and child stayed back home in Shandong province. The two practitioners returned to China yearly for reunions with their respective families during the Spring Festival. Why would they continue to return to Nairobi, I queried? The woman doctor explained that they had patients who needed them. She was very serious when she said that she had a sense of duty towards them (*you gongzuo shiyexin* 有工作事业心). She presented her life as caught in between kinship ties, personal ties to her teacher and strong ties to her African clientele. It was a real meshwork. This dwarfed the issue of economic incentives, although it did not entirely eliminate it. It also gave me a visceral feeling of the devotion that forced her to live a life of mobility and connectedness.

Another Chinese medical practitioner was similarly eager upon my first visit to show me the various certificates he had obtained. These were not issued by the PRC but by US and Kenyan authorities. One hung in a frame on the wall. It read: 'This is to certify that Aierkon granule (Aikechongji 艾克冲剂) complies with the relevant labeling section of FDA 05-08-98'. Dr Xiong from Northeast China vehemently denied that he had come to Africa to do business. He was in Kenya for idealistic reasons, and on his way to rich Botswana to conduct further research there. He first went to Tanzania (in 1991), and later settled in Kenya (in 1994) in order 'to do research on AIDS'.

In this case too, Dr Xiong acted out of an obligation towards his teachers. They had entrusted him with the anti-HIV/AIDS formula that they had developed within the Sino–Tanzanian project at Muhimbili hospital in Dar es Salaam during the early 1990s, a group which, he said, had since dissolved. 'My teachers are over 70 and 80 years old now, I am 48 years old', he said in December 2001. 'I am the second generation working on Chinese anti-HIV/AIDS drugs.' He claimed to have modified the ingredients of 'Aikechongji' (the formula originally developed by his teachers at Muhimbili hospital), and prescribed those small granules together with a large medicine bolus (his own formula) for his HIV/AIDS patients.

Several photos on the wall of AIDS patients before, during and after treatment recorded several very visible instances of the success of his treatment. He knew that biomedical researchers would call these few success stories anecdotal. However, what mattered for him was, he said, that one recovery was better than none. Several photos showed him and one patient at different events that they had both attended. Furthermore, although he did not say so, the happiness on his face in one photo with one of his much chubbier patients, after only a few months of treatment, spoke to an emotional bond with the success story's co-producer and their re-convalescence from acute AIDS.

One detail caught my eye years later, as I looked at the photos of Dr Xiong and his successfully treated HIV/AIDS patient, whose face was eminently bright and spirited. It was not only the big smiles on the faces of patient and physician as they looked into the camera, but also their heads pressed together, the bare skin of cheek touching cheek. This practitioner was clearly emotionally connected to his patient(s) and involved in dynamics of healing on multiple sensory levels. Their success story of Chinese medical treatment resulting in a newly regained sense of wholesomeness evidently did not happen overnight, and it was clearly celebrated as a joint project of joint craftsmanship. The photo emphasised the we-relation.

In March 2003, Dr Xiong showed me a master's thesis by a student at the University of Nairobi, Department of Pharmacy, conducted under Prof. Anastasia Guantai, which identified the quantity of various chemical ingredients in his formula. Dr Xiong was serious about being on the forefront of research on herbal treatment of HIV/AIDS. He was excited by it. There is little doubt that his motivation for being in Africa was AIDS research, born out of a sense of obligation to his teachers. He evidently combined both doing research and doing good. He did not say so, but it was apparent that he was emotionally invested in the patients who committed to his treatment.

In this context, it is worth noting that while in their narratives, only a few practitioners presented their profession as a vocation, as did Drs Cheng and Xiong, several interviewees emphasised *yide* 医德, a physician's morality, ethics and commitment to care for their patients. Practitioners regularly said that one of their main aspirations was to be a 'good doctor' (*hao yisheng* 好医生): one noted that although he found it hard, he continued his habit of reading every evening, another emphasised conscientiousness (*renzhen* 认真) and work ethics (*shiye xin* 事业心), and a third responsibility (*zeren xin* 责任心): 'I had a patient who was diagnosed with and treated for rheumatism since 1996, and then I realised it was lupus, swollen joints – sometimes I cannot sleep because I'm thinking about a patient.' These instances all highlight the practitioners' multiple ways of articulating care for the patient, undeniably within a *Thou*-relation that grows out of the now of the face-to-face encounter.

Incidentally, the two practitioners who mentioned loyalty to their teachers also had visibly close ties with their patients. They did not say this of themselves during the interview, but it became apparent to me before and after the more formal part of my visits to their practices. I spent many hours in Chinese medical practices, in different localities and in different roles. I saw professionalism, concentration and deep care paid to hygiene; I experienced humorous moments and others of heartfelt compassion. I very rarely saw instances of brash impoliteness, and none of outright misconduct, nor of medical care delivered with evident negligence. However, in a few cases, particularly when it came to the selling of medicine pots, a medical practitioner sometimes transmuted into a trader and started adopting the morals of the marketplace (see below).

## *Motives for Mobility: Summary*

In scale, the motivations to become mobile varied: some were specific to Kenya, some to Chinese medicine, and others applied to Chinese mobility in general. Most respondents had come from Shandong province to Kenya, motivated by the prospect of collaborating with the gatekeeper, Dr Lai, who had been on a former Chinese medical team to Tanzania, but got too involved with (local) politics and had to step down. Events specific to China's political history were mentioned in all life histories, although barely anyone would foreground this in their narrative. Respondents instead said: 'The climate here is good' (*Nairobi qihou hao* 内罗毕气候好), alluding to lifestyle. Economic incentives were a readily mentioned motivation in Tanzania, which at the time attracted many businesspeople from Northeast China, but not in Kenya. Education for one's offspring was given as main motivation. This indirect mode of elite schooling in the global South in order to secure tertiary education for one's offspring in the global North has so far not been much discussed (e.g. Biao 2011). Finally, loyalty to one's teacher(s) was an explicit motivation for at least two practitioners.

## *Mobility and New Encounters*

When telling their life histories, Chinese medical practitioners mentioned three groups of people in Kenya with whom they made connections: their fellow Chinese, representatives of Kenyan authorities and their patients.

## Encounters with Fellow Chinese

Some doctors had fairly close relations to other Chinese – fellow practitioners or other businesspeople – while others had barely any. Some would phone each other on a regular basis or have lunch together in an internet café, or their wives would visit each other for a chat. Most were involved in some kind of mutual transaction of material goods, be it a computer or a car, books, magazines, newspapers or videos. Some also cooked for each other, particularly if someone fell ill. Emotions were expressed through the idiom of food; the gift of food expressed polite or heartfelt care, and comments on its quality varied; sometimes they appeared to concomitantly reflect the quality of the friendship. Some wrote letters for businesspeople with lesser educational backgrounds, including love letters, for instance to a prospective partner found on the internet. In general, the life histories elicited conveyed that they enjoyed the relative autonomy they had in Kenya. Most were not eager to have closer relations with other Chinese.

Having said this, most practitioners in Nairobi had contacted a representative of the Ministry of Commerce at the Chinese embassy. Apparently, one of them had suggested the idea that this representative should write letters of recommendation for them to facilitate access to the relevant Kenyan authorities for opening a medical practice (e.g. the City Council and the Department of Culture). However, several doctors were already well established when this happened, and they did not depend on the Chinese embassy's letter of recommendation; several made clear that the fewer relations with any officials, the better.

There were, of course, also conflicts between the practitioners, which went beyond the usual competition in a commercialised health field, and they involved backbiting and boasting. Interestingly, although cheating and fraud were involved, the Chinese migrants were more inclined to solve these problems among themselves than to report them to the local authorities. Common problems concerned the delivery of promised and prepaid medicines. The magnitude of the finances involved in these cases was sometimes quite considerable. For instance, a practitioner who was an employee of another practitioner and wished to return to China instantly after a dispute managed to sell vital assets of his colleague, namely his new car, in order to buy an aeroplane ticket. Such a dispute between two practitioners could also result in one depriving the other of important documents, like passports or work permits, by either burning or stealing them.

There was also a lot of trading going on all the time that an ethnocentric analysis would call cheating and lying. It was known to be particularly rampant in the food industry and less evident among medical practitioners, of whom most had a strong work ethic, although the gist of one such commerce-oriented negotiation between a local pastor and a Christian Chinese practitioner is given at the very end of this chapter. Sometimes, the cheating was so blatant, it was surreal. For instance, when on a special occasion I ordered bamboo shoot and Chinese [shiitake] mushroom, which in oyster sauce makes a characteristic Chinese dish, for a guest, she was served green asparagus sprouts and sliced champignons, both from a tin and stir-fried together. When I thereupon complained loudly and pointed to the asparagus, saying, 'This is not a bamboo shoot', the restaurant owner responded with poise: 'Sorry, this is bamboo shoot. Enjoy!' He knew that the occasion did not allow me to pursue the issue, and my guest duly praised this Chinese emperor's new clothes by eating it.

## *Encounters with Kenyan Authorities*

Chinese medical practitioners did not openly complain about the attitude of the Kenyan government towards their practice, perhaps because of their uncertainty about my status and perhaps out of habit. It was evident that there were problems. Many Chinese (but not all) were selling an insignificant number of Western medical drugs that had been produced in China (aspirin, penicillin and sulphonamides in particular), and they knew that the government did not approve of TM/CAM practitioners selling biomedical pharmaceuticals. In September 2002, there had been a meeting of TM/CAM practitioners, that is, Chinese medical practitioners and Kenyan healers and diviners, with representatives of the Kenyan Ministry of Health. Certificates for opening 'traditional medicine' practices in the past had been issued by the Department of Culture, as 'traditional African medicine' was comprehended as an aspect of 'traditional African culture'.[13]

In future, these certificates were to be issued by the Ministry of Health. This development was similar to that in other nation states, such as the PRC, where until the mid-1950s the Bureau for Chinese Medicine was under the jurisdiction of the Ministry of Commerce, which regulated the purchase and selling of the Chinese *materia medica* (*zhongyao*), before it came, in 1957, under the jurisdiction of the Ministry of Health (Lampton 1977: 48–49; Taylor 2005: 131). The difference was that the Chinese government had been more favourable to the development of traditional medicines then than the Kenyan government was in the early twenty-first century.

A Chinese practitioner commented: 'There are three points that the biomedical doctors of the Kenyan health authorities do not understand: first, they have not had first-hand experience of our traditional medicine, and have prejudices against it; second, they think Western medicine can solve all health problems, without the help of traditional medicines; third, there is also a question of competition between traditional and modern medicine on the health market that should not be underestimated.' He formulated the problem of TM/CAM and its legitimation very concisely.

At the meeting in question, health officials had declared that each chemical substance in a 'traditional medical' *materia medica* should be tested for its efficacy according to modern Kenyan rather than traditional Chinese medical standards before coming onto the market in Kenya. Chinese medical practitioners were in agreement that regulations should be put in place regarding TM/CAM but the procedures suggested were clearly unreasonable. Given that Chinese practitioners were selling up to a hundred or more different ready-made formula drugs, each constituted of several 'natural' Chinese *materia medica* (*zhongyao*) that each contained several hundred chemical substances, it is clear that such a decision would render their business impossible. In a series of smaller follow-up meetings, it also became clear that the Kenyan government did not have the facilities to carry out the necessary tests. In this situation, some TCM promoters pushed for the criterion of the *safety* of formula medicines to take priority over testing their *efficacy*.

Debates were protracted. Some emphasised the regulation of the *education* of TM/CAM practitioners as being more important than surveillance of the chemical ingredients they worked with. However, several senior biomedical physicians who advertised themselves as TCM practitioners would thereby be put in a difficult position. Furthermore, Kenyan regulators would have to recognise more than one single Chinese qualification and educational standard for the different forms of TCM care on offer in Kenya. Chinese health provision had great potential to assist primary and palliative care. This, however, required collaborations between the Kenyan and Chinese health bureaucracies that at the time were unthinkable.

There was no institutionalised continuing education of any kind in place. The work ethic of the practitioners was that their work experience in their private practice was educative and allowed them to improve their medical skills. However, there was a danger that those who had once received a reasonable education were not maintaining their professional standards. Another risk was that well-trained TCM professionals would avoid immigrating to Kenya. Indeed, there was a trend in the commodified late-liberal health markets to increasingly attract minimally educated entrepreneurs into the informal sector. They were not practitioners of what was once highly refined medical learning, but drug sellers.

To conclude, although Chinese medical doctors felt marginalised, none was keen on setting up an association. First, the mere idea of becoming organised for a political purpose was unappealing. Second, any regulatory body would have to include some practitioners but exclude others. The variation in medical specialisation and the differences in educational levels, as seen above, was remarkable. Third, practitioners' opinions about each others' medical practices, competence and ethics were strong and not always good. Despite the obstacles they faced from the Kenyan government and the advantages that a union might have brought, therefore, all Chinese medical practitioners interviewed in 2001 and 2003 upheld the maxim that each should care for their own business and not meddle with that of others. Many did not mind living on the margins.

## *Encounters with Patients*

The people whom Chinese medical practitioners encountered on a daily basis were their patients. They were mainly Kenyans and also, quite frequently in some practices, refugees from Somalia or Sudan. As already noted, Chinese doctors treated their patients with respect, and as they told me, they valued the respect that their patients gave them. Simultaneously, they were also interested in selling their medicines. As in other 'traditional' medical settings, prescriptions and the prices of prescriptions fluctuated depending partly on the practitioner's evaluation of the patient's spending power. Some encounters with patients were warm and very friendly, and over time, people had become very familiar with each other.

A few practitioners had made one or two close Kenyan friends. They considered them unpretentious (*meiyou zhongguoren name xuwei* 没有中国人那么虚伪) and true (*shizai* 实在), praised their good-heartedness (*xin hao* 心好) and humour (*youmo* 幽默), and emphasised their 'good company'; others admired their culturedness and politeness (*hen wenming* 很文明). While some Chinese practitioners who had lived in Kenya for over a decade did have close friends among Africans and South Asians, most claimed to have barely made any local friends. 'Africans', one Chinese doctor commented, 'what should I say about them, I don't really know them . . .'. He marvelled at the Kenyan government's complete lack of social responsibility, and over authorities who, he felt, simply did not care about the people, and he inferred that individuals too lacked social responsibility. He admitted to having very little insight into African cultures and kinship relations, and it is conceivable that over time, his opinions would change. He expressed admiration for the optimism with which common people countered difficult life situations, with no money, no job, no anything, and yet their comportment was good-humoured. Nevertheless, although he said this with a certain admiration, it reminded me of the paternalistic view of colonisers towards the happy-go-lucky African. 'They make no plans, all happens in the moment.' This made it difficult for him to form friendships with them. Among the Chinese of the older generation, marriage was not considered an option, but several younger Chinese practitioners apparently had local girlfriends, 'despite the AIDS scare', as their colleagues who told me about this said. Some of the Chinese teenagers dressed like their schoolmates and insisted on wearing Kenyan hairstyles; sooner or later they would entertain intimate friendships, likely not exclusively with Chinese.

In general, the medical anthropological literature emphasises – as do biomedical ethics – the services that doctors provide for their clientele. My research among the Chinese medical practitioners in East Africa demonstrates, however, that patients can also have lasting effects on their doctors. Medical practitioners sometimes need to come to terms with difficult life situations and acute and chronic illness, in themselves, their dependants and their parents.

Moreover, patients may affect practitioners more than is generally assumed.

## *Mobility and Conversions to Christianity*

One senior Chinese medical practitioner, a Chinese Communist Party member, underlined how impressed she was with the faith of her patients in God and the inner strength that this gave them to cope with their illness. 'Africans are plain (*pusu* 朴素)', she continued in an appreciative tone, 'they got a Christian education.' She implied in this way that Christianity provided guidance for them; for her as a Marxist it went without saying that religion was opium for the people. She herself was complicated in character (*fuza* 复杂), like Chinese generally are, and therefore, it was impossible for her to believe in God. However, she was impressed by the physical and psychological strengths that the belief in God engendered in her patients.

Another Chinese practitioner commented: 'I think the church is good, if there were no African church, the Africans would develop into bad people, just like the Chinese have in recent years.' If I were to go there – China – again, he said, 'You would not be able to adapt, I myself cannot adapt. Can you imagine, young Chinese people now think the elderly ought to die, they have no conscience whatsoever (*genben meiyou liangxin* 根本没有良心).' His outrage reflected deeply engrained Confucian filial piety, although he was not an intellectual (*zhishifenzi* 知识分子). Rather, he said that he was a Buddhist. He had read the Bible, had been given many booklets by Christian missionaries and had heard his patients speak of God, but he decided against converting. This does not mean that he had reserved a spot for incense-burning on the floor in the waiting room of his practice – or in front of a scroll onto which the deity Guanyin was painted, as another Chinese medical doctor had done – nor did his ideas about deities strike me as particularly Buddhist. Yet it seemed that the Christianity of his patients had reinforced his awareness of, and adherence to, his own religion (which the literature calls 'Chinese folk religion'; see Shahar and Weller 1996).

In this context, it is important to remind ourselves that not all physical strength was thought to be derived from religious belief and spirituality. As noted above, the physicality of African bodies was considered extremely healthful, and some Chinese medical practitioners prescribed a reduced dosage of antibiotics; when I raised with them the danger of such practices causing microbial resistance, they insisted that their dosage was adequate. Interestingly, a Russian biomedical anaesthetist who had worked in an international team in Somalia for over a year commented that in her profession it was common not to provide anaesthetics prior to surgery in the usual dosage; it was considered an outright overdose for Africans. Was she embracing a colonialist prejudice (e.g. Littlewood and Lipsedge 1982: 26–60)? Chinese medical practitioners too seemed to embrace this in their practice: some admitted to prescribing Chinese formula medicines and *materia medica* at a dosage that was reduced in comparison to that prescribed to their Chinese clientele. They guessed that this may have been due to genetic adaptation over thousands of years, reasoning along the lines of bodies becoming habituated to the medicines they consume, and the medicines therefore becoming less effective over the millennia. In summary, African bodies were generally considered healthful, both due to people's capacity for having faith in God and also for biologistic reasons.

Kenyans are Christians of many different denominations, and in Nairobi my respondents mentioned a fellowship of specifically Chinese Christians. In 2001, members apparently numbered in the twenties. They met at least once weekly, on Sunday afternoons, in a meeting room in a hostel. In 2003, two among the eighteen doctors I interviewed in Nairobi had converted to Christianity and were members of that Christian fellowship. Independently, they had also become neighbours in a downmarket suburb of Nairobi, but otherwise their life trajectories were very different.

Dr Bell was from Hunan, the son of a worker (*gongren* 工人) and the nephew of a Chinese medical doctor who had opened a practice in Nairobi before he emigrated to the United States in 1995. He followed in his maternal uncle's footsteps, and called himself the same Anglicised name: Dr Bell (he was the only practitioner to use an Anglicised name). He had been a regular student at the Hunan TCM college, in a special class that only lasted four years instead of five and was devoted to 'integrated Chinese and Western medicine'. He worked for one year in his hometown at the hospital, then transferred for two years to a Red Cross hospital in another province, and thereafter opened a private clinic (*getihu* 个体户) back home. He was one of the few Chinese medical doctors in Kenya who had undergone regular training and had at least five years of work experience before moving to Africa. His contacts with other Chinese seemed fairly limited. He was one of the only Chinese practitioners in East Africa who became seriously involved with an African woman – they cohabited and had a baby, then married and had another child. Many but not all of his patients were living with HIV/AIDS, he said, and he prescribed them a medicine called 'Marvel' that he had apparently developed himself. He came across as a quiet and reserved person, and he also practised calligraphy, as various poems on the walls of his practice showed; he certainly appealed to his Kenyan clientele through his exoticism and his rootedness in Chinese cultural practices.

Dr Bell converted to Christianity in 2001, as he told me then in Chinese, because his African girlfriend wished him to do so. In 2003 he was married to her and a father of two children, and his practice had moved away from the little lone house by the roadside into a shopping mall. He instantly recognised me when I visited him for the second time. I admired his calligraphy in Chinese ink on rice paper, which he had hung up prominently on the walls of his practice, although he also had photocopied certificates of his training. His lifeworld was clearly oriented to the ancient Chinese arts, of which he understood medicine to be one, and he was obviously on a life trajectory other than that of most of my respondents.

During both our conversations, an episode of his life stood out clearly: his father's death in 1999. When telling his life's story the first time, in Chinese, he said that he had gone back to China in that year, but when he returned to Nairobi, his uncle's clinic in the city centre, in which he had worked for four years, had been rented out to another Chinese medical doctor, a woman from Shanghai. So, he opened a new clinic in a suburb. When I visited him again fifteen months later, he is tape-recorded to have said in English: 'When my father was very sick, I wanted to go back to China and sell my clinic, but I did not sell it and in that year my father passed away. So I stayed here. . . . Had I gone back in that year, I would not have become a Christian.' While I suppose that he was more accurate about the physical movements he had made when speaking to me for the first time – that is, he did indeed go to China and back to Kenya – he was more explicit about his feelings the second time. In 2003, he emphasised how very important his conversion to Christianity was to him, whereas his narrative of 2001 underlined tactics of the everyday with a view to the future. His conversion to Christianity was an aspect of the process of getting married and becoming Kenyan, as the founder of a Kenyan nuclear family. Interestingly, although his conversion happened, as he said in 2001, so that he could have a future with his girlfriend in Kenya, he foregrounded in 2001 a life crisis in China, his father's death. Meanwhile, the narrative in 2003 of the converted Christian expressed a retrospective gaze and imposed a linear timeline, by allocating the suffering and death to within the first part of his life, and emphasising new beginnings thereafter.

The other Christian convert, Dr Bing, had in respect of his life history much more in common with many other Chinese medical practitioners I spoke to. Together with five others, he had come from Northeast China to do 'medicine as business' (it is important to know that 'doing business' was in Dengist times very much encouraged, as it was seen to work towards increasing the prosperity of the nation; e.g. Pieke and Salaff 2007; Biao 2013). They had originally planned to move to a hospital in Equatorial Guinea, but another group of doctors was apparently quicker in occupying the premises, so they got stuck in Nairobi – but after four months only, the group disintegrated.

Dr Bing had all the attributes of a petty entrepreneur: he was likeable and friendly, had connections (his aunt was a senior doctor in town) and was always wanted on the mobile phone; he could hold no conversation without being interrupted. He had minimal training in Chinese medicine and medicine in general, although the first time we spoke in 2001, when he was not quite certain about my status as interviewer, he claimed to have been a regular TCM student between 1978 and 1982 (this cohort was the first to consist of students who had passed a nationwide exam after none had been held for twelve years, and hence included the nation's best brains). From 1982 onwards, he had worked as a clerk in his father's work unit for a long time, before trying his luck as a businessman in 1991. His business failed: he was cheated, he said, and he had been unemployed for two years before he decided to emigrate to Africa in 1997. This was the narrative I elicited from him in 2001.

By 2003, Dr Bing had converted to Christianity, and his narrative, which as previously was given in Chinese, had changed: he mentioned very early on that his mother had died when he was in high school. After graduation (which apparently was in 1976), he worked for two years in the countryside (*xiaxiang* 下乡), then became a soldier and stayed for three years with the army. Thereafter, he reverted to civilian status and started working in his father's work unit, the Heilongjiang TCM University. He had a younger brother who needed caring for, 'So I could help' (*rang wo bangzhu* 让我帮助), he said. After a year, he decided to take evening classes at the work unit while he worked there as a clerk. In 1991, he opened his own clinic. 'For how long?', I asked in a routine way. One, two, three, four, five ... he counted his fingers in front of me. 'For five years', he said and smiled amicably at me (when I knew that this was a blatant lie in light of the narrative provided in 2001). However, the government did not allow him to set up a private enterprise, he said, so he emigrated. He did not mention that he had been unemployed and got into all kinds of troubles before leaving the PRC, but instead said that he had become a gambler.

Dr Bing's life history had changed drastically. Most obvious was that he now emphasised emotional aspects of his life: his mother's death while he was an adolescent and the care that his younger brother required. As in Dr Bell's case, Dr Bing's awareness of traumatic life events seemed to have been a recently learned aspect of telling one's biography. Evidently, the narratives of both converts were transformed so as to emphasise emotionally moving crisis points in their lives, a self-awareness that they had both probably acquired in their Christian community. Interestingly, the narrative convention of emphasising trauma, particularly in one's relations to one's parents, is generally identified as a characteristic of psychoanalysis, as famously formulated by Sigmund Freud in *fin de siècle* Vienna. In Nairobi it reconfigured in a strange, if not estranged, way how lives lived in China would be told (cf. Zhang 2007; Hsu 2013a).

Events in Dr Bing's life were in passing mentioned to me by another doctor, who suggested that he had indeed joined the People's Liberation Army in his youth, rather than becoming a regular university student. His first narrative was certainly meant to cover up educational inadequacies, while it was more accurate about his business failures. In 2001, he made hints that during his last few years in the PRC, he got into complications with both his comrades and local authorities (debts, fraud, theft, prison, petty crime), and that during his first few years in Nairobi he had worked in the textile trade rather than in medicine. The narrative that he gave of himself as a Christian convert emphasised that he had been a gambler (who would have spent well-earned money) and that the Chinese authorities were to blame for his business failures (the 'government'). The former epitomised the view of many people in Africa, expatriates in particular, of 'the Chinese' as gamblers, and the latter typified an anti-communist stance that Christian narratives tend to have. The Christian narrative allowed him to present himself with more confidence, but perhaps less honesty, as a capable businessman and doctor. To my surprise, however, Dr Bing also expressed the wish to become a pastor. He was waiting to be permitted by the leaders of his Christian community to enter a school that provided two years of training for pastors in Singapore. If he were to become a pastor, he said, he would return to China as a Christian missionary. In that case, Dr Bing's conversion to Christianity ultimately would not work to his 'empotment' into Kenya.

## *Mobility and Transmuted Traders*

In Republican and Communist China, Christian converts were met with a prejudice that they were good merchants rather than devout believers, given that their conversion won the trust of foreigners and opened doors to international trade. Dr Bing's conversion to Christianity certainly opened new doors for him as trader. I once overheard a conversation between him and a Kikuyu pastor who dropped in on Dr Bing's practice. They were neighbours; their 'friendship' began on the street through talking about religious belief, and this in turn provided the grounds for them to develop into business partners.

The pastor had patients suffering from serious conditions, like cancer, although he stressed that he was a Christian pastor and not a *mganga*: 'When someone is a *mganga* in Africa', he explained to me in English, 'you do some funny funny things so that the native is able to get a feeling . . . but when you do something funny, something which is not visible, something people cannot be able to understand . . . because a lot doing is basically something of the imagination'. However, in the medical practice of his Chinese friend he was seeking advice on medical prescriptions. His visit revealed that some Christian pastors inhabit a grey zone between the churchman and the medical doctor, the secular and religious (which is not uncommon; e.g. Krause 2011).

The pastor was looking for a medicine that reduced 'swellings' caused by cancer (*tumor* in Latin means 'hill' or 'swelling'). Dr Bing offered him a Chinese formula medicine, Mocrea, well known for its boosting of the immune-system, which Chinese doctors primarily prescribed for treating HIV/AIDS in the early 2000s (Simmons 2006). Dr Bing, in line with few other Chinese medical colleagues, offered it to treat 'cancer'. Meanwhile, the pastor considered the 'swellings' diagnostically relevant. He had observed that the rheumatically caused 'swellings' of some of his patients who had used large anti-rheumatic plasters from Chinese doctors had been drastically reduced. So, he asked for two such plasters. There followed a palaver over the price of the medicines, which was KES 100 for each plaster and amounted to twenty times less than the cost of Mocrea (KES 2000). Dr Bing seemed to understand that the pastor had lumped cancerous and rheumatic swellings into one category, that of 'swellings', but made no effort to rectify this. Even the pastor himself seemed to be aware this. Eager to present himself as a rational customer, he kept on saying: 'If it works, I'll keep coming.' He seemed to justify his use of rheumatic plasters for the treatment of a tumour as a form of legitimate 'trying out'.

This episode highlights how religious affiliation can indeed pave the way for new trade relations. Christian Kenyans with minimal spending power who seek treatment from Christian Chinese may affect the future of Chinese medical practices in unusual ways.

## Reflections: Mobility and Connectedness (*ling* and *tong*)

The theme of 'mobility and connectedness' elaborates on Stafford's (2000) *Separation and Reunion*, which in turn draws on John Bowlby's attachment theory. This chapter comments on these themes through the actors' own narratives. Rather than ethnicising them as specifically Chinese matters, it presents 'mobility and connectedness' as more general phenomena that mark the livelihoods of these transnational individuals. To be sure, the words *ling* and *tong* were not verbally expressed in the practitioners' life histories, but they emerged as relevant from the co-production of ethnographic knowledge. As argued here, *ling* 灵 (flexible, always ready to adjust, quicksilver-like, with virtuosity, magical or miraculous) and *tong* 通

(striving for connectedness, togetherness, equality, alikeness) referred to dispositions valued in ancient Chinese cosmology (see also Hsu 1994, 2013b).

Whyte and Siu (2015) also speak of connectedness in their discussion of the uncertainty that HIV/AIDS patients who had 'second chances' experienced, in the context of introducing 'contingency' as a concept to sharpen one's analysis. Contingency denotes the uncertainties about what may or may not happen in the future, they argue, yet it directs one's attention to specifics and, in particular, to (specific) connections (ibid.: 19). The contingent may be experienced positively, as possibility, chance or opportunity that arises out of being related and connected, but contingencies can also be negatively experienced, as in the case of apprehension, worry, lack of control and growing insecurity.

The terms *ling* and *tong* may of course be understood to refer to a pragmatic individual's 'navigating' and 'networking' within late-liberal health markets that due to their utter fluidity are marked by contingency. Indeed, the embodied movement that *ling* affords is agile and flexible, but it is also 'virtuous' and positively evaluated (see Farquhar 1994), in contrast to profit-seeking selfishness. It is a movement defined by the self's openness to, or at least its willingness to be open to, the world and its disposition to seek a connection with the world, and to connect (*tong*).

The concepts of *ling* and *tong* were developed in a cosmology that underlined that the flow of life depends on a self that defines itself through its – *Thou*-oriented – connectedness to the surrounding world, which would always imply a sensitive responsiveness. The spaces of the surroundings are always already textured such that the navigation of these spaces cannot be random, but demands the connecting self's virtuous responsiveness to their sensory affordances. For sure, the mobile Chinese medical experts discussed above had all kinds of intentions and motivations, but if one discusses their mobility from the vantage point of the cosmology within which *ling* and *tong* are virtues, their movements were also instantiating a very basic curiosity, sensitivity and openness (willingness to connect) fundamental to all organisms that strive to stay alive (e.g. Ingold 2011). The phenomenologist Alfred Schütz insisted on this very basic orientation towards, and also curiosity about, the you as fundamental to being human.

Finally, the question that motivated the research presented in this chapter, 'who are these practitioners and why have they come to us?', can now be partially answered. We found that 'freedom' and boredom, played a role, alongside ideology and idealism – which I propose to interpret as primarily to reinforce the we-relation with those in need in the two cases discussed, alongside a sense of duty and loyalty to teachers and patients. Meanwhile, the most pervasive desire that the foreign practitioners, and also the local paramedical professionals, expressed (see below), was to provide a route to education for their offspring. In this case, the concept of self with which they were working was one that spanned several generations; that is, their parents may for reasons of education have moved from rural to urban areas, while they themselves became transnationals along a South–South trajectory in order to bring their offspring into the desirable higher education of the northern hemisphere.

Finally, a note on those who were arguably 'victims' of the Dengist reforms is warranted. Several had been urged to go into early retirement, as they occupied senior positions while lacking education due insufficient training during the Cultural Revolution. Yet given their resourcefulness, their capacities of being *ling* and *tong* (which albeit only very rarely resulted in an extremely lucrative business), it is hard to perceive them as losers.

In the late 1990s, the spending power of the middle-class clientele started to wane, and one couple running a Chinese medical practice was quick – *ling* – to build up another business, which was possible because they were openly disposed to others and well connected, *tong*. They identified the existence of old equipment from a firm back home in Shanghai and imported it to East Africa. On the premises of a plot of land that they bought in a suburb for their own residence, they then drilled a well down to the groundwater level and a pavilion with facilities for bottling drinking water. This made it possible for them to start selling 'purified drinking water' to affluent businesspeople and the city council's offices. During my fieldwork, their adverts, which were a designer product, dotted the urban textures of the inner city. The financial breakthrough that they experienced with their drinking-water firm reverberated across all the Chinese communities in the region, as it was enormous. However, it had not come overnight. The couple had tried out several businesses before making this 'big money', which had a profit margin much higher than any Chinese medical practitioner would even dream of.

## More Ethnography: The Paramedical Professionals

Auxiliary staff and paramedical professionals, specifically the laboratory technicians and linguistically able interpreters, also had life stories that revealed a search for education; education entitled one to a higher salary, socio-economic status, and more. However, researchers tend to overlook paramedical professionals, and auxiliary staff are notoriously undervalued (Davies 2007). It was only in the second part of my fieldwork, between 2004 and 2008, that I elicited narratives from nine different individuals. The interviewees comprised in total two receptionists (both female), three lab technicians (one male, two female) and four interpreters (all male) working in Mombasa, Moshi and Dar es Salaam. I also had memorable informal discussions with a local drugstore owner on Lamu in 2007 and a drugstore employee in Kampala in 2008.

### *Difference Makes a Difference*

One receptionist had worked for seven years in a Chinese medical practice in urban Kenya when I interviewed her in 2005. She had high school education (Form 4) and she had attended one year of medical school but then dropped out. She was married and had two children, whom she and her husband decided to send to a private school as they both received a good monthly salary, topped up by generous bonuses, after the Chinese practitioner observed her able handling of interpersonal crisis situations at work. She was given the trust to act more or less as the manager of this Chinese medicine business. As manager, she ensured that the practice's ethos attracted middle-class clients with good spending power.

A laboratory assistant in Dar es Salaam was of similar respectable social background, having received, after high school (Form 4), two years of vocational training. She had worked at various private biomedical hospitals over the past ten years, which opened and closed at an only slightly slower rate than the Chinese medical clinics that shifted across different neighbourhoods. Every time her workplace closed down, her large pool of friends and family working within the medical field introduced her to another private clinic. For her, there was no fundamental difference between working for locals or 'the Chinese', she said, nor did she mind 'the Indians'. Yes, the Chinese did request her to work seven days a week, but it was small money and not very hard work. Sometimes she had three tests to do in a day, sometimes twenty, she claimed. She was married to a lawyer, and had three children of 5, 6 and 15 years old. 'I was very interested to look into this microscope', she said, 'from childhood on.' And what about her future? As in the narratives of other paramedical professionals, education was given as a primary concern: her wish was, eventually, to study for three more years to become a fully qualified laboratory technician. Her husband was in support of this.

Education was also mentioned as the most central goal in the life history of a laboratory microscopist, who discussed opportunities for education alongside failures to realise them. He was from Mbeya region, the only and eldest son, with six younger sisters. In his childhood, his parents moved to the region of Tabora. They were looking for land to grow a cash crop, tobacco, but ended up growing subsistence crops like maize and rice. He started his education there, in Tabora. After completing primary school, Standard 7, he made the selling of fish between Tabora and Kigoma into a business and learned Ha in this context (he spoke five languages: Nyamwezi, Mara, Ha, Swahili and English). In this way he earned the money to finance secondary school. He completed Form 4 and then worked at the regional hospital for one year as a medical laboratory microscopist. He started working for missionaries 'who chose me'. He worked in Xinyanga for seven months, and was on the cusp of being translocated to Rwanda:

> I filled in the form, I asked for leave, but my parents in Tabora said no, in Rwanda there is war. I told my boss, and went to Mbeya instead. I took several exams, I always failed, the third time I passed, but I had no money, so I failed. I even went to the missionaries to ask for support, I failed. Then, I went to Kigoma hospital, worked there as a microscope lab technician, not more than six months, then I stopped working, the salary was too low, then I came to Dar es Salaam, to ask the Chinese. They said we have no job, but let us have your telephone number; in Dar I had no relatives, no friends. I stayed for sleeping there, in a local dispensary. Then, after two months I got a call. The Chinese medical doctor and the interpreter interviewed me. They offered TZS 2,000/day, which makes TZS 60,000 a month. I wanted to learn to become a lab technician. All my sisters and my mother depend on me. (Notebook no. 4)

His father had passed away, and he was helping his sisters to get schooling. In addition, his wife cared for their 6-year-old back home in Mbeya. He wore conspicuously good-quality leather shoes, as did his Chinese boss; he clearly had not bought them himself, but received them second-hand as a bonus. Did he like the Chinese?

> I like them, but not all of them, some treat us like a slave. I have to do reception, do the cleaning, be interpreter and do the lab; two days ago I said I can't do the cleaning. (Ibid.)

What were the main differences between the Chinese and the local lifestyle?

> The Chinese life is very cheap, but Tanzanians, their life is very complicated. They [the Chinese] eat very simple, but we eat rice with beef as a lunch [which is expensive], TZS 400. These Chinese, they like to stay in a good accommodation house, we just rent rooms. Tanzanians have huge marriage ceremonies, and spend a lot of money. But these Chinese, they like money more than anything. If a patient has no money, they can't give him any medicine. (Ibid.)

There followed a brief silence; I was busy jotting down what he had said, and was evidently moved by it. I felt for him; I remembered that I had noted him already on one of my first visits to that clinic. Was it a certain sadness in his eyes or his silent attentiveness, observant in the background? To me he had always exuded intelligence and humility in one. He then said that he had bought a bicycle. He explained that the *dalla dalla* cost him TZS 300/day and TZS 9000/month; the bike cost TZS 40,000 and he had used it for a year now. In this way, he felt that he had become a bit Chinese.

Interpreters also had remarkable life histories to tell. One had studied engineering in China for five years, and after he retired in his forties, he had time to act as interpreter for a Chinese medical practitioner. Yet another interpreter, who had also graduated in engineering at a Chinese university, had come back with a speech defect and hence had difficulties with finding employment. His speech defect, which became aggravated when he felt stressed, was not usually a problem when he worked as an interpreter. Finally, there was the army fighter pilot, who had been trained in China for two years. After leaving (he did not say 'defecting' from) the Tanzanian army at a fairly young age – he said it was when he was scheduled to serve in Zimbabwe – he found himself able-bodied and on the job market. He applied to become a pilot in civil aviation, to do balloon flying and to build up a private company. All failed. So he agreed to work for the Chinese.

There was also a bright young interpreter in the TCM clinic in Moshi who spoke excellent Chinese. Where had he learned it? Not far from where he was stationed, he said. He had joined Buddhist monks who regularly held sessions for reading the scriptures, praying and meditating. He did this for some time, and excelled in it. Then, he was asked whether he would like to transfer to Taiwan and become a Buddhist monk. This required him to go to South Africa for two years to train as a novice and learn Chinese. He did go to South Africa, and he underwent intensive training, but then he could not imagine himself leaving African soil. He ran away: 'I could not leave my mother.' He returned to Moshi in Tanzania.

## *Living in the Limen*

Relations between the Chinese medical practitioners and their support staff were generally friendly, and some were characterised by affectionate joking; only very rarely were interactions ostensibly cordial and warm or tactile. Chinese medical practitioners were aware of their total dependency on loyal receptionists, and their visible efforts to strengthen their connectedness with the latter consisted also of financial incentives. By contrast, lab technicians were considered easily exchangeable. As noted in Chapter 1, lab technicians usually rented a room in the Chinese practice and brought with them the microscope and chemicals, financially working on a separate budget. They ran their own businesses.

As in every business, there were also employment issues: the monthly salary, financial bonuses sporadically paid out, good will, if a staff member or one of their dependents got ill. Working hours with the Chinese were notoriously long; Sunday work was expected with no extra pay; communication was difficult due to the lack of linguistic skills (usually, in English) on the part of the practitioner. One staff member commented: 'The doctor himself is good at heart, but his wife is not, she bosses everyone around.' Moreover, 'they want you to read their face, and whatever you do – they say – must come from the heart.' Or, 'you are important whenever you are of use to them.' One employee asked me: 'You do research on Chinese culture? You like it?' I did not wish to be offensive and said nothing. Then, I admitted that I liked Chinese food. 'I don't eat this food', he commented.

There was also outright hostility, aggression and assault. I have already mentioned manslaughter, if not murder, of at least one Chinese medicine practitioner. There were also instances of violence and robbery. Among them belonged assaults at gunpoint that could happen at any time of the day or night, particularly in Nairobi. Violent assaults were more frequent in Nairobi; robbery was ubiquitous. Chinese people only went by car to socialise in restaurants and bars, or casinos, after dusk, which in equatorial latitudes is at 6 p.m.

To understand the violence of which Chinese medical practitioners were aware, let me recall one episode that affected a family I had become friendly with during the early years of my research. This family was adamant to emigrate long-term to Dar es Salaam, with the paternal grandparents, parents and infant lodging on the premises of the Chinese medical practice. However, they were forced to return to China due to their necessary documents not being reissued. Their visa and business permit were close to expiry in 2005. They had a Tanzanian patron whose situation however became more precarious over the years, leading to his eventual death at the age of fifty ('from malaria'). Moreover, there were issues with this practitioner's practice. His patients said that he had sold fake antimalarials, and his Chinese colleagues that he was insufficiently experienced. So, after several years of residency, the family's efforts proved a failure; they could not renew their papers and had to pack up and return to the PRC. Apparently, on the day before they boarded their flight, bundles of cash tucked away in their luggage, their lab assistant knocked on their flat's door at dusk. He was escorted by a group of young men. They had come to rob the family. The practitioner's father tried to stop them by barring their entry, stretching out his arms wide, only to collapse onto the floor, which was quickly turning blood-red, as he had been injured by the blow of a machete to his thigh. He was instantly hospitalised, but the wound prevented the family from flying until a week or two later.

When darkness fell, many Chinese did not feel safe, either in the streets or in their homes. In the course of conducting research on the Chinese noodle-makers in Zanzibar and Mombasa, I found that one Chinese community had the ingenuity to use gambling establishments as a place of protected socialising after dusk. I was surprised to find that the easiest way to locate my interview partners was by going into a gambling establishment after supper, when it was dark, around 7–8 p.m. Here, all assembled, were the elders whose parents had emigrated to Mombasa and Zanzibar between the World Wars and soon after the Second, in Republican times. They came from one single Chinese community in Guangdong province: Shunde 順德. They had a separate alcove of the enormous gambling palace all to themselves. They were scattered in groups of three to four, ostensibly disorderly and arranged around small tables, with genders segregated but not strictly.

The assembled community was playing bingo while making small talk in Cantonese. Some ordered just one soft drink over the whole evening (the consumption of one item was compulsory on every visit). As I was introduced to the different members of the different groups in the room, I was told by each and almost every person that over the years (several decades), they had won a very large sum of money at least once. They were interested in telling me that everyone had been a winner, rather than being precise about the differences in exact gains. The room was filled with chatter, as they had developed extraordinary skills in talking with each other, and with me, and simultaneously responding with great agility to the fast-changing numbers on the screen. No photos were taken after this initial introductory meeting; we were on the premises of a gambling institution, after all, which, with its internal rules of conduct, evidently not only provided physical protection for those at leisure on its premises but also assured their anonymity.

## Notes

1. Frank Pieke was interested to hear in 2001 about the wave of migration out of Northeast China into Africa; a corresponding research position was created at the University of Oxford (see Biao 2013).
2. 'There may be one individual who maintains high levels of homeland contact and is the node through which information, resources and identities flow' (Levitt and Glick-Schiller 2004: 1009).
3. The population researched for this study was small, but almost all members were known to me.
4. This section draws on Elisabeth Hsu. 2012a. 'Mobility and Connectedness: Chinese Medical Doctors in Kenya', in Hansjörg Dilger, Abdoulaye Kane and Stacey Ann Langwick (eds), *Medicine, Mobility and Power in Global*

*Africa*. Bloomington, IN: Indiana University Press, pp. 295–315. Used with permission.

5. See Shimazono (2003).
6. I say this in awareness that 'economic migrants also engage in projects of the self and indulge in an ongoing search for a better quality of life and lifestyle' (Green 2014: 147).
7. He used the word 'medical team' (*yiliaodui*) because that invoked prestige, but he was not one of the government-selected physicians from Shandong province; he was a member of a medical team working for TAZARA.
8. He was not the only Chinese medical doctor to have been robbed at gunpoint; it happened with very few exceptions to all of those interviewed in Nairobi.
9. On the gendered role of women as earners of residence permits, see Ong (1999: 127–29). Ong describes men as 'astronauts' in mid-air, shuttling across borders on the trans-Pacific business commute, whereas the movements of Dr Ming and his wife were more weblike.
10. Parkin points out the minimal objects of refugees, and also migrants, who engage in a more general process of 'self-inscription in non-commodity' (1999: 313).
11. The PRC never dispatched any medical teams to Kenya, as diplomatic relations were not as close as with socialist-oriented states like Tanzania and Zambia.
12. He explained that injections and 'the drip' were not exclusively provided by Western medical doctors, but also by traditional doctors in the PRC (see also Hsu 1992; White 1998; Chen et al. 2020). They were not merely a modern medical technology, but part of 'integrated Chinese and Western medicine'. TCM practitioners who had the training, he argued, should be permitted to give injections.
13. On the precarious position of the 'traditional medical' doctors, *waganga*, since colonial times, and the wish of some to return to the jurisdiction of the Ministry of Culture, see Nichols-Belo (2018). See also Bruchhausen (2006), Luedke and West (2007) and Langwick (2011).

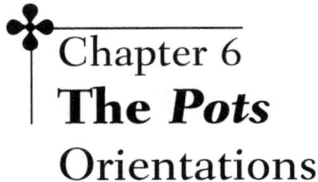

# Chapter 6
# The *Pots*
# Orientations

## Synopsis

This monograph comprises three parts and nine chapters that each have an ethnographic core, an introductory section on ethnographic methods and a concluding section on reflections that was added ten to twenty years after fieldwork was conducted.

Part I concerns the practico-sensory realm of space. Chapters 1 and 2, on the interface of medical, sensory and linguistic anthropology, highlight how I gained access to the field, first by paying attention to the sense-perceived topographies of space and second by attending to recurrent patterns in the linguistic exchanges and conversations held in these spaces – specifically, as fieldwork revealed, to 'phonemic misunderstandings', which I then interpreted as creating spaces for personal reflection.

Part II forms the core of the book. Chapters 3–6 are concerned with a very old, but specifically medical anthropological, message, which has always been emphasised by the literature on medical pluralism, namely that the medical encounter is not merely one between patient and practitioner. Rather, as argued here, the medical encounter enfolds patients, practitioners and so-called pots into a process of probingly making a place (PPP in ppp: Patients, Practitioners and Pots engage probingly in processes of place-making). Accordingly, as shown in Chapter 3, treatment aims not only at a narrative 'emplotment' (Good 1994; Mattingly 1998), but also – and importantly, at least for East Africa – at an 'empotment' of patient and practitioner into a new place, as proposed here, even if each is entangled in a different long-term trajectory. In Central, Northeast and East Africa, healing has been described as a process of emplacement that reconnects the patient to their ancestral lands (Green 1996; Davis 2000; Geissler and Prince 2010a, 2010b; Fayers-Kerr 2018, 2019). This finding directly puts in line sensorial and sensory anthropology with sensory medical anthropology in that it moves one's analytic gaze away from embodiment to emplacement (Howes 2005: 7; Pink 2011); or, as suggested here, to 'empotment'.

Healing appears accordingly as part of a long-term retexturing dynamics, aimed at 'making whole' through a material and spatial 'empotment'. To achieve this, practitioners bring into use different 'techniques of transformation' – Dr Wu had a wide range of instruments for wound-healing, and Dr Wei for obstetrics and family planning, while Dr Wang, who was evidently on the move, entangled different 'African' localities into what she perceived as a weblike mobility, in which she could partake with the small, light acupuncture needles that she always had at hand. She, like others, defined herself as flexibly connected (*ling* and *tong*) to a similarly mobile cosmopolitan clientele that through the therapeutic procedures of individual transformations contributed to the shaping of East Africa's urban textures.

Chapter 4 asked: who were these practitioners' patients? I interviewed about thirty patients, whenever possible in their homes, in the urban areas of Dar es Salaam and Mombasa, and on rural Pemba: ninety patients in total. Those in Dar es Salaam I interviewed twice, the second interview six months after the first. These cases highlighted the wide range of complaints and serious diseases (e.g. TB, stomach ulcers, STDs) that the mostly East African clientele brought to the Chinese practitioners. They also underlined the importance of malaria, widely recognised at the time as a major 'burden of disease'. As with most infectious diseases, those living in informal settlements and 'poor' living conditions were most affected. Yet interestingly, the patients whom I interviewed generally defined themselves as 'middle-class'. Indeed, their ethos was found to be that of enterprising individuals, mostly men but also women. They were upwardly mobile, searching and probing, aiming to forge their destiny as is expected from members of the middle class (in this respect they differed from another thirty patients of a local healer whose education was mostly 'Standard 7'). However, these self-identified members of the 'middle class' did not have the financial spending power of the people usually termed 'middle-class' in the Africanist literature.

Chapter 5 concerned the narratives of the people who became migrant Chinese medical doctors and of the paramedical professionals – interpreters, laboratory assistants, receptionists and cleaning personnel. I elicited life histories from twenty-one practitioners in Kenya and from nine paramedical professionals throughout urban East Africa, and I found that regardless of whether they were Chinese or local, one of their main motivations for doing the work they did was 'education'. Among the Chinese practitioners who had received higher education in the PRC, the motivation was in particular to enable their offspring enrol in university studies in North America. The healing they offered thus had to do with the will to learn on several levels.

Chapter 6 – this chapter – forms the core of the book, and presents interconnected reflections on how to account for the materiality of the different sorts of pots brought into play in a medical encounter. In doing so, it will address issues concerning the perception of the environment (e.g. Ingold 2000) and the anthropology of life (e.g. Haraway 2016). It will also explore forms of cohabitation, symbiosis and symbiogenesis among plants and animals, fungi, and Protista, with a view to the textured and texturing ways of making whole that are experienced as healing among human beings.

Part III will focus on investigating the materiality of the *pots* that are co-constitutive of a medical encounter. Chapters 7–9 will discuss three domains of medical services for which, as my ethnographic fieldwork suggests, Chinese practitioners were mostly sought and to which they catered. Since I undertook no quantitative surveys given the difficulties of researching these practices, I cannot claim that the Chinese medical health provisions discussed are representative of the whole of Africa. However, my fieldwork observations regarding general practice, preventive medicine, public health and primary care, as well as self-care and enhancement medicines for the self, are not entirely random either. Among other aspects, I discuss medicines for the postcolonial disorders of 'sugar' and 'pressure' (Chapter 7); gender-specific enhancement medicines (Chapter 8); and 'depression' and 'malaria', as recognised by 'hospital-medicine', which patients sought to treat with the 'Chinese antimalarial' (Chapter 9).

Rather than being fixated on the continued study of (traditional) medical treatment and its *efficacy* in respect of an assumed *homo rationalis*, motivated by rational choice and RCT results, this exploration of the textured medical practices that facilitated the refinement of certain therapeutic techniques – such as those for 'generating synchronicity' by flouting Grice's maxim of manner, 'empotting' the self into kaleidoscopically-transformable urban textures, 'incorporating' one's healer's substances, titillatingly teasing and deceiving self and other, and overall adopting an 'as if' stance – speaks to a *homo ritualis* (Hsu 2011).

## *Space*

Merleau-Ponty (1962: 243) is explicit in saying that 'Space is not the setting (real or logical) in which things are arranged'. Rather, space is best conceived as an enabling power for making connections to other people and things: 'Rather, we must think of it as a universal power enabling them [the things] to be connected' (ibid.: 243). Merleau-Ponty later addresses specifically the methodological problem contained in the above statement. The 'spatiality' he talks about is neither analytically useful as defined through its 'physicality' or 'materiality' ('things in space'), nor as a dimension or a 'medium' ('spatializing space'; ibid.: 248). In other words, it makes no sense to conceive of space either as a thing or as a context. Instead, 'we have to look for *the first-hand experience* of space and the hither side of the distinction between form and content' (ibid.: 248, italics added). This very sentence reads to me as inviting us to think in terms of *pots* as being directly perceived; and through this – their sensory perception, enabled through body techniques that make them perceptible – they become part of social relations.

'Space always precedes itself' – it is 'always already constituted' (Merleau-Ponty 1962: 252). As Merleau-Ponty put it, 'being is synonymous with being situated' (ibid.), and 'since every conceivable being is related either directly or indirectly to the perceived world, and since the perceived world is grasped only in terms of direction, we cannot dissociate being from oriented being' (ibid.: 253). My body is not to be understood as 'a thing in objective space, but as a system of possible actions, a virtual body with its phenomenal "place" defined by its task and situation' (ibid.: 250). This understanding of the self in the world is non-materialist and could be called 'spatialist'; it entails that 'My body is wherever there is something to be done' (ibid.: 250).[1] Sense perception, inclusive of its affective dimension, plays into orienting the body that is entangled in a meshwork of relations, as a 'system of possible actions'.

It might be helpful in this context to remind ourselves of the figure–ground image presented in the first chapter of this book (Figures 1.3 a and b). If you squint your eyes such that the white interstices are foregrounded, you can perceive two differently shaped white pots. They each have a bulging belly and aesthetically pleasing rims of different widths around their necks, and the shapes of these directly affect the facial features of the two human figures in black that are facing each other.

So, sense-perceived *pots* are not things that have been rather randomly placed into a three-dimensional, empty container of space. The thing perceived as a 'pot' in a Euclidean space becomes a *pot*, as referred to here, after having been perceived and engaged with intersubjectively by the self and by the other – say, by the patient and the practitioner, as well as by myself, the attentive and responsible fieldworker-*cum*-co-author – who all are 'squinting their eyes'. *Pots* will always have, at the very least, an affective effect on those who sense-perceive them, known as their 'demand character' or 'affordance'; and they will be experienced as either attractive or repulsive. *Pots* are therefore known by how they affect the perceiver, that is, by what we might call the 'sensory experience' of an 'object' of 'material culture' – three terms that do not quite express the issues I am trying to convey here.

First, we must get away from the idea that sensory perception arises due to stimuli that the body is passively exposed to. Rather, sensory experiences are elicited through the way in which I project myself and move into my spatial surroundings. They are elicited through the 'body techniques' that I apply to things. Particularly in efforts towards effecting a reconfiguration of wholeness, these techniques tend to be part of 'intercorporeal' (Csordas 2008) procedures. They are often aspects of processes, more than 'objects', and rather than reducing them to 'material culture', they are best comprehended in terms of an 'ecology of materials'.

So far, so good. However, what about squinting at the figure–ground image in a way that puts the white interstices between the two black figures into the background, letting the two human figures appear as if they are encountering each other in a featureless, empty space? I refer to this interstitial space in the background as *pots* too. However, I do not consider these background *pots* featureless, as it is in Figure 1.1. This background space actually has 'archi-textures' (Lefebvre 1991: 218), as demonstrated in Figures 1.2 a–b. In other words, the medical encounter is neither a disembodied nor a non-embedded event, but takes place in 'archi-textures'.

Accordingly, both the material 'pots' (as comprehended from a Cartesian point of view) – that is, the vase in the foreground – and the therapeutic places (i.e. the interstitial space forming the background) become *pots* as they become enmeshed in the meshworks of patients and practitioners (and also the researcher). This inevitably raises the question of what is gained by defining *pots* as embracing both the medicines that are transacted during a medical encounter (seen when squinting such that the white vase/pot is foregrounded) and the places in which this happens, such as the Chinese medical consultation room (seen when the white interstitial space becomes a background).[2] The answer is that it allows us to account in a non-Cartesian but social-relational way for 'new materialities' like *qi* that Chinese medicine practitioners work with.

Langer (1953), Ingold (2000) and Kapferer (2004), along with authors who have written on autopoiesis and sympoiesis, automorphic symmetries and self-similarity, do not locate agency in clearly bounded individual actants. Rather, they point to patterned movements and textures. Accordingly, agency is not in the person[3] or thing, but in the 'rhythm' (Ingold 2000: 197), or in 'the building up and resolution of tension' (Langer 1953: 126, quoted in Ingold 2000: 197), in 'a complex interweaving of very many concurrent cycles' (Ingold 2000: 200). The efficacy of a medical treatment depends on what is in the 'pots', surely, but as the 'pots' become comprehended as *pots*, sensed and handled in spatial practices and interactions, questions of medical efficacy are minimalised while those concerning relational interdependencies that give rise to wholesomeness become more important.

## Sedimentation and Articulations

Merleau-Ponty comprehended the body as the emergent 'interface' of the self moving through space.[4] He underlined that sensory bodily perception is pre-objective (we are not born with a representational idea of, say, a table), while no one is born as a pre-cultural being (i.e.

everyone is born to a 'mother' and 'father', and into a kinship group). He thereby gave the body-self historical depth, and the spaces it moved through a texture. He spoke of 'sedimentation'. One's predecessors' movements through the world are 'sedimented' within the body-self, the spaces it inhabits and the pots that it handles.

Merleau-Ponty's notion of sedimentation implies a responsiveness to the environment that reminds us of the process of perceiving that the phrase 'learning to be affected' also expresses, something that Vinciane Despret (2004) foregrounded and Bruno Latour (2004) also took up in his seminal article about 'articulations' (citing Despret; both judiciously omitted reference to the philosopher Baruch Spinoza as they likely built on insights of another thinker). When asking 'How to talk about the body', Latour productively amalgamates insights from different thinkers – and also, although unacknowledged, from Merleau-Ponty and his understanding of the body arising at the interface of the self's movements through space.

> One way I have found to talk about those layers of differences is to use the word *articulation*. . . . The main advantage of the word 'articulation' is not its somewhat ambiguous connection with language and sophistication, but its ability to take on board the *artificial and material* components allowing one to progressively have a body. (Latour 2004: 209–10)

When Latour speaks of progressively having a body, he draws directly on Merleau-Ponty.

> Thus body parts are progressively acquired at the same time as 'world counter-parts' are being registered in a new way. Acquiring a body is thus a progressive enterprise that produces at once a sensory medium *and* a sensitive world. (Latour 2004: 207)

Evidently, Latour's discussion of articulations hinges on insights gleaned from the phenomenology of perception and sensory anthropology. While Latour speaks refreshingly in his own language, what he actually says is not much different from Merleau-Ponty – for instance, his claim that the perceiver is always in motion. The body is 'what leaves a dynamic trajectory by which we learn to register and become sensitive to what the world is made of' (Latour 2004: 206). When Latour speaks of *layered* set-ups 'to make my nose sensitive to differences' (ibid.: 208–9), he seems to be drawing on processes of perception implied by Merleau-Ponty's concept of 'sedimentation'.[5]

> An articulate subject is someone who learns to be affected by others – *not by itself*. . . . Articulation thus does not mean to talk with authority . . . but being affected by differences. (Latour 2004: 209–10).

Latour also draws on philosophers other than the unacknowledged Merleau-Ponty when developing his argument regarding 'articulations'. Important for us here is that thinking in terms of 'articulations', just like thinking along the lines of Merleau-Ponty, allows the researcher to make generalisations that are not reductionist. Rather:

> Generalization should be a vehicle for travelling through as many differences as possible – thus maximizing articulations – and not a way of *decreasing* the number of alternative versions of the same phenomena. (Latour 2004: 221)

In summary, the Latourian project of layered articulations comes very close to Merleau-Ponty's ideas about the process of 'sedimentation'.

## *Autopoiesis*

The continuity between the habitus of living organisms and their habitat has long been posited by biologists. Hermann Weyl (1952) went so far as to claim that organisms reproduced 'automorphic' symmetries. Needless to say, this continuum is marked by non-linear variability, where automorphic symmetries reconfigure chunks of materials that have been fractured, reassembled and are again re-fractured. Lynn Margulis (1997) makes a related point when she speaks of re-assembling prokaryotes within a process that she calls 'autopoiesis'.

To be sure, the term 'autopoiesis' has many facets of meaning (see Clarke 2012). The sociologist Niklas Luhmann wrote prolifically from the early 1960s on complex social systems, in ways that he later proselytised through articles like 'The Autopoiesis of Social Systems' (1986). Meanwhile, the biologist Francisco Varela and his colleagues (1974) spoke of autopoiesis in respect of 'the organisation of living systems'. Lynn Margulis (1997) contrasted, as an explanation for evolutionary change, 'physiological autopoiesis versus mechanistic neo-Darwinism', while Pier Luigi Luisi (2006) used the term autopoiesis to explain 'the logic of cellular life'.

I mention the concepts of autopoiesis and automorphic symmetries together here because they both suggest that there is a spontaneous organising principle within the organism itself. Questions regarding the efficaciousness of certain healing procedures will certainly need to take account of the automorphic symmetries, autopoiesis and self-similarities intrinsic to the constellations of these procedures.

In many ways all of the above authors' thinking dovetails with the mathematician Benoit Mandelbrot's fractal geometry, introduced into anthropology by authors such as Mosko and Damon (2005), for whom 'The term "fractal" refers to phenomena of self similarity, or the tendency of patterns or structures to recur on multiple levels or scales' (Mosko 2005: 24). After all, living organisms are never on their own but are always related, and anything they do will involve others too. Each with their own understandings of self-organising principles, the above researchers all appear to be gesturing towards an organism's predilection to be actively involved in its own making and in the making of its surroundings.

## *Symbiogenesis*

In her research on the Protista (unicellular eukaryotic organisms that started to populate the waters of planet earth over 1.2 billion years ago), the evolutionary theoretician and microbiologist Lynn Margulis studied one such event triggered by textured spatiality. Specifically, Margulis explored how parts became constitutive of newly emergent wholes. This was when she spoke of holobionts (whole living beings) living in a variety of different ways together in interdependency. Symbiosis was a mutually beneficial form of cohabitation. For instance, lichens that appeared to be autonomous organisms were in fact a composite of symbiotically cohabitating fungi and algae.

There is a fine line between symbiotic relations, such as those between trees and mycorrhiza (e.g. Tsing 2012), and parasitic relations. Contrary to general opinion, orchids living in the sunny habitat of the trees' canopies are not parasites, just epiphytes (ibid.). Among the organisms that biologists study, there are many other organismic interdependencies and forms of cohabitation, most not very well understood, as they vary in degree and strength, quality and number. Studying them more closely may provide a source of inspiration to anthropologists interested in figurations of sociality. Inter-organismic interdependencies need not only be metabolic, but often are also structural, architectural or spatial: for instance, organisms that produce cellulose can put others into a structurally elevated position, as in the case of epiphytic orchids on tall trees.

Margulis proposed to speak of symbiogenesis as arising after an extended period of symbiosis or, say, as co-habiting interdependencies between two holobionts that eventually fusion and give rise to a new organism (Margulis 1991). Among those holobionts that were formed through symbiogenesis belong what are today the mitochondria of animal and human cells and the chlorophyll organelles in plant cells. Margulis knew that Russian geneticists had already noted at the turn of the twentieth century that the mitochondria had a different genetic make-up from that of the nucleus of a eukaryotic cell. As the interdependencies between the prokaryotic holobionts were reinforced, so her story goes, they started to live not only in a symbiotic relation with each other. Rather, as holobiont became organelle, they began to reproduce themselves as part of a whole, namely the eukaryotic cell.

Margulis's opponents consider symbiogenetic changes to be restricted to the above, historically unique cases, but Margulis aimed to generalise the term and spoke of symbiogenesis as a principal driving force of evolutionary change and becoming (by fusioning rather than by branching out). Margulis's generalised concept of symbiogenesis is diametrically opposed to the neo-Darwinian insistence on mutation and fierce competition over scarce resources, sexual partners and territory, as the main driving forces for evolutionary change (Margulis 1998).[6]

To explain symbiogenesis, Margulis notably does not use a vocabulary of violence and voraciousness, as would be used in the case of saying that a host cell imbibed a refuge-seeking guest. Her point is that the protection-providing holobiont, that is, what was to become the eukaryotic cell, was also transformed through the process. Guest and host eventually became a new whole, namely a eukaryotic holobiont that could not live without its organelles. The yet-to-be eukaryotic cell was providing shelter, and in the course of doing so was eventually fundamentally transformed itself. Margulis speaks of 'the intimacy of strangers' (see also Haraway 2016). The holobiontic 'strangers' had unusual capabilities, and by eventually giving up their status as holobionts, they transformed into parts of a greater whole. Margulis's interpretation of evolutionary change through symbiogenesis imbues 'the stranger' with the potential of being key in effecting a fundamental change of the status quo. This resonates with some of the insights of Simmel ([1908] 1950b) and Schütz (1971: 91–105).

## Intimacy with Strangers

Margulis did not deny that there was competition for resources, mating partners, offspring, and so on, between organisms, and that this competition affected evolutionary change. However, any biologist who learns about co-evolution will query the Hobbesian view of every individual being in combat with every other on all fronts. Even if organisms may be seen to be driven by self-interest, this does not mean that they have an innate drive to profit-making (Adam Smith), as profit-making is a historically specific, learned behaviour. The nineteenth-century view of humankind being involved in cutthroat competition on an overcrowded planet (Thomas Robert Malthus), permitting the 'survival of the fittest' only (Herbert Spencer), is the rhetoric of a dated ideology. Yet it reinforces the view of human beings as ruthless by biologising their egotism and selfishness, and provides the basis for contested claims such as the 'selfish gene' (Dawkins 1976) or a 'culture of greed' (which is, in fact, not naturally given; Hinde 2015).

'Symbiogenesis' is a concept that is used to explain specific aspects of the evolutionary quantum leap from prokaryotic to eukaryotic organisms. The eukaryotic cell is about one hundred times larger than a prokaryotic cell, such as one of the class of archaeobacteria that are thought to have populated the planet since about 3.5 billion years ago. The eukaryotic cell has a cell wall and cell plasma. Together these provide a nurturing and protective milieu for the organelles that a eukaryotic cell typically houses.

The plant-cell plasma in a leaf, for instance, provided a habitat for a green organelle filled with chlorophyll, which with the energy provided by sunlight could turn $CO_2$ and $H_2O$ into glucose and oxygen. Glucose provided energy for the cell and oxygen dissipated into the atmosphere, thereby transforming it [the atmosphere] into an aggressively oxygenating one. Prokaryotic holobionts sought protection from oxygen in what was to become the eukaryotic cell. According to the hypothesis of symbiogenesis, the green organelle nowadays lodged in the eukaryotic cell would have been a prokaryotic holobiont that sought refuge in the eukaryotic cell plasma from the aggressive oxygen that it itself had produced.

Margulis gathered evidence lifelong for symbiogenesis as a general principle of evolutionary change. With this in mind, let us turn to the discussion of the pots, 'pots' and *pots*, and to the dynamics that an 'intimacy with strangers' may lead to reconfigured wholeness.

## Towards an Ecology of Materials

When Ingold (2000: 352–54) discusses 'skills', he critiques Mauss's body techniques. However, while Mauss can indeed be read as a Cartesian who elaborates on Plato's 'controlling mind and subservient body' (ibid.: 352), the book edited by Nathan Schlanger, on which my understanding of Mauss's discussion of techniques and technology hinges (Mauss 2006b), was to be published six years after *The Perception of the Environment*. In my reading, Mauss outlined an approach that his students would develop into a more full-blown ecological understanding of technology (Hsu 2019), and he did not only adopt the utilitarian approach that continues to be read into his texts.

Meanwhile, Ingold's (2000: 289–319) discussion of skills has obviously influenced my reading of Mauss (2006b) on techniques and technology. I understand Mauss to have made an effort to provide a non-dualist, non-representational, more down-to-earth and lastly more modest account of the concrete diversity of the 'toings and froings' (and what we now call 'doings') that define 'culture' (a concept that preoccupied him).[7] Indeed, as Ingold (2000: 352) skilfully put it, a craftsman's hands and eyes, alongside their tools, 'are not so much used as *brought into use*'. They are patterned by the already given 'dextrous activity', he says: 'intentionality and functionality . . . are . . . immanent in the activity itself, in the gestural synergy of human being, tool, and raw material' (ibid.). Or, in the vocabulary we developed above, a movement's propensities have a texturing effect both on the movement and its surroundings.

So, what happens if we think in terms of an entangled interdependency between Chinese medicine patients, practitioners and pots? One ingenious way to think of similar interdependencies, regardless of whether they are human or non-human, is in terms of a triangle of actants on a quasi-equal standing, each with their own agency and intentionality in the bay of Saint-Brieuc (e.g. Callon 1986). Another way, beyond ANT (actor–network theory), may be Tim Ingold's study of SPIDER (Skilled Practice Involves Developmentally Embodied Responsiveness; 2011a: 89–94). As noted by Ingold (2000: 352–53), such conceptualisations of ontological interdependencies are ultimately indebted to Gregory Bateson (1973b), who in the discussion of what he meant by skills – say, the skills involved in felling a tree – emphasised that one had to account for the system in which they had an effect, such as the triad of man–axe–tree as a dynamic (ecological) system.

Such an ecology of a triadic relatedness is in this monograph projected into the figure–ground image (see Chapter 1, Figures 1.1–1.3; this fascinated gestalt psychologists, though for different reasons), insofar as the shape of the two figures, say in black, is interdependent with that of the white space in between. As repeatedly emphasised, the spaces in between would not be blank and empty. Rather, the white space between the black figures (of patient and practitioner) would refer either to the materiality of a vase (e.g. a medicine pot and its contents) in the foreground or of the 'architextural' stuff in the background (e.g. the spatiality of a consultation room).

## New Materialities

By considering the in-between spaces of the figure–ground images as forming not a vacuum but a space filled with textured and texturing materials – or what people tend to call 'stuff' (in German, *Stoffe*; Ingold 2012: 439) – the well-known paraphrase is brought to mind of the all-pervasive *qi* as 'stuff', which constitutes and actively affects the medicines and the bodily processes they modulate:

> We might define [*qi*] – or at least sum up its use in Chinese writing about Nature by about 350 – as simultaneously 'what makes things happen in stuff' and (depending on context) 'stuff that makes things happen' or 'stuff in which things happen'. (Sivin 1987: 47)

Sivin found in 'stuff' a concise term that accounts for the nondualist experience of 'matter' as being imbued with an intrinsic agency. This understanding of matter is fundamental to Chinese medical theory and practice, still today. So, tactually ascertained events, such as *qi* movements in pulse diagnostic contexts, will be seen to testify to 'materialities'. Vice versa, the 'materialities' I speak of in this book are known to exist due to their tactile sense perception: among people who have learned to pay attention to them, they are socially recognised and bodily sensed phenomena. For our purposes here, the figure–ground image in its entirety is to be comprehended as a whole constituted by such, admittedly contested stuff.

There were two ways according to which I observed people to relate to the material aspects of medicine pots: either as 'pots' (the 'Cartesian' understanding of pots) or as *pots* (as handled and sensed). The *pots* thus referred also to the stuff or materiality with perceived 'affordances' that shaped the relatedness between patients, practitioners and the *pots* themselves. By paying particular attention to salient sensory aspects of the *pots*, that is, the Chinese formula medicines, I aim to provide an account that socialises the medicine pots' material aspects.

In a figure–ground image, it is important to treat 'the interstitial space' – that is, both the material pot or vase in the foreground and the stuff-filled background space – 'symmetrically', in Descola's (2013b) terms, that is, with the same respect and attentiveness towards each of them and ourselves, and as constitutive of the whole situation. We are reminded here that 'humans and nonhumans are different but are not to be regarded as *ontologically* distinct' (Witmore 2007: 546, as cited in Ingold 2012: 430). Accordingly, the figure–ground image depicts an ontological whole within which any modification of the two persons or 'figures' is intricately affected by the modification of the vase or pot. Gestalt psychologists worked with differences in shape, but in what follows, interdependencies in material constitution will be in focus.

Latour (2000a), of course, has long made this point; in his piece on the Berlin key, he highlighted so compellingly that specifics of technology are entwined with specifics of sociality. He showed that the shape of the key was central to shaping the profile of the social relations between the janitor of a housing complex and its inhabitants, for the key was designed such that the housing units could not be locked by their inhabitants, but only from the outside by the janitor. I propose to transpose this sort of social interlocking between janitor, inhabitant and door key onto patients, practitioners and pots. My discussion focuses on the materials of which the Chinese medicine pots were composed and the techniques of applying them, with similarly interlocking social implications.

It is ironic that a schema from the psychology of form (gestalt psychology) will here be used to explain an anthropology of matter and 'new materialities' (cf. Hicks 2010: 73–79). The figure–ground schema is of course too black and white, and too static and schematic, to capture the transformative potential that these new materialities have. Grasseni (2007) proposes thinking *through* materials, Farnell (2000, referred to in Ingold 2012: 437) speaks of 'thinking *from*, rather than *about*, the body', and Ingold (ibid.: 434) underlines that 'materials are not *in* time; they are the stuff of time itself'. The figure–ground schema reminds us that we as researchers also have to become actively involved with what we look at (e.g. by squinting our eyes).

## Technique as Efficacious Action on Matter

Marcel Mauss defined matter through the efficaciousness of the technique that affected it. He interlinked social action, technology and matter through the prism of efficaciousness. This is a compelling way of defining matter, particularly for the fieldworker. As Jean-Paul Warnier (2009) explained, Mauss recognised that matter is socialised through technology that is considered efficacious.

To make this point, Warnier started with a critique of once-dominant ways of thinking about efficaciousness. He first critiqued Claude Levi-Strauss for 'restrict[ing] efficacy to belief, speech, and [the deprivation of] social and emotional support by the group', with the effect that 'Material and bodily techniques/cultures are not taken into consideration' (2009: 463). This critique need not be laboured here, as it has also been made in various guises in medical anthropology (see Chapter 8).[8] Warnier (ibid.: 463) then went on to critique the narrow understandings of technology adopted by the adherents of 'cultural technology' (e.g. Robert Cresswell), as they worked with a narrow and materialist definition of techniques and technology. They embraced an approach opposed to that of Mauss's two outstanding students André Haudricourt (1911–96) and André Leroi-Gourhan (1911–86). It is in this context that Warnier proposed returning to Marcel Mauss himself, whose definition of technique and technology is much broader and more inclusive, and hence very much up to date.

> I call technique an act which is traditional and efficacious (and you can see that, as such, it is no different from the magical, religious or symbolic act). (Mauss [1936] 1950: 371, trans. Warnier 2009: 460)

This definition that links technique to matter is basic to Warnier's (ibid.: 465) insight: 'A subject is a subject-with-its-objects in motion'. It is also basic to the argument of this monograph that treats what Warnier calls 'objects' as *pots* that have a texture and propensity to change in some directions and not in others. Accordingly, what in Warnier's vocabulary causes 'efficacious action' is the reconfiguring of PPP, the patients, practitioners and *pots*. Mauss considered the technical arts, magic, sacrifice, sorcery and shamanistic practice to be mutually associated with one another and to result in tangible effects. For the medical anthropologist interested in accounting for the materiality of traditional medicines through the study of their *pots* with tangible effects, and their otherwise sensed and reported efficaciousness, this broad Maussian definition of technique and technology is indeed very useful.

Warnier needs to be acknowledged for having identified the merits of Mauss's above definition of the technique as 'efficacious action', and for explaining how it differs from 'cultural technology' approaches. In contrast to Warnier, however, who is fascinated by the cognitive sciences, I take a phenomenological anthropological approach to the body. By this I mean that I take peoples' intersubjective appreciation of the medicine *pots* and their tangible effects as starting point for my analysis of the *pots'* sense-perceived efficaciousness that often pertains to non-Cartesian 'new materialities', like *qi*.

Warnier's (2009: 460) rendering of Mauss's technique as 'traditional and efficacious action on matter' is an insightful translation, it opens up research into the 'new materialities'. Brewster's translation reads:

> I call technique an action which is *effective* and *traditional* (and you will see that in this it is no different from a magical, religious or symbolic action). It has to be effective and traditional. There is no technique and no transmission in the absence of tradition. (Mauss [1935] [1973] 2006a: 82)[9]

The definition of 'matter' as that which is affected by the 'efficacious action' of a 'technique' is not mentioned in Brewster's translation. It is a definition that is not easy to grasp. In my understanding, this definition socialises our comprehension of the material world, and allows us to extend the notion of matter to include the 'new materialities'. And it changes our modernist attitude to techniques and technologies, which is to separate them from mainstream concerns and let them be investigated by 'specialists' in 'specialist' departments. Mauss tells us that we engage with techniques in the everyday, and underlines that our technological managing of the everyday is cosmogonic, that is, it generates the cosmos and culture. Mauss's definition of technique works not only with a broad concept of matter, but also with a very inclusive concept of efficaciousness.[10]

Mauss (2006a, b) makes techniques and technology into an instrinsic aspect of the total social fact. On the one hand, he deferred to his uncle, Emile Durkheim, as one of the founders of our discipline (James 1998), but, on the other hand, his work contains a critical edge as well. Hence, he can be read as being in dialogue with his uncle when he says:

> The point however which never has been sufficiently developed, is the degree to which all of social life depends upon techniques. (Mauss [1927] 2006b: 51)

Clearly, Mauss is not a materialistic Marxist here, for whom technology is part of the means of production constitutive of the economic base in a triply tiered social system. For, in another context, Mauss ([1920] [1953] 2006b: 47) explicitly says that the foregrounding of economic pressures is but a very recent development in human history. Rather, the above quotation seems to be responding to his uncle and further developing a train of thought that he had begun earlier. It concerned the themes and topics worth studying for the sociologist-anthropologist:

> The notion of class or genre is mainly juristic; . . . the notion of time [Hubert] . . . the notion of the soul [Durkheim] and . . . too little noticed, the notion of the Whole are mainly religious and symbolic in origin – none of these arguments mean to say that every other kind of notion has had the same kind of origin. We do not believe that. There remain to be studied many other categories . . . . (Mauss [1927] 2006b: 50)

Mauss then goes on to praise Frank H. Cushing's (1892) article on 'manual concepts'. So, when he says that 'social life depends upon techniques', he aims to widen the remit of 'that general sociology whose basic outlines Durkheim formulated quite early' (ibid.: 50).[11]

Mauss's highlighting of the importance of techniques and technologies in order to make sense of cultural change contrasted with the then-predominant explanations drawing on the essentialised 'systems' of religion, language and society. If one worked with such systems of representation, the 'translations' and 'transfers' across their marked boundaries would always be *defective* in comparison to the original. However, in Mauss's view, when it came to techniques and technologies, there had always been mutual borrowing, copying, modifying and re-borrowing. Techniques and technologies easily moved across cultural boundaries. Their movement was, Mauss surmised, in order to bring an artefact to *perfection*. This technical effort was also part of an effort to excel in both the individual's and the social body's doings.

> Techniques are eminently liable to borrowing . . . The human actor identifies himself with the mechanical, physical and chemical order of things. He creates and at the same time creates himself. He creates at once his means of living, things purely human, and his thought inscribed in these things. Here is true practical reason being elaborated. (Mauss [1927] 2006b: 52–53)

It is important to see here that 'efficacious action upon matter' is considered both part of self-creation and part of art and artefact-creation, and that the creation of the artefact and the self cannot be separated from one another. Mauss had what might today be called an embodied understanding of technology (as noted earlier, on the basis of entirely different evidence, by Crossley 2005).

When developing this line of argument, quite intentionally, I suppose, Mauss made no allusion to the connection between matter and form, *hyle* and *morphe*, but reminded us instead of that between *hyle* and *silva*, a connection that Sir James Frazer and Lucien Lévi-Bruhl both had apparently made earlier. He commented on this 'highly interesting' connection, saying among other things: '*Silva* is the germinative power' (Mauss [1939] 2006b: 143). Evidently, Mauss was here emphasising a non-Cartesian understanding of matter, contrary to the then and still predominant view of matter as inert and passive.

So, if one put the material wood (*hyle*) in connection with the living woods (*silva*), Mauss implied, one could see that immanent to *hyle*, matter, are the germinative powers of *silva*. The seemingly dead material *hyle* contained within it the germinative powers of *silva*.

# Part III: Preview

I will use the word *pot* to refer to the ground, that is, both the 'background' and the 'foreground', in a figure–ground image (see Introduction, Figures 1.1–1.3), where the black profile of two people stands out against the white ground, or vice versa. As repeatedly said, this ground, as background, is not to be taken as an empty vacuum but as an animated space filled with tangible things. Or, by the squinting of the eye, a vase or pot can be foregrounded, surrounded by either a black or a white ground. Again, the pot or vase should not be seen as being placed in a vacuum, but as part of a space that is material and animated. Now, if one superimposes the two figure–ground images onto each other, one can note that as the shape of the vase changes, the profile of the two people changes as well. This suggests a direct interdependence between the shape of the pot and the profile of the two people. The pot is now no longer merely a thing transacted from practitioner to patient, imbued with metaphoric and metonymic meanings. Rather, it is part of an efficacious relatedness, where the ground affects the textures of the *entire phenomenal field* thereby reconfigured.

Part III of this monograph explores the material aspects of Chinese medical practice, that is, the pots. It starts by asking: what were the materials with which the Chinese medical practitioners were working? Thus, Chapter 7 discusses different Chinese medicine 'pots' from the viewpoint of biochemistry. It reports on legal and regulatory routines regarding (1) how the information on the packaging related to 'the contents' of the medicine 'pots' and (2) the ways in which the Chinese formula medicines, which epitomised 'integrated Western and Chinese medicine', flouted the principles of a purificatory modernity.

It has been proposed, as Tim Ingold (2012: 434) notes of David Pye (1968: 47) that he opposed objectively known 'properties' of materials to subjectively experienced 'qualities'. He considered sensory experience to be individual and subjective. This view is no longer tenable. 'Signatures', *rasa* (juices) in Ayurveda or 'flavours' (*wei* 味) of the Chinese *materia medica* are 'intersubjectively' known (e.g. through somatic modes of attention; Csordas 1993). Yet even if we compare the so-called objectively known with the intersubjectively known (rather than the subjectively known), the comparison comes close to repeating Whitehead's bifurcation of nature, which Latour (2004) deemed *uninteresting*.

Indeed, as we will see, to focus on the question 'What is matter?' is unproductive insofar as it locks us into a Cartesian account of materials as passive and inert. In this context, the Maussian idea to link matter to efficacious social action and relatedness, caused by an active projection of the body into the world by means of a tangible, technical or technological intervention, promises a more *interesting* analysis.

Chapters 8 and 9 draw on Marcel Mauss's understanding of the technique as efficacious action on matter, which intrinsically socialises matter. In Chapter 8, I ask: how was the different Chinese formula medicines' efficaciousness brought about and perceived? A participant observer can account for tangible effects and other sensory experiences of the medicines' material aspects, and what their respondents say about them. Anthropologists generally work backwards from what they observe in the field. How was the Chinese formula medicines' 'materiality' experienced and perceived?

Chapter 8 treats the Chinese formula medicines as *pots*, that is, as an aspect of what is generally subsumed into a nexus of technique, matter and metaphor that affects an intersubjective, bodily felt sensory dimension. Existent research on the efficaciousness of medicines in East Africa has highlighted, first and foremost, that *distance* enhances their perceived efficaciousness, regardless of whether the distance is cultural, geographical or life-style dependent, and regardless of whether the medicine is a commodity or a force, like *uchawi* (witchcraft/magic).

Potency- and fecundity-enhancing Chinese formula medicines were found to be particularly desired by the Chinese practitioners' East African clientele. What kind of *distance* did they embody? Rather than aiming to explain their perceived efficaciousness through the placebo effect or through homeopathic or contagious 'magic', and rather than studying sound and colour 'symbolism', I propose to expand on languageing events) to explore the extent to which the *materialities* of sound and colour explained their efficaciousness. I will also identify indirectly implied (if not secretly transmitted) and imaginative (if not fantastic) narrative alongside a 'good sense' of the world that the local clientele engaged with in everyday life.

Chapter 9 will focus on 'the Chinese antimalarial', which in 2001 made up more than 50 per cent of over-the-counter transactions. I will first present it as a biomedically known 'pot' and subsequently engage in an analysis that foregrounds important relational aspects of it as a medicine *pot*. Chinese practitioners claimed in a tongue-in-cheek manner that its manufacture was no different from that of other Chinese formula medicines. However, this claim is historically incorrect, as artemisinin was 'discovered' by scientists pursuing a military task (e.g. Zhang [2006] 2013) and not in what looks like a playful 'ethnochemistry' within the field of integrated Chinese and Western medicine. I demonstrate how 'the Chinese antimalarial' changed in chemical composition in accordance with commercial developments in the 'playing field'. My discussion highlights that the regulatory and legal developments of late-liberal health markets affected not merely the *social* but also the *material* lives of drugs. There are, accordingly, close interdependencies between the materiality of the medicines and the historically evolving playing fields in which they play a social role.

# Notes

1. Merleau-Ponty defines life not in the modernist, biologistic sense as the span of a single organism between birth and death. Rather, life is a 'general project', marked by a 'blind adherence to the world' (1962: 254).
2. A Cartesian would have us see material things ('pots') in a space conceived as an empty container, within which the material things are arbitrarily assembled. However, in the context of trying to explain the sensory efficaciousness of medical treatments in terms of 'empotment', the usefulness of this Euclidean conception of space is queried.
3. Autopoiesis is discussed at greater length below in regard to 'holobionts'. Automorphic symmetries are discussed in a separate section in the Introduction as relevant to all spatial texturing, irrelevant of size and scale, animateness or inanimateness. Sympoiesis, which expands on autopoiesis (Haraway 2016), and self-similarity as discussed in anthropology (Mosko and Damon 2005), also called fractal geometry, are not much developed here.
4. 'The outline of my body is a frontier which ordinary spatial relations do not cross' (italics added, Merleau-Ponty 1962: 98).

5. Latour (2004: 205–14) misleadingly uses the word 'phenomenological' as though it designates 'subjective experience' (contrasting with objective knowledge and 'physiology'), for instance when he contrasts the 'physiological' and the 'phenomenological' body (ibid.: 208). This is confusing. Latour also speaks of 'subjective embodiment' as 'the phenomenological body' (ibid.: 207) and of 'the trough of ordinary "body talk", broken into physiology and phenomenology . . .' (ibid.: 214). In these phrases Latour seems to reproduce and reinforce the dualistic understanding of the Cartesian body. This misrepresents and belittles the philosophical project(s) of phenomenology.
6. In line with earlier critiques, Lynn Margulis (1998) points out that the phrase 'survival of the fittest', to which Darwinism is often mistakenly reduced, is a) pleonastic and b) Herbert Spencer's, not Charles Darwin's.
7. As an anthropologist, Ingold is naturally also concerned with cultural issues; his concern has been to break down dualisms between culture and nature, animals and humans, innate 'instincts' and learned skills, and so on. I use the term 'technique' (mostly in the sense of Ingold's 'skills') because the literature uses it not only in a narrow sense (as Ingold 2000: 352 deplored), but also in a more embodied and inclusive sense (see Crossley 2005).
8. The difference between healing through narrative and interpretive efforts (affecting the mind) and curing through surgery or pharmaceuticals (affecting the physical body), which initially brought focus into the project of medical anthropology, is today experienced as a club foot by researchers who aim to understand medical efficaciousness beyond the dualistic lens, for instance as a ritual dynamics affecting textures and figurations.
9. Mauss's perspicuous definition of matter, technology and efficacious action is however followed by a rather conventional view: 'This above is what distinguishes humans from animals: the transmission of their techniques and very probably their oral transmission.' (Mauss ([1935] [1973] 2006a: 82). This view is widely queried today (e.g. Ingold 2000).
10. The importance of considering efficacy as a key aspect of health systems was already recognised by Kleinman (1980), but in medical anthropology, the way in which the efficacy of healing technologies has been assessed has insufficiently problematised matter and materials as an aspect of sociality.
11. Note that Mauss speaks of studying 'social life' in place of 'culture' and 'collective representations'.

# Part III
## Pots, 'Pots' and Pots

# Chapter 7
# What Is in a 'Pot'?
## Industrially Produced Chinese Formula Medicines

## Fieldwork: Tackling Prickly Issues

Questions of efficaciousness cannot be reduced to a matter of biomedically approved evidence, and research into them also needs to account for social and cultural, as well as epistemological and ontological orientations. As argued so far, both practitioner and patient are entangled in reconfigurative (ritual/medical) dynamics with *pots* that 'work' on a *homo ritualis* more than a *homo rationalis*. Therefore, insights from gestalt psychology, Merleau-Ponty's phenomenology of perception and anthropological approaches to sensory experience matter.

During fieldwork at the turn of the millennium, Chinese medical practitioners mostly sold industrialised 'Chinese formula medicines' (*zhongchengyao* 中成药) to their East African clientele. These were both reviled (by many biomedical health professionals) and revered (by some of the Chinese practitioners' patients), yet they were easily confused with the Chinese *materia medica* (*zhongyao* 中药) made of 'natural' herbal, animal and mineral constituents. They were all called *dawa ya Kichina*.

Ethnographic research on these medicinal substances was a prickly issue throughout fieldwork. Issues of contention pertained (i) to the packaging: Tanzanian customs inspectors were impeded in conducting routine quality control of imported medicinal commodities as the Chinese script on the packaging was illegible to them. They thus requested a repackaging and relabelling of the imported medicines, or otherwise would confiscate them. Furthermore, (ii) before ARVs became widely available, Chinese-manufactured Western and Chinese medicines, or hybrids, for the treatment of HIV/AIDS – all also called *dawa ya Kichina* – were popular. Finally, (iii) health officials insisted on maintaining a boundary between the medicines dispensed by 'traditional' healers and those prescribed by 'modern' licensed biomedical professionals. So, (i) make-belief through packaging, in particular, for enhancement medicines, (ii) longterm pharmaceutical provision for AIDS care and (iii) the treatment of post-colonial disorders with 'alternatively modern' medications in a health field aiming at 'purification' required considerable navigation skills from TCM practitioners.

To conduct field research in this situation on those prickly issues, I took recourse to the anthropology of material culture and its methods, which included:

(a) *Collecting and photocopying the leaflets in and the text on packaging.* However, no matter where I have done fieldwork, in Africa or China, my friends have granted me the permission to photocopy and photograph only very hesitantly. Photocopies and photographs produce an iconic similarity that qualifies as legal evidence. They are easy to decontextualise. Their thinginess affords quick transmission, reminiscent of the stuff of witchcraft, but it was their serial reproduction and mechanistic propagation that caused the most anxiety.

(b) *Taking photographs of the medicines on display.* I did not make use of this method frequently, as I felt it was too intrusive. Usually, I took a portrait of the practitioner with the medicine shelves in the background.

(c) *Recording in handwriting each medicine's name, indication, ingredients, therapeutic function and recommended dosage, as given on the leaflet or packaging (or both).* This method was awkward but rewarding. Handwritten texts are the fieldworker's personal belongings and not the practitioner's responsibility. I made use of this method only once, while sitting in a clinic's waiting room for a whole week; I recorded over a hundred formula medicines on display in this way. These recordings were not easy to understand, and they started to make sense to me only after I discussed my handwritten notes with

Chinese medical practitioners, in particular one who had a postgraduate master's degree (*shuoshi*).

(d) *Discussions with biomedical professionals and patients* were also valuable.

## Purificatory versus Alternative Modernities

This chapter problematises the modernist biomedical professional's insistence on establishing a boundary between traditional and Western medicine, and on dividing the health field in an effort towards what Latour (1993) has called 'purification', with the aim to marginalise health- and care-oriented practices outside the purview of the modern nation state. Not only TCM practitioners, but also CAM practitioners and local and regional prophets and TM healers were sensitively affected by this (e.g. Nichols-Belo 2018). Transnationally, the insistence of biomedical professionals on maintaining a clearcut boundary between tradition and modernity has been remarkable, and tangibly so (e.g. Ferzacca 2002; Langwick 2006).

The Chinese formula medicines (*zhongchengyao*) were grounded in Mao's socialist vision of 'integrated Chinese and Western medicine' (*zhongxiyi jiehe*) and clearly advertised what has been defined as an 'alternative modernity' (e.g. Knauft 2002a). Manufactured in line with the socialist ethos of integrated medicine as progressive and advanced, they challenged the usual 'purificatory' preoccupations of government officials, who were insistent on being modern by separating traditional from modern medicine.

Packaging, shape, form and appearance are much-discussed topics in the anthropology of pharmaceuticals (e.g. Nichter 1980; Van der Geest and Whyte 1989; Moerman 2002; Pordié and Hardon 2015). Indeed, problem number one encountered in fieldwork was the packaging. For health inspectors it was paradoxical that a 'traditional' medicine was presented in 'modern' packaging, like that of biomedical pharmaceuticals. For customs officials, packaging had to do with trade and commerce, but for Chinese practitioners it also affected medical efficacy. For patients, medicines in hi-tech packaging with glossy materials, such as aluminium foil, plastic, cellophane and the like, were more authentically Chinese. They were more than modern: they were 'advanced' and prestigious. This made them 'more powerful', at least, more so than the white plastic tubs with Swahili labels commonly used by drug sellers on the market. Finally, for the commerce-driven Chinese manufacturers, the capitalist principle of augmenting sales by presenting the same old wares in ever more novel packaging was lucrative. However, if one shipment brought a medicine in one packaging and the next the same medicine in another, practitioners found it difficult to convince patients that it was indeed the same medicine. This is a well-known problem for health professionals (see the authors mentioned above).

Chinese *materia medica* (*zhongyao*) were, in addition, used by a few practitioners who occasionally prescribed traditional formulas composed of ten to fifteen different ingredients. However, this also raised problems. For one thing, the 'natural herbs' were not fresh from the field; *zhongyao* are in fact 'cultural artefacts', as they have been handled and processed in many ways (Hsu 2010b). The Chinese *materia medica* on offer in East Africa had been deep-frozen and ground to a powder. As they were stored in plastic tubs, they did not appear to be a natural product. Second, biomedical regulators required a chemical identification of each chemical compound contained in a medicine. But these requirements were impossible to meet, as already noted, as Chinese *materia medica* are derived from 'natural' organisms constituted by hundreds of chemical compounds. Since Chinese medical prescriptions required practitioners to import a stock of over one hundred different tubs of *materia medica* powders yearly, how should customs carry out quality control?

In this situation of inventing new routines for customs control, stochastics (Lave 1998) provided a practical solution! If the Chinese *materia medica* powders stored in transparent plastic tubs were classified in regard to colour – say eight to twelve colours, which would group the more than one hundred tubs accordingly into eight to twelve groups, customs officers would not feel overwhelmed by their task – it was doable to check a dozen of times a dozen of pots, more so than handling a single load of over one hundred in one go. This ingenious invention by a Chinese TCM practitioner and customs officer who had made friends was a matter of stochastics more than of an empirical research-based or rational classificatory effort.

Colour enabled some sort of quality control; if there was a leakage that led to the growth of mould, or if acid gases got inside the tubs, the colour of some materials would change. However, every Chinese medical practitioner would tell you that while the colour of Chinese *materia medica* does indeed affect its signature, the colour of these powders was, in general, irrelevant. The quality control of Chinese *materia medica* powders according to colour was thus bogus. Given that bureaucratic regulations often made little sense or were impossible to follow, which likely spurred corruption, some practitioners made practical problem-solving via ingenious cheating into a sport.

## Western Medical Physicians Working as TCM Practitioners

A major issue of contention among TCM practitioners, a third of whose education had involved studying Western medicine, was that the selling of Western pharmaceuticals was strictly prohibited for traditional healers. African nation states represented no exception to this international ruling (e.g. Last and Chavunduka 1986; Bruchhausen 2006). However, biomedically trained Chinese practitioners[1] who had extensive clinical experience preferred not to sit the requested exam – hinting at red-tapism.

For this reason, they opened TCM practices instead. This required them to obtain a document from the Ministry of Culture acknowledging their status as 'traditional healers', and a permit from the city council for opening a private business. Accordingly, they were permitted to sell 'natural herbs' but not biomedical 'pharmaceuticals'. As the following subsection will show, most TCM practitioners abided by these rules, although many kept a very small number of pharmaceuticals for strategic use in stock. There were, however, two 'TCM' practitioners in urban East Africa who visibly dispensed large quantities of pharmaceuticals. The respective Ministry of Health officials were well aware of this, and quietly supported them in their endeavour. Why?

Both were biomedical practitioners who called themselves TCM doctors. They had both been trained in the PRC and had many decades of clinical experience. One physician was very welcoming the first day I met him, while the other was more cautious. I passed by the latter's premises many times before he finally permitted me to get a glimpse of the practice; it was for thirty minutes only, as he was very busy. He was a middle-aged Chinese man who had worked in a leading position in a Western medical hospital and then gone into early retirement. His clinic in Dar es Salaam was heaving with patients, mainly women with gynaecological problems, many of whom he treated with sulfonamides. I saw him take the pulse of every patient,[2] mostly however without writing its quality into the patients' notebooks as a traditional Chinese medical doctor would do.[3] Nor did this biomedically trained physician ask his patients to open their mouths and poke out their tongues, as a standard diagnostic procedure of the four methods in TCM would require. He called himself a TCM doctor, yet had access to antibiotics in large quantities (large plastic containers of the generic drugs were openly stacked on his consultation room's shelves). He was permitted to purchase them from Tanzanian health authorities. He explained that his business was co-owned by a Western medical health professional. He did not say that this person was a Tanzanian, but he gave me the impression that he wanted me to believe this. In this case, the Ministry of Health was well informed about his dispensation of biomedical pharmaceuticals, but no health official intervened. He was evidently delivering primary health care in a highly effective way, and health officials approved of it. Every time I passed by briefly to say hello, his waiting room was filled with up to forty mostly female patients.

While sitting by his side during the half hour that I was granted in 2007, I was struck by his authority and professionalism: the friendly manner with which he addressed his female patients and the conversation that he struck up in good Swahili as he gave each patient just about the seven minutes of a standard NHS consultation (in that half hour period). I was also interested in his competencies. They struck me as basically biomedical. So, I asked him again the question that I had asked him previously, which was whether he was a trained TCM practitioner, and this time he said no. He treated mostly STDs – not necessarily HIV/AIDS – with antibiotics, of course, but these were not the only complaints for which he was sought out by patients of both genders. Interestingly, his reputation was not that of a Western medical expert, but that of a TCM practitioner.

This was not bogus, nor outright cheating, as the term *dawa ya Kichina* was inherently ambiguous. This Western-trained physician acted as a *homo ritualis*: he put his patients and himself into an *as if* situation. Had he insisted on the crass truth, he would have acted according to the texturing given for a *homo rationalis*. Meanwhile, *homo ritualis* has a propensity to create and participate in *as if* situations that cannot be further reduced. A doctor who acts also as a healer will particularly appreciate the benefits of this. Whatever ritual procedure *homo ritualis* engages in will have an *as if* dimension, and the dynamics of healing depend on the physiognomic appreciation of a given *as if* situation in its complexity as a whole. This is not to say that there is no deception, lying or falseness, but like 'true' love and 'complete' commitment, for *homo ritualis*, statements like 'I am a Chinese medical doctor' take on an *as if* dimension in a ritual procedure that is not to be further queried.

The other Western medicine practitioner who offered TCM services ran a public health clinic in Kampala (mentioned in Introduction). In the brief interview that he very kindly granted me when I passed by his practice for the first time, he explained that he had been sent as a state-sponsored Ugandan medical student for five years to Western medical training in the PRC in the 1990s, and thereafter stayed a few years longer to enrol in a master's course in TCM. He said that this was because during his medical studies, he had been intrigued to witness – with his own eyes – that many patients were successfully treated by traditional medicine. In the ten or so years since, he had built up a private health care centre not far from the main bus station in Kampala. It was packed with health personnel and patients. At the time of my interview in January 2008, he was preparing to transfer from the cramped facilities near the bus station to more spacious premises in another ward of the city.

In this primary care centre, TCM was offered as one among many health care interventions, most of which were biomedical. TCM's efficacy was treated as a matter of fact and not queried. This clinic was known to the health authorities and very much supported by them; it aimed to implement the Maoist vision of 'integrated Chinese and Western medicine', alongside a family planning unit, an immunisation station and other public health services.

Other biomedically trained Chinese practitioners who worked as TCM practitioners were considered to work within the emergent TM/CAM field of the urban South. They treated a wide range of disorders, as their medicines on display showed, and their work amounted to public health interventions. However, health authorities in East Africa did not treat them as biomedical professionals.

## Western Pharmaceuticals Displayed as TCM Formula Medicines

In what follows, I go into the prickly issue of TCM practitioners having pharmaceuticals in stock. Almost all Chinese practitioners displayed medicines on open shelves, usually behind lockable glass doors. In some practices the medicines in the show cabinets numbered fewer than forty, and the practitioners in charge had drugs in stock in other cabinets all over the clinic, for use but not on display. In other practices, the drugs on the shelves were fairly representative of the medications in stock. They included, in many cases, a very limited amount of biomedical pharmaceuticals. Rather than being hidden away in drawers, the pharmaceuticals were openly displayed on the shelves alongside the Chinese formula medicines, sometimes in glass bottles with no labels. The hope was that a health inspector would overlook these.

After repeated visits, one practitioner in Tanzania and two in Kenya gave me permission to record all the medicines that they had on open display. The formula medicines, *zhongchengyao*, in those three clinics ranged between seventy and one hundred different kinds. In addition to formula medicines, another two practitioners in Kenya displayed about two hundred different kinds of traditional *zhongyao* in powder form in plastic tubs. The deep freezing of the dried *materia medica* reduced their potency, I was told, but made them fit for the tropics; they were less prone to rot and grow mouldy. Finally, there were also two practitioners on Zanzibar – one on Unguja island, the other on Pemba island – and they too allowed me to record the formula medicines on display in their practices; their stocks of medicines were not as impressive, however, and numbered at most forty. All these practitioners admitted to stocking a small number of Chinese-manufactured biomedical pharmaceuticals. These were generally not dispensed on their own (they were often more expensive than the other brands available in East Africa), but tended to be strategically utilised in combination with the formula medicines.

In what follows, I discuss just one practitioner, who set up a practice in a popular neighbourhood. She even allowed me to photograph her entire stock on display. In her practice, almost all drugs were offered in locally sourced white plastic bottles, with handwritten or typescript labels. They provided the name of the medicine, the condition for which it was indicated, dosage and expiry date. She had repackaged the medicines, she explained (in April 2003), because it would enable her to sell them in small quantities affordable to her clientele. The packaging and appearance of the Chinese formula medicines she sold was thus very similar to that of the usual pharmaceuticals one can get in the informal sector elsewhere, at bus stations and markets. Unlike other Chinese practitioners, she felt that this similarity in presentation was advantageous, as her business was thereby familiar to common folk.

The medicines on display she had grouped as follows (according to labels in Chinese stuck onto the shelving): medicines for treating diabetes; for enhancing (male) *yang* potency; for treating asthma, stomach ulcers, obesity, skin problems, rheumatism, coughs, women's problems, toothache, athlete's foot, liver inflammations, heart problems, colds, high blood pressure, epilepsy and malaria; 'supplementing medicines' (*buyao* 补药), such as ginseng and immune-system boosters for treating HIV/AIDS; drugs for urinary tract infections; and anti-inflammatory drugs. Several medicines were Chinese formula drugs, while others were Western pharmaceuticals. Yet others were Western alternative medicines, such as a bottle of evening primrose and a cream of aloe vera.

Furthermore, this TCM practitioner sold vitamin C, aspirin, No-flu, Ceez Cold, various Western biomedical antimalarials, herbal soaps, Viagra and Venegra (sildenafil citrate, which also treats erectile dysfunction). The evening primrose, Ceez Cold and Venegra she sold on behalf of an 'Indian woman', she explained, who worked at a herbal health care centre nearby. From studying the photos that she allowed me to take, one can guess that she displayed about 120 different medicines. Of the thirty-three medicines that I recorded, she commented that about sixteen were Western medical pharmaceuticals. It was difficult to gauge the ratio of traditional versus Western medicines among the remainder.

This was the only practice among the thirty to forty practices that I visited in Kenya and Tanzania that had so many Western medical drugs on display, considering that most Chinese practitioners had between fifteen and twenty different kinds of pharmaceuticals, unlabelled, among around one hundred different kinds of formula medicines on display. This is said in awareness that neither the display on a shelf nor the number of over-the-counter transactions can give a conclusive answer regarding any practitioner's use of the medicines, as that depends on their treatment style.

## Simple Procedures for Multiple Morbidities: Unregulated Non-Biomedical Treatment of Chronic and/or Terminal Diseases

Members of the Tanzanian Ministry of Health, which at the time was building up a Traditional Medicine Bureau (Langwick 2010), informally expressed a concern with 'traditional healers' in general. This was because they dispensed unregulated drugs for the treatment of chronic and terminal diseases, such as HIV/AIDS. However, traditional medicine doctors working in the urban health field alongside the Chinese medical practitioners saw their role differently. Patients turned to them in desperation, they said. Modern medicine was either out of their reach, financially or geographically, or had failed them, being unable to cure terminal and chronic conditions. Traditional medicine practitioners did not speak of doing 'palliative care', but often gave it.

Some Chinese practitioners explained that they dispensed different kinds of medicines acting on multiple levels. For instance, they explained that their formula medicines were not merely boosting the immune system – say, in order to cause a proliferation of T-cells. Importantly, they said, their medicines strengthened and supplemented the centre (*bu zhong* 补中). In Chinese medicine, the centre (*zhong* 中) refers to the digestive system, and in the Chinese language more generally it refers to the centre of one's existence and personality. Western medicine was good for combatting infections, often in acute emergency situations, while Chinese medicine was good at strengthening the centre, which aided particularly the weakened and depleted, and which ultimately would restore a patient to an enduring level of good health.

The formula medicines that strengthened the centre and self of the chronically or terminally ill were said to be gentle and sweet. They typically contained licorice (*gancao* 甘草), literally the 'sweet herb', which in pre-twentieth-century Chinese formulas had the status of a homogeniser and mediator (Bensky et al. 2004: 732–34). When writing prescriptions, physicians tended to mention it last, after listing around ten *materia medica* that made up a traditional formula, and they generally prescribed it in small quantities. Licorice was not unlike what Koen Stroeken (2008) described regarding Sukuma poly-'naturals' as a 'semantic marker' or a material 'meaning-maker', providing a signature or punctuation mark at the end of a composite bouquet of flavours.

Meanwhile, a newly designed formula, called 'Mocrea', was known to contain very large quantities of licorice (see this Chapter, below). Mocrea was one of the most popular Chinese-manufactured medicines sold in and outside Chinese medical clinics. Some Chinese medical practitioners said that it was a formula medicine, while others vehemently denied this. In the early 2000s, it was in the inventory of Southeast African drug sellers and healers on the streets (e.g. Simmons 2006), but in 2007, towards the end of my fieldwork, it was no longer on offer; very occasionally, however, large dried parts of licorice plants in vacuum-sealed packaging were tucked away, out of reach, in a cupboard, indicative of their scarce use.

## Miti *and Decoctions*

As fieldwork in the suburb of Manzese, Dar es Salaam, in March 2002 revealed, people sought out local traditional healers for all kinds of reasons, and HIV/AIDS was not usually mentioned during a consultation. For instance, to keep skin rashes under control, patients might seek out a healer in the neighbourhood. The healer I worked with was from Morogoro, but he worked in Manzese. His house was inhabited by his numerous wives and their children, and on one side, its corrugated roof provided shelter for his clientele, who would sit on an earthen bench alongside the house's wall while they waited. They would be given big chunks of tropical medicinal hardwood (*miti*) to 'boil in water'. In Chinese medical terms, they were asked to make 'decoctions' of the *miti* at home, and to fuel the charcoal fire at their own expense. This routine of preparing a decoction came close to those undertaken for the 'traditional' *zhongyao* in China, while *zhongchengyao* were generally consumed like the 'modern' biomedical pharmaceuticals. The initial phase of most treatments that this healer delivered, whether patients suffered HIV/AIDS or not, consisted of patients being washed with such a decoction, and it was custom to also drink a few sips of this water before or after washing oneself with it.

Some patients had the procedure done in the healer's compound, while others would repeat it over several days at home before returning the chunks of wood, *miti*, to the healer. Some took shortcuts, bringing several bottles of rose water from a nearby stall by the roadside. The bathing procedure, which worked against bewitchment (as the healers hinted; see also Wreford 2008), had a visible effect on the body, for instance when rashes were visibly reduced, at least temporarily. The boiling and the washing amounted to a cleansing technique. This was a simple procedure for multiple morbidities. It alleviated bodily ailments, and achieved its effects not through make-belief alone. It was a non-biomedical treatment of chronic or terminal diseases, but to call it unregulated would be to miss the point.

### Mzisi *and the Divinatory Tool Kit*

Professionalised traditional African healers, who catered to a more educated clientele, had often been subject to the 'purificatory' processes of modernity. They were adamant that they relied on healing routines quite separate from *uchawi* (witchcraft), and were intent on producing medicine pots that met bioscientific standards. According to Langwick (2008), whose fieldsite was in rural southern Tanzania, *uchawi* was of the past and no longer existed. Likewise, some members of African traditional medical associations made clear that *uchawi* was not the way in which their practices achieved success in treatment.

One such traditional healer invited me to his practice in downtown Dar es Salaam in March 2001. He showed me not only shelves and shelves of clean laboratory utensils, neatly aligned for a laboratory test, but also, hidden away in a solid hardwood box, his divinatory toolkit. When I was slightly puzzled and asked how he thought his medicines worked, I learned for the first time about *msizi*, the ancestors and their ancestral powers. This reminded me, importantly, that *uchawi* was only one alongside many other 'spiritual' powers that could arise from the transgression of social mores and taboos, the evil eye, struggles for authority between elders, moral retribution, ancestral presence, divine powers inherent to a place, and the like. The *msizi* were perhaps invisible, but they were not immaterial; their powers were constitutive of the places they inhabited.

## The Ethnographic Focus: The Chinese Formula Medicines (*zhongchengyao*)

TCM practitioners in urban East Africa were a small and heterogeneous group in the early 2000s. Their activities, in a grey zone of legality due to the above regulations, contributed to 'medical pluralism' (Nichter and Lock 2002). They played on a hybridity that African practitioners kaleidoscopically refractured, mirroring the acronym of TCM in 'modern traditional clinics' (MTCs; see Chapter 1). However, while research into medical pluralism and hybridity plays an important role in countering public health conceptions of the 'traditional' as a bounded entity, it has surprisingly little to say on the specific procedures and materials enacted in 'traditional' medical treatment (cf. Langwick 2010, 2018).

In this section, we explore the rationale underlying the manufacture of the Chinese formula medicines. As we will see, the intention was to recombine different materials and substances, regardless of whether they were derived from 'natural' plant, animal or mineral materials or synthetic chemical compounds produced in the laboratory. The revolutionary Maoist ethos had been transformed into a probing 'ethnochemistry', recombining, trying out and tinkering with different *materia medica* and chemical substances. This heterogeneous composition of the industrially produced formula drugs ostensibly flouted the distinction between the modern and traditional that the regulators so energetically advocated.[4]

Biomedical regulators and many laypersons assumed that 'authentic' 'traditional' medicines were the most likely to be efficacious. The Chinese formula medicines, however, were modernised traditional medicines. Although no one on the street recognised in them an 'alternative modernity' (Gaonkar 1998; Knauft 2002b), they were grounded in a socialist vision of integrated medicine, and their manufacture, distribution and consumption obviously required novel regulatory and legislative procedures. When conducting fieldwork in the 2000s, I did not recognise that the field was in the early stages of a reformulation regime (cf. Pordié and Gaudillière 2014) – or perhaps not a 'regime' in Foucault's sense, but rather a 'regulation multiple' (Quet et al. 2018). Reading these scholars' work ten years later was an eye-opener, *tout court*.

## Asian Reformulation Regimes

Pordié and Gaudillière (2014) opened up entirely new avenues for discussing the materiality of poly-'natural' pharmaceuticals, among which category the Chinese formula medicines belong, as they interfaced with regulatory systems, innovation research and global health markets. Where previous research into Asian medicines had foregrounded epistemological issues, Pordié and Gaudillière shifted the gaze onto the techno-scientific sector. They also mobilised social theory and insights from science studies in illuminating ways.

Pordié and Gaudillière (2014) start by pointing out that the pharmaceutical industries, in countries of both the Global North and South, have experienced a 'crisis of innovation', wherein the screening for new drugs has slumped. They present this crisis as coinciding with a period in which an existent, medium-sized South Asian pharmaceutical industry, in place since the early twentieth century, is experiencing a surge in innovative developments. They speak of recombination practices, standardisation and the dynamics of property rights and patenting routines:

> [W]e examine the social dimensions of the drug-object in association with the technical dimensions of the drug-in-society and use reformulation practices as a prism to do so. (Pordié and Gaudillière 2014: 59)

The products in question are internationally marketed as food supplements and alternative and complementary medicines, or so-called TM/CAM. Medical anthropologists taking a 'social life of medicines' approach are now encouraged to research traditional 'polypharmacies' in the context of drug development, that is, in the laboratory, marketing research institutions, regulatory offices and so on. The focus of anthropological fieldwork regarding the 'complexity of herbal substances and learned knowledge of Ayurveda' is now no longer the bedside, the clinic or the hospital. Nor is its primary aim to account for a 'holistic' approach to illness by documenting how patients, their social entourage and health professionals interact (Pordié and Gaudillière 2014: 59). Rather, based on what has been called 'reverse engineering', a 'reformulation regime' has arisen 'in order to create new "traditional" medical drugs for the biomedical disorders of an international as well as [local] Indian clientele' (ibid.).

This is not a matter of 'integrating' traditional medicines into biomedicine, nor of 'adapting' traditional practices to contemporary routines. The reformulation of a drug involves a recomposition that is based on unique knowledge-prospecting mechanisms and singular industrialisation schemes for the remedies. Thus understood, drug 'reformulation' redefines knowledge and preparation practices, focusing on the properties of complex medicinal materials produced and sold on a mass scale for uses in which medical cultures are mixed.

An essential aspect of reformulation is that it feeds the emergence of an autonomous 'pharmacy' (in the sense of a world exclusively devoted to therapeutic substances) that breaks with Ayurvedic clinical practice, both from a sociological point of view (preparations are no longer made by doctors, but by persons specialising in medicinal plants and their manipulation) and from an epistemic point of view (formulations are ready-to-use mixes for specific indications, no longer *ad hoc* mixes that are part of an individualised treatment regime).

> [T]he mass production of drugs thus tends to simplify and depersonalize the act of healing. This process objectifies medicine by placing the drug at the centre of the clinical relationship (Pordié 2010). These changes coincide perfectly with the needs of the market (Pordié and Gaudillière 2014: 63).

The reformulation regimes under discussion depend on an interlinked national and international drug market, and arise in particular kinds of economic, regulatory and mobility contexts. They make it possible to see that the textures of the 'playing fields' of the medicine pots on sale also affect the material composition of these very medicine pots, and accordingly their perceived efficaciousness. Rather than narrowly focusing on the patient–practitioner dyad, patients and practitioners are in this way viewed as part of a wider nexus within which the materiality of the *pots* is seen to have a transformative effect on the textures of human bodies that are part of the urban landscapes of which they are constitutive.

There was a dearth of anthropological research on the material aspects and the materiality of mass-produced compound drugs in the early 2000s when I conducted fieldwork in East Africa, and in their opening statement, Pordié and Gaudillière (2014) reaffirm this (with regard to South Asia):

> In so-called traditional medicine in South Asia, substances have not ordinarily been prescribed or consumed in isolation, yet the transformation of compound formulations have been comparatively little studied from any position within anthropology or history. (Ibid. 57)

Indeed, by 2014, just a handful of medical anthropologists, apart from Pordié (2008), had written their doctoral theses on the industries effecting the transformation of compound formulations, namely Ayo Wahlberg (2006, 2008a, 2008b, 2012), Ma Eun-Jeong (2008, 2015), Stephan Kloos (2010), Martin Saxer (2013) and Jan van der Valk (2017, then still underway). In addition, there was, particularly in regard to the anthropology of Tibetan medicine, extended discussion on the placebo, precious pills, potent substances and the rituals for empowering them (see Introduction, 'Review of Some Key Texts').

Inspired by this burgeoning research on the new materialities of medicine pots, my research in East Africa – which framed the problem of *Wanderung* (migration) as one of *Wandlung* (cultural reconfiguration), as Marcel Mauss ([1929/30] 2006b) once put it – was from the beginning designed so as to examine the nexus of patients, practitioners and *pots*. My notebooks are filled with detailed information on the materiality of these drugs, as assessed from at least two epistemological viewpoints – Chinese medical and biomedical ones – complemented by occasional jottings relating to the affective dimensions and sensory experiences they afforded. My drawers overflowed with photocopies and leaflets about them. Yet what I lacked was the social theory that would assist me in making sense of my field notes.[5] Pordié and Gaudillière provided it.

## *'Sensory Properties', 'Signatures' and 'Scents'/'Flavours'* (wei)

Pordié and Gaudillière (2014) not only account for the material aspects of the substances that they discuss in pharmaceutically informed and biomedically accurate ways, they also record traditional medical knowledge and knowing. They mention the controversies among their consumers regarding phyto- and synthetic lab-produced molecules; they highlight controversies arising from intellectual property rights, bioprospecting, conservation and biological heritage; they point to the transcriptions and the translations between scarcely identifiable equivalents; they discuss the hurdles leading to the formalisation of economic profit with local communities, benefit-sharing and unequal consequences; and they draw attention to transnational flows of techno-scientific goods and market-building, biotechnological invention and investment strategies. To this needs to be added – for East African ports and harbours in particular – the navigation of corruption (Meier zu Biesen 2018). The materiality of the medicine pots arises from this entwinement of often-contested, if not highly politicised, relationships and social mobilities. However, Pordié and Gaudillière's discussion does not stop here. They also address the problem of the human body and its sensory dimensions. For instance, in the context of discussing the mechanisation and standardisation of manufacturing procedures, they raise the question of how to deal with *rasa*, 'the taste' of traditional medical remedies.

> The issue here is not only to standardize the organoleptic judgement for industrial quality control . . . but to stabilize relations between therapeutic activity and sensory properties. (Pordié and Gaudillière 2014: 74)

In the conventional jargon of a history of science that differentiates between objective tastes and smells, the organoleptic judgement would pertain to the 'properties' of the material aspects of the remedies as opposed to their subjectively perceived 'qualities' (Pye 1968). When Pordié and Gaudillière (2014) use the term 'sensory properties', they are creating an oxymoron, and this hybrid term, in my reading, signals that they disagree with the conventional Cartesian understanding of the sensed world. Taste is not merely in the mind of the individual and 'subjectively' experienced, it is a culturally modulated matter of social disposition (Bourdieu 1984) and, as further specified here, an 'intersubjectively' experienced 'somatic mode of attention' (Csordas 1993).

Accordingly, the *rasa* in Ayurveda (or *wei* 味 in Chinese medicine), approximated in English translation as 'tastes' or 'smells', are socially recognised, even if sometimes only among a small group of learned scholars. They are thus 'intersubjectively' experienced, as a phenomenologist of the body, following Merleau-Ponty, would put it (see also Chapter 6). They are furthermore matter defined by supra-regionally recognisable, but culturally specific, healing techniques:

> These properties are used not to determine the drug's composition but as signatures for specific therapeutic action. (Pordié and Gaudillière 2014: 74)

Pordié and Gaudillière thus arrive, at the very end of their landmark publication, at a point that I will take up as the starting point for our theoretical considerations that follow. The sensory experience of tastes and smells, as just noted in the previous quotation, need not be instrumentalised and reduced to a device that provides information on the Cartesian, biomedically recognised 'properties' of chemical substances. Rather, the sensory is socialised. We learn that 'tastes', that is, *rasa* (or *wei*), are used 'as signatures for specific therapeutic action' (Pordié and Gaudillière 2014: 74). The term 'signature' reminds the reader of medieval astrology and alchemy, and of the interface between so-called 'modern scientific' and 'premodern scientific' chemistry. Like the TCM 'distinguishing pattern' (see Chapter 1) or the 'taskonomy' contained in any 'illness label' of common folk (Nichter 1996), a 'signature' contains information on treatment strategies and tasks for future therapeutic action; these strategies and tasks are both medical and social.

A 'signature' makes the relation between therapeutic activity and sensory experience a social one. In scholarly language, the efficaciousness of traditional medicines is comprehended according to how their 'flavours' or 'signatures' affect the mindful body. To understand the materiality of tastes, smells and flavours, which in Chinese medical terminology are all called *wei* 味, requires therefore research into what they can afford and effect. We need to find an ethnographic approach and a language that can account for these subtle relations.

## Zhongyao *and* Zhongchengyao, *and the Effects of Their Odoriferous Substances*

By working backwards from intersubjectively experienced effects to the techniques of applying the flavours used, one may glimpse how the efficaciousness of these materials was socially produced and experienced. A TCM practitioner, based on the four methods of Chinese medical diagnostics, would inspect the complexion (*wang se* 望色), and the tongue and tongue coating; take the pulse (*qie mai* 切脉); listen and smell (*wen* 闻); and speak with the patient (*wen* 问). They would then write out an individually tailored formula with the right selection and dosage of the components specific to the patient's condition at the moment of diagnosis – the so-called 'distinguishing pattern' – for which a formula would be prescribed, composed of several (around eight to fifteen) Chinese *materia medica*.

As already noted, the Chinese *materia medica* are derived from living matter, mostly from plants and occasionally also from animals and minerals, but those are then subject to a series of highly culture-specific procedures, such as, for instance, harvesting the right parts of the living matter at the right time; physically transforming them by cutting, rasping or pounding them, and sometimes by then drying them in the sun, shade or oven; chemically affecting them by roasting, frying, parboiling or cooking, or occasionally by burning them into ashes; and sometimes adding chalk, lemon, honey or other foodstuffs. The 'poly-naturals' or so-called 'natural' *materia medica* of a decoction were thus crafted, a cultural artefact in themselves (Hsu 2010b). They involved know-how, skill and coordination of complicated procedural steps (Hsu 2014).

A Chinese medical diagnosis of a specific 'pattern' can change within a few days, particularly if the medicine 'worked'. Therefore, practitioners writing out prescriptions would want to see the same patient again within a week, and acupuncturists every other day. Treatment by means of Chinese medical decoctions required time and energy from the patient or the patient's carer at home: the dried *materia medica* first had to be soaked in cold water, then brought to the boil, and finally simmered over a small fire, usually for twenty minutes or up to half an hour. Only then could the medicinal liquid be decanted and ingested. It would typically be drunk while it was warm. The affinity to the boiling of the tropical hardwood – *miti* – is striking. However, since the dried traditional Chinese *materia medica*, as sold throughout China and Southeast Asia, were generally not available in East Africa, people were unaware of them.[6]

The industrially produced Chinese formula medicines, which came in pills and tablets, capsules and boluses, were hygienically packed, and sometimes had a faint odour, but nowhere did they lead to the sense events effected by a Chinese medical decoction. The dried plant and animal parts, and the crumbled minerals, have an odour, sometimes indistinct and sometimes very distinctive. To reiterate, they cannot be called raw materials, but should be regarded as cultural artefacts at an early stage of their social lives when they are still on display in the market stall or in the wooden drawer of a traditional pharmacy.

The odours can be reinforced or modified as the dried materials are soaked in cold water and thereafter brought to the boil, with the steam escaping from underneath the lid of, ideally, the earthenware in which they are decocted. The vapours then spread throughout the entire dwelling and can also linger on for some time. The smells of a decoction signal to the family, or other inhabitants living in the cramped dwellings, that someone is ill, and some inhabitants would know how to read different odours as signatures of specific disorders. Home-based care might accordingly be mobilised and the patient forced to take on a 'sick role'. The penetrating odours of a decoction that is brought to the boil make it impossible for patients to hide even a slight distemper or unwellness, let alone a serious illness or terminal disease.

For this reason, some young women would rather take the scentless 'modern' Western medical pills and tablets in order to not be known to have taken medication. The 'alternatively modern' 'natural' Chinese formula medicines, which came in pill, capsule or tablet form, or sometimes as granulates, and which were in appearance often indistinguishable from the 'purificatory modern' Western pharmaceuticals, would be a desired choice, for instance to combat period pains. In the late 1980s young women would not attend class during their periods, which thereby were inevitably made into a social event, but whether or not they experienced period pain, they preferred not to broadcast it.

Vice versa, the odours of a decoction can be experienced as purifying and uplifting. I also observed that they can be experienced as uplifting by the patient when very ill, but once the patient recovers, the very same scent can be experienced as repulsive. The smells of *materia medica* also differ from the taste of ingesting the decoction. Sweet wormwood (*A. annua* L.) has a very sweet smell, but an infusion of its dried leaves (made by pouring hot water onto them) tastes very bitter. Fever-reducing and antimalarial plant preparations are expected to taste bitter by most practitioners of any phytotherapeutic medical practice (e.g. Etkin and Ross [1983] 1997). Furthermore, the taste of Chinese decoctions is in most childhood memories one of unbearable bitterness. I found that admixed to the 'scars of experience' of having survived an episode of being seriously ill was the memory of sensory events marked by bitterness – scars effected by odoriferous substances that, as Lock (1980) noted long ago, have immense social significance and demand compassion and attentiveness from the social surroundings.

## *Material 'Properties' and Chinese Medical 'Qualities' of New Materialities*

A few TCM practitioners had the training to diagnose Chinese medical 'distinguishing patterns' and prescribe medication accordingly, but most attended to common symptoms or to diagnoses that patients had received in local outpatient clinics, often of chronic conditions like hypertension or diabetes. Chinese formula medicines were considered effective for managing 'pressure' (cf. Strahl 2003, 2006) and 'sugar' (cf. Ferzacca 2004), although peoples' understanding of these conditions was sometimes quite idiosyncratic. In conversation, the colloquial reference to these conditions occasionally included a tinge of personal life experience irrelevant to the diagnosis. In other words, patients presented complaints mostly in biomedical terms, but some meanings central to the semantics of the biomedical term were lost, while new meanings had been added, attuned to the patient's 'local' or 'situated biology' (Lock 1993; Niewöhner and Lock 2018).

The formula medicines were manufactured according to a wide range of therapeutic strategies. Some had been produced on the basis of well-known formulas (*fangji* 方剂) from the scholarly Chinese medical archive. Others claimed to be based on age-old formulas that have to this day remained family secrets. Some were based on age-old formulas but contained innovative elements. Some were entirely new formulas, developed in consideration of either Chinese or Western medical rationales. Some contained herbal extracts that were not further identified, like 'saponins', from one single Chinese *materia medica*. This was rarely the case, as most Chinese medical formulas are composites. Finally, some formula medicines contained a mixture of Chinese *materia medica* and synthetic chemical substances produced in the laboratory; these in particular raised the hackles of the modernist regulators.

In what follows, we shall first investigate, within a Cartesian framework, the (immaterial) information given on the packaging about the (material) contents of the Chinese medicine 'pots'. This information will be given in terms of both biomedical and TCM terminology, based on my handwritten recordings and discussions of them with knowledgeable practitioners. It pertains to what a historian of science might conventionally call the 'properties' and 'qualities' of a formula medicine's material aspects.

The eleven Chinese formula medicines that I discuss below are each exemplary of a different rationale of their reformulation, a rationale identified in discussion with practitioners in a sample of well over one hundred recordings. The list is not exhaustive, nor does the order of presentation reflect any ethnographic reality. Some had the same name, but the ingredients indicated on the packaging were not entirely identical. In other cases, the names differed but their ingredients were identical. The diversity of reformulations was mind-boggling.

Before embarking on details, a caveat is warranted. This is that a reliable account of Chinese formula medicines was rendered difficult because it was not possible to know their exact ingredients from reading the labels and inside leaflets alone. Often, just a few ingredients were mentioned, and dosages were generally not indicated. Intentional misguidance and safeguarding of the secrecy that surrounded some formulas posed further problems. In this context, Chinese practitioners emphasised that formula medicines were commodities to which market rules applied, such as protecting one's 'secrets of commerce' (*shangye mimi* 商业秘密).

The formula medicines 1–11 will now be discussed along a somewhat arbitrary gradient from 'traditional' to 'modern' medical properties and qualities (the numbering is also arbitrary). I first indicate their composition (information I obtained from my expert respondents) and then list the *materia medica* that they contain (information gleaned from the packaging; botanical identification based on Jiangsu Xinyi Xueyuan [1977] 1986). Thereafter, I discuss each of the eleven exemplary formula medicines in more detail, with the aim of understanding the rationale of their composition more clearly.

1. A well-known age-old Chinese medical formula:
   *Liuwei dihuangwan* 六味地黄丸 (Six-flavour Rehmannia pill)
   Composition:
   - *shu dihuang* 熟地黄 (*Rehmannia glutinosa*)
   - *shan zhuyu* 山茱萸 (*Cornus officinalis*)
   - *gan shanyao* 干山药 (*Dioscoria opposita*)
   - *danpi* 丹皮 (*Paeonia suffruticosa*)
   - *fuling* 茯苓 (*Poria cocus*)
   - *zexie* 泽泻 (*Alisma orientale*)

2. A folk recipe that has remained a family secret:
   *Liushenwan* 六神丸 (Six-spirits boluses)

3. An age-old formula with some new ingredients:
   *Sanjinpian* 三金片 (Three gold tablets)

Misleading information given on packaging:
- *jinyinggen* 金樱根 (*the root of Rosa laevigata,* not a standard *zhongyao*)
- (but: *jinyingzi* 金樱子, the seed of *Rosa laevigata*, is a well-known *zhongyao*)
- *haijinsha* 海金沙 (*Lycopodium japonicum*)
- *jinshateng* 金沙藤 (a local herb not listed in TCM textbooks)

Chinese medical doctors who used it suggested its active principle was:
- *shiwei* 石韦 (*Pyrrhosia sheareri*)
- [*guan*]*mutong* [关]木通 (*Aristolochia manschuriensis*)
- *huangbo* 黄柏 (*Phellodendron amurense*)

4. An entirely new formula, developed according to Chinese medical rationale:
*Sanjiu weitai* 三九胃泰, called 'Weitai 999' (Stomach health 999)
- *sanyaku* 三桠苦 (*Folium et ramulus Euodiae leptae*)
- *jiulixiang* 九里香 (*Folium et cacumen Murrayae*)
- *baishao* 白芍 (*Paeonia lactiflora*)
- *shengdi* 生地 (raw *Rehmannia glutinosa*)
- *muxiang* 木香 (*Saussurea lappa*)

5. Entirely new formula, developed according to Western medical rationale:
Mocrea (immune-system booster for HIV/AIDS patients)
- *renshen* 人参 (*Panax ginseng*)
- *danggui* 当归 (*Angelica sinensis*)
- *gouqizi* 枸杞子 (*Lycium barbarum, L. chinense*)
- *gancao* 甘草 (*Glycyrrhiza uralensis*)

6. An extract of a single Chinese *materia medica*, chemically not further identified:
*Danggui jingao pian* 当归浸膏片 (tablets made from *Angelica sinensis* plant extract)

7. An extract from one single plant used in a folk recipe, not further identified:
*Leigongteng jingao pian* 雷公藤浸膏片 (tablets made from *Tripterygium wilfordii* plant extract)

8. Partially purified substances extracted from one single Chinese *materia medica*:
   *Di'ao* 地奥 (Mystery of earth)
   - *zaiti zaodai* 甾体皂甙 (steroid saponins)

9. A chemically produced substance that was originally extracted from dead animals:
   *Niuhuang jiedu pian* 牛黄解毒片 (cow bezoar poison-dissolving tablets)
   - man-made *niuhuang* 牛黄 (bovis gall-stone of *Bos Taurus domesticus*)

10. An extract of a chemically modified *materia medica*:
    *Sanhuangpian* 三黄片 (Tablets of the three yellows)
    - *dahuang* 大黄 (*Rheum officinale*)
    - *yansuan huanglian su* 盐酸黄连素 (berberine hydrochlorid, berberine extracted from *Coptis chinensis*)
    - *huangqindai* 黄芩甙 (baicalin, a chemically modified baicalein extracted from *Scutellaria baicalensis*; a glucoside group has been added)

11. A combination of Chinese *materia medica* and Western medical substances:
    *Fufang luobuma pian* 复方罗布麻片 (Apocynum compound tablets)
    - *luobuma* 罗布麻 (*Apocynum venetum*)
    - *yejuhua* 野菊花 (*Chrysanthemum indicum*)
    - *liusuan shuangjing taiqin* 硫酸双肼酞嗪 (dihydralazine sulphate)
    - *qinglu saiqin* 氢氯噻嗪 (hydrochlorothiazide)

Having listed eleven formula medicines above, which exemplify different rationales of drug composition, the following gives a more detailed account of each in the same sequence. *Liuwei dihuangwan* 六味地黄丸 (Six-flavor Rehmannia pill, no. 1) is a well-known Chinese medical formula that is nowadays available as an industrialised formula medicine. The main ingredients are *shudihuang* 熟地黄 (*Rehmannia glutinosa*), *shanzhuyu* 山茱萸 (*Cornus officinalis*) and *ganshanyao* 干山药 (*Dioscoria opposita*), which all have supplementing effects (*buyao* 补药), in particular on the Chinese medical kidneys (*shen* 肾, not to be confused with the biomedical kidneys, which are also called *shen*; see Sivin 1987: 373–77). The TCM textbook on *The Study of Chinese* Materia Medica (*Zhongyaoxue* 1984: 214, 233, 255) says that these ingredients nourish blood (*yang xue* 养血), solidify roughness (*gu se* 固涩) and enhance *qi* (*yiqi* 益气). The formula also contains *danpi* 丹皮 (*Paeonia suffruticosa*), *fuling* 茯苓 (*Poria cocus*) and *zexie* 泽泻 (*Alisma orientale*), which have discharging effects; they clear heat (*qingre* 清热), disinhibit water (*lishui* 利水) and discharge heat (*xiere* 泄热) (ibid.: 47, 95, 96). As a Chinese doctor commented, *Liuwei dihuangwan* 六味地黄丸 was an ancient formula (*gufang* 古方), based on the Chinese medical principle of 'threefold supplementation and threefold discharge' (*sanbu sanxie* 三补三泄). In this case, the drug's galenical form had been modernised, but its composition had not changed. Both the 'properties' of its biochemical make-up and the Chinese medical, intersubjectively experienced 'qualities' of the industrially produced formula medicine were considered identical to that of the traditional herbal formula.

According to Chinese medical rationale (*Fangjixue* 1985: 104), this formula was to be used for treating the following distinguishing pattern: *ganshen yinxu* 肝肾阴虚 (liver and kidney *yin* depletion). However, the instructions on the package of this drug did not refer to Chinese scholarly medical patterns. Indications for therapeutic usage were given in colloquial Chinese and Western medical terminology, in this case, *shenyin kuisun* 肾阴亏损 (kidney *yin* deficit), which is a colloquial Chinese term. Furthermore, the following symptoms were enumerated: *touyun erming* 头晕耳鸣 (dizziness and tinnitus), *yaoxi suanruan* 腰膝酸软 (the waist and knees feel sour and soft), *guzheng chaore* 骨蒸潮热 (bone steaming and hectic fevers), *daohan yijing* 盗汗遗精 (night sweats and semen loss) and *xiaoke* 消渴, which literally means 'wasting and thirst' and is often considered to be caused by different kinds of *yin* 阴 deficiencies, of which some tend to be equated with diabetes.

*Liushenwan* 六神丸 (Six-spirits boluses, no. 2) was also a frequently encountered Chinese formula medicine. It was said to be derived from a common folk recipe rather than from a scholarly medical family tradition. It was used for treating headaches and sore throats, but the package provided no information on ingredients (a folk recipe is generally kept secret). It was very popular with Chinese and African clients alike. Apart from praising its rapid medical effects, patients also commented on its packaging and appearance. Tiny black-coated pills were contained in a small plastic bottle, and the patient was to take about ten twice or thrice a day. It seemed as though the manufacturers were aware of the 'meaning response' that the more pills, the more efficacious the medicine (Moerman 2002: Chapter 5).

Some scholarly medical families' formulas were also kept secret. One was popular with patients who suffered from urinary infections. It was called *Sanjinpian* 三金片 (Three gold tablets, no. 3). The packaging mentioned the names of three herbal ingredients that in their Chinese names contained the term 'gold' (*jin* 金), namely (a) *jinyinggen* 金樱根 (the root of *Rosa laevigata*), which does not actually belong among the standard Chinese *materia medica* (but *jinyingzi* 金樱子, the seed of *Rosa laevigata*, does (Zhongyaoxue 1984: 256); (b) *haijinsha* 海金沙 (*Lycopodium japonicum*: ibid.: 101); and (c) *jinshateng* 金沙藤, a common herb that does not belong among the standard ones listed in TCM textbooks. However, the practitioner with whom I discussed this formula medicine noted that the ingredients given on the packaging were misleading. They were not important for explaining the efficacy of the formula medicine in Chinese medical terms. He explained that this medicine was likely to contain *shiwei* 石韦 (*Pyrrhosia sheareri*), *mutong* 木通 (*Aristolochia manschuriensis*) and *huangbo* 黄柏 (*Phellodendron amurense*), which disinhibited water and dried out dampness (*lishui shenshi* 利水渗湿). These explanations were to the point and reflected standard TCM textbook knowledge very well: *shiwei* and *mutong* disinhibit water and enable urination (*lishui tongshui* 利水通水), and *huangbo* clears heat and dries out dampness (*qingre zaoshi* 清热燥湿) (Zhongyaoxue 1984: 42–43, 99, 101). The packaging did not provide information on the Chinese medical qualities of the formula medicine, but instead gave as main indications biomedical nosological entities, such as pyelitis (*shenyu shenyan* 肾盂肾炎), infection of the bladder (*pangguangyan* 膀胱炎) and infection of the urinary tract (*niaolu ganran* 尿路感染), expressions that evidently border on colloquialisms. Since formula medicines of the kind were based on a secret formula, it was difficult to know whether any new ingredients had been added. There were several industrially produced variants of this formula on the market.

Some formula medicines were new formulas, but were composed according to a standard Chinese medical rationale, as in the case of *Sanjiu weitai* 三九胃泰, advertised as 'Weitai 999' (Stomach health 999, no. 4). This was used for treating stomach ulcers and other intestinal inflammations, and was extremely popular with Chinese and African clientele alike. It was said to have the effect of eliminating inflammations and stopping pain (*xiaoyan zhitong* 消炎止痛). Notably, this Western medical idiom was given in the format of four syllables, which echoes that of the four-syllabic distinguishing patterns in TCM. The packaging stated, as a therapeutic strategy, that it ordered *qi* and strengthened the stomach (*liqi jianwei* 理气健胃), which is a typical Chinese medical idiom.

Furthermore, this formula medicine was ingenious in that it recombined two well-known herbs that the Chinese practitioners referred to as folk remedies (*caoyao* 草药, *minjianyao* 民间药) with three standard Chinese *materia medica* (*zhongyao* 中药). The folk remedies were called *sanyaku* 三桠苦 and *jiulixiang* 九里香 – that is, Folium et Ramulus *Euodiae leptae* and Folium et Cacumen *Murrayae* – and they were combined with the following three very commonly known Chinese *materia medica* : *baishao* 白芍 (*Paeonia lactiflora*), known for its blood-supplementing qualities; *sheng dihuang* 生地黄 (raw *Rehmannia glutinosa*), known for its heat-clearing qualities, or, as people might say, its anti-inflammatory effects; and *muxiang* 木香 (*Saussurea lappa*), a *qi*-ordering drug considered to reduce bloating (*zhang* 张) and stomach pain. (*Zhongyaoxue* 1984: 45, 120, 234).

Other Chinese formula medicines were newly designed formulas following a Western medical rationale while making use of Chinese *materia medica*. Mocrea (no. 5) was a case in point. Mocrea was a very popular immune-system booster among HIV/AIDS patients in the early 2000s – sold at a price of about TZS 15,000 in bottles that lasted for a fortnight – but it had disappeared from the East African health markets by 2007. Its packaging indicated that it contained *renshen* (*Panax ginseng*), *danggui* 当归 (*Angelica sinensis*) and *gouqizi* 枸杞子 (*Lycium barbarum, L. chinense*; see Zhongyaoxue 1984: 209, 232, 241). As a TCM practitioner explained, its peculiar quality and therapeutic effects resided in its material make-up: it contained unusual amounts of *gancao* 甘草 (*Glycyrrhiza uralensis*). Although licorice, which supplements the centre (*zhong* 中), was not mentioned on the packaging, other TCM practitioners confirmed that Mocrea contained it in large quantities.

Mocrea was arguably not a reverse-engineered Chinese medical reformulation. A Chinese practitioner commented that it contained Chinese *materia medica* but was grounded in a Western medical rationale. In biomedical colloquialisms, it was an 'immune-system booster'. In China it is common grassroots knowledge that ginseng supplements *qi* and Angelica supplements blood. Simultaneously, ginseng and Angelica are treasured Chinese *materia medica*. They are both known to supplement the kidneys, liver and spleen (in this sequence). Strictly speaking, Mocrea was not a reformulation of a well-known Chinese medical formula. Rather, it assembled three well-known supplementing Chinese *materia medica* (*buyao* 补药), and added licorice as a fourth. However, while licorice otherwise works as a harmoniser, and is often added as a semantic classifier in small quantities to a given formula, it was the main constituent of Mocrea. This cocktail of herbal ingredients was sold as a much-sought-after 'immune-system booster'.

Some medicines on offer were constituted of the chemical ingredients contained in one single Chinese *materia medica*. They were called *danfang* 单方. The Chinese formula medicines classified as *danfang*, which means 'simple formula' or 'formula made of only one ingredient', paradoxically formed a rather complicated, heterogeneous group in regard to their chemical make-up. They might contain the plant extract of one single Chinese *materia medica* – as in the case of *danggui* 当归[7] – but they may also contain one single class of chemical substances or one single purified chemical substance extracted from a single Chinese *materia medica*, which thereupon is sometimes slightly chemically modified. *Danfang* were generally considered new formulas (*xinfang* 新方). While single-ingredient formulas do feature in China's medical history (e.g. Hsu 2006a), the *danfang* plant extracts on offer in East Africa had been produced by modern technology. Perhaps, this modern technology was derived from and further developed in 'traditional' European phytotherapy, perhaps not. More research is needed.

*Danggui jingao pian* 当归浸膏片(tablets made from *Angelica sinensis* extracts, no. 6) was one such *danfang*, consisting of an extract of a well-known Chinese *materia medica* (*Zhongyaoxue* 1984: 232–33). It was used for regulating the menses (*tiaojing* 调经) and was indicated in cases of irregular menses (*yuejing butiao* 月经不调) and painful menses (*tongjing* 痛经).

Other *danfang* were derived from folk recipes and locally used plants. One such example is *Leigongteng jingao pian* 雷公藤浸膏片 (tablets made from *Tripterygium wilfordii* extracts, no. 7). It was often seen on display in Chinese medical clinics, and was in high demand. Chinese practitioners used it mostly for treating arthritis and other forms of rheumatism. The fact that it was derived from popular knowledge rather than from the Chinese medical canon did not bother them or undermine their perception of its efficaciousness.

Each of the two *danfang* (nos. 6–7) were derived from dried plant parts from one single Linnaean species. However, the appellation of them as simple formula is misleading as each of these plants contained many hundreds of chemical substances. In general, only a few substances in these plant extracts are known by their precise chemical or molecular structures. For the East African health regulators, plant extracts that contained substances not further identified did not qualify as modern biomedical drugs, as Western medical pharmaceuticals contain one purified chemical substance only, the molecular structure and kinetics of which are known. To what extent single-ingredient formulas may be instantiations of a Westernisation, insofar as a traditional European phytotherapeutic practice may have been implemented as a modern Chinese technology, deserves further research.

Some formula medicines that consisted of only one group of chemical substances were strangely not referred to as *danfang*, such as *Di'ao* 地奥 (Mystery on earth, no. 8). This was known to contain only steroid saponins, *zaiti zaodai* 甾体皂甙. It was on display in more than one medical clinic and was used for treating patients with chronic heart disease, but few practitioners had anything to say about it.

There was also the case of a Chinese *materia medica* (*zhongyao*) that is nowadays said to be man-made (*rengong* 人工), that is, synthetically produced, not from scratch but from bovine bile; it has thus become classified as a Chinese formula medicine (*zhongchengyao* or *chengyao*). This is *niuhuang* 牛黄 (*calculus bovis*, the gall stone of *Bos Taurus domesticus*, no. 9), which is the main ingredient of *Niuhuang jiedu pian* 牛黄解毒片 (cow-bezoar poison-dissolving tablets). Even though this substance was man-made, the drug was not classified as a modern biomedical medicine, as bezoar is not constituted of one single purified substance. Its yellow pills, which looked just like No-flu, were used – just like No-flu – for treating colds.[8]

Furthermore, there were formula medicines that contained purified chemical substances extracted from Chinese *materia medica* that had then been chemically modified. One of these was called *Sanhuangpian* (tablets of the three yellows, no. 10). It also looked much like No-flu, and was also used mainly for treating colds. This formula medicine combined specific material aspects of three well-known Chinese *materia medica*, namely *dahuang* 大黄, *huanglian* 黄连 and *huangqin* 黄芩 (Zhongyaoxue 1984: 41, 42, 70), which all contained the term 'yellow', 黄, in their name. The traditional *materia medica* called *dahuang* (*Rheum officinale*; ibid.: 70), generally used for inducing an evacuation of the digestive tract, was used in combination with others that were entirely new. It was combined with berberine hydrochloride (berberine being extracted from the Chinese *materia medica* called *huanglian* 黄连; often substituted by the herbal *Coptis chinensis*: ibid. 42) and baicalin (which contains a glucoside group on the substance baicalein that in turn is extracted from *huangqin* 黄芩; *Scutellaria baicalensis*: ibid.: 41). In other words, the plant extract from rhubarb (*dahuang* 大黄) was mixed with two chemical substances (extracted from *huanglian* and *huangqin* respectively) that had undergone further chemical modification: from berberine to berberine hydrochloride and from baicalein to baicalin.

Finally, let us turn to the main target of Western medical polemics: industrialised reformulations that combined Chinese medical drugs with substances commonly used in biomedicine – for instance, *Fufang luobuma pian* 复方罗布麻片(*Apocyneum* compound tablets, no. 11). This contained at least two Chinese *materia medica*, namely *luobuma* 罗布麻 (*Apocynum venetum*) and *yejuhua* 野菊花 (*Chrysanthemum indicum*; see Zhongyaoxue 1984: 29, 204), but the combination of them represented a new formula. To the powder of the above two *materia medica* were added two chemical substances, namely dihydralazine sulphate, which is a Western medical drug known to reduce blood pressure, and hydrochlorothiazide, which facilitates urination and can thereby also reduce hypertension.

Health officials in East Africa were concerned about the safety of such 'integrated Chinese and Western medical' combinations. However, the Chinese medicine practitioners with whom I discussed this formula medicine were extremely positive about its efficacy. In their view, it enhanced the medical effectiveness of known Chinese medical treatment, on the one hand, and reduced the side effects of biomedical drugs, on the other. In general, Chinese medicine practitioners were inclined to praise the 'integrated Chinese and Western medical' formula medicines as the most remarkable achievements of contemporary Chinese medical research, as did several of their patients, who reported striking therapeutic effects.

It is important to keep in mind that the composition of the Chinese formula medicines was not entirely new, nor entirely fluid. A dynamic, creative and playful 'ethnochemistry' was reassembling already-known bits and pieces of existent formulas and Western medical pharmaceuticals. We could, on the one hand, speak of a transfiguration and point to the unstable states of balance and fluidity of Chinese medical rationales as they shaded into common, folk-medical and Western medical knowledge and practice. On the other hand, the material culture change instantiated by these medicinal reformulations could also be interpreted as a kind of kaleidoscopic refraction. Solid materials fracture, and the Chinese medical formulas seemed to have broken into groups of different substances that were reconfigured in reverse-engineered reformulations. Their reconfiguration was at least in part symmetrical.

To recapitulate, the above has presented examples of reformulations of 'traditional' Chinese medical formulas. Specifically, I discussed formula medicines produced on the basis of well-known Chinese medical formulas (see no. 1) and age-old family secrets or secret folk recipes (no. 2). Furthermore, some formula medicines were derived from age-old formulas, but contained innovative elements (no. 3). Some were entirely new formulations, developed in accordance with either Chinese (no. 4) or Western medical rationales (no. 5). Some consisted of extracts from the plant parts whence the Chinese *materia medica* was derived. Some contained a variety of substances within one chemical class (nos. 6–8), while others consisted of a synthetically produced chemical substance commonly used in place of the identical chemical substance in a naturally occurring *materia medica* (no. 9). Yet others were constituted of purified, chemically identified substances contained in a plant extract of a Chinese *materia medica*, which then were chemically modified (no. 10). This chemical process was apparently instigated to stabilise the compound or to make it easier to absorb in the digestive tract. Finally, some formula medicines consisted of a combination of Chinese *materia medica* with purified synthetic compounds commonly used in Western medicine (no. 11). This list is not complete, but it gives a gist of the playful inventiveness with which Chinese medical formulas were kaleidoscopically reconfigured.

As is evident from the above, the Chinese formula medicines were a very diverse and heterogeneous group of medicines that exemplified adherence to non-purificatory practices and were derived from a socialist ideology of integrated medicines. They blatantly flouted the regulatory efforts of biomedical health professionals. The chemists who produced these reformulations had evidently engaged in practices of selective borrowing and recombining, trying out, testing and probing. I made recourse to scientific Western and Chinese medical terminology, which, I stress, provided me not with 'objective' versus 'subjective' knowledge, but with a description of these formula medicines' Cartesian properties and their Chinese medical 'intersubjectively recognised' qualities.

## *Material Variability Due to 'Substitutions'*

Reformulation regimes face multiple tensions when commerce has already shaped intellectual property rights, contractual trade agreements and the like. Although the above formula medicines were sold mainly in the informal sector, many were considered effective, as indicated by the many patients who kept returning to Chinese medical clinics. The above eleven formula medicines were not cheap, but neither were they so expensive as to be beyond the spending power of upwardly mobile, middle-class men and women (the price of Mocrea sought for trreating HIV/AIDS was exceptionally high).

In what follows, I will first briefly mention how the material constitution of these reformulations was closely tied up with issues pertaining to the ethos of their marketing. Then, the variability of the material aspects of these formula medicines will be in focus. This variability provided difficulties not only for their purificatory regulators, but also for the anthropologist interested in their efficaciousness.

A dilemma regarding the ethos of marketing was raised vis-à-vis the reformulation called PartySmart in South Asia (Pordié 2015). The private company that produced PartySmart was acutely aware that excessive alcohol consumption belonged in a moral greyzone, particularly among the TM/CAM clientele. Hence it was looking for new playing fields in which more aggressive marketing could be implemented. By slightly modifying its components and chemical profile, a new version of PartySmart was developed to treat certain side effects of diabetes. The tweak in chemical constitution allowed the company to market the revised version more confidently, not as PartySmart, but as a liver-strengthening product in Mongolia. Where drinking, overweight and diabetes were prominent public health issues, the reformulation could be marketed with an ethos of doing good.

The industrial mass production of Asian medical reformulations led to other problems too. Age-old formulas may include rare, expensive and even illegal *materia medica*, which have names and other features that spurn the imagination and may thereby enhance their potency. The pragmatic solution in those cases is called 'substitution'; one substitutes one ingredient with another. This is an age-old practice. Rhinoceros horn can be substituted with water buffalo horn, bear bile with coptis, cow bezoars with synthetically produced molecules of deoxycholic acid. However, substitution can capture neither the powers of metaphor and figurative speech nor the name's materiality of sounds and colours, nor other communicative technologies at play, or issues to do with the variability of the materials that practitioners and patients become engaged with. Samnor, one of the most successfully marketed reformulations of *sowa rigpa*, prompted the following reflections after a jointly held workshop with forty *amchi* (healers) from Tibet, Nepal and China as well as extended fieldwork experience.

> Alternatives to three of Samnor's most problematic components were discussed: two for rhinoceros horn, two for musk and five for elephant bezoar. Almost all of these were accepted by those present as having similar properties to the 'originals', despite their varied sources. Few, if any, of the assembled *amchi* were using the original materials and there was unanimous acceptance of the urgent need to agree upon the most appropriate substitutes for universal use. By combining the three originals and nine substitutes discussed at this workshop alone, 54 variants of Samphel Norbu could be made. The possibilities extend much further given that other materials besides these three may also be substituted, and many of the components can also be varied proportionally or omitted altogether. Thus, several hundred Samnor avatars can emerge from a single written formula. (Blaikie 2015: 14)

Blaikie et al.'s (2015) discussion was motivated by biomedical concerns regarding the medical efficacy of a pharmaceutical. The practice of 'substitution' not only plays to the imagination, but also to material aspects of the medicine and its efficaciousness. Needless to say, the Cartesian rationale that motivates the application of GMP standards was alien to the Tibetan doctors and healers who engaged for centuries in the social pragmatics of 'substituting' *materia medica*; and so have been the principles underlying Chinese medical treatment evaluation by means of RCTs (Scheid and MacPherson 2011).

Meanwhile, the 'substitution' of ingredients in a medical formula, 'traditional' or otherwise, also raises more fundamental anthropological questions. If healing is a technology of a project aiming to reconfigure wholeness, its efficaciousness will be related to how the nexus of communicative technology, materiality and (manual) technique is brought into play. How do those dimensions of lived experience affect the perception and practice of the patients and practitioners, and the materiality of the *pots*? This is a question that we will further pursue at length in the following chapter. However, before embarking on that enterprise, let us pause here and reflect more generally on modernity's texturing of sensuous experiences.

## Reflections: On The Sensory Affordances of Traditional Medicines

In 'Medicines and Men of Influence', David Parkin (1968) commented on an era of rapid change in post-independence economic, political and social life, when cash crops became the 'modern' thing to do. In that article, he discussed inter alia how changes in sociality were entwined with those affecting the materiality of the commodities that became constitutive of new economic playing fields; this, at least, is the reading I give the article some fifty years later.

Among the Giriama on the East African coast, men of influence – that is, the elders – were well known to have a long-standing habit of making use of medicines (*dawa*) to assert their sociopolitical authority (Parkin 1968).[9] But the Witchcraft Act forbade 'the poison' already in colonial times. Its abolition sensitively affected the elders in their efforts to ensure the 'social order' as inherited from their ancestors.[10] As the power of the poison waned after independence, new medicine pots gained potency, namely those acquired from outside the community by those who had the necessary monetary spending power.

The medicines of the Giriama elders had always been deployed for both the purposes of healing and harming. Efforts after Kenya's independence in 1963 to bring these occult practices under control resulted, as Parkin (1968) noted, in an outright 'cleansing' of non-ethnic Giriama healers from the Michikeni district adjacent to the city of Mombasa. Parkin notes that this politically motivated cleansing of powerful elders in Giriama territories was carried out in the idiom of *dawa*, medicine and medicines.

By comparison, the Cultural Revolution (1966–76) in China, which happened at about the same time, and which to a certain extent also arose from intergenerational tensions over political authority, was not carried out in the idiom of medicines. Rather, the Red Guards youth humiliated the veterans of the Revolution of 1949, thereby forcing many into committing suicide (fieldwork, 1988–89). My point is that generational tensions over political authority are common, but their texturing is place-specific. In East Africa, medicines as *pots* seem to have been central to intergenerational conflict, far more visibly than in China (and perhaps other regions of the world). To uphold their authority, men of influence depended on the efficaciousness of their medicines – or at least, as Parkin remarked, they depended on the perception of them as efficacious. However, in the social anthropology of the late 1960s, the theme of 'materiality', and the materiality of medicine *pots*, as sensed and perceived, was not as fashionable as it is today. Rather than investigating how it was possible for the materiality of the new medicines to advertise a new era, Parkin (1968) foregrounded the tensions between men of different ages over sociopolitical authority.

## *Where Did Sensuality Go? Continuities between Post-Independence and Late-Liberal Economics*

In his monograph *Palms, Wine and Witnesses*, published only a few years later, however, Parkin (1972) did foreground how a newly emerging economy involved a change of the materiality of the goods traded, even if their source of production (or, in Marxist jargon, their means of production) – that is, the palm trees – remained the same. To be sure, the Giriama's palm groves did not remain exactly the same over the period of several generations in the twentieth century, and the ecological belt of the palm groves very visibly widened after independence. It had always been wedged between one ecological belt in the coastal area, butting onto the sea, where fishing shaped Giriama livelihood, and another one inland, with grazing grounds for cattle. The reason for the palm groves' expansion into palm plantations was economic: trading with the copra of coconuts enabled the Giriama to become implicated into the rapidly growing capitalist market economy, which was, at least in the short term, lucrative.

I will now ask a question that Parkin did not formulate in this way at the time. This is whether and how the materiality of copra differed from the materiality of the goods previously derived from the palm tree. Copra, which is the white fat that grows hard on the inside of a coconut's shell, was, as a capitalist economy requires, a commodity that was easy to store and accumulate, easy to handle by unskilled labour, and easy to transport and distribute afar. We remind ourselves here that, incidentally, we identified earlier in this chapter precisely these attributes – ease of accumulation, distribution, dispensing and consuming – as attributes of the Chinese formula medicines that in the early twenty-first century were in circulation in urban East Africa.

The good for which the Giriama's palm groves were created in the first place was palm wine, not copra. Palm wine was made from the sweet and protein-rich sap that was taken from the palm's blossom. This wine was required for ritual purposes, for celebrations and parties, in large quantities at a time. This required the owners of the palms to have access to manpower in large numbers at specific, regularly and irregularly given times; men were to be skilled in climbing the palms and taking the sap, women in regulating its fermentation. As Parkin notes, this system of producing palm wine was extremely laborious, required know-how and involved gender-specific, closely coordinated skills following each other in quick succession. In fact, the magnitude of human labour required at some points in time was unpayable. As Parkin points out, marriage politics ensured that the necessary labour would be in place when needed, the implication being that you could ask sons or nephews and their wives to work for you in a way you could not with a waged labourer. In this way, the economic problem of palm wine production was experienced as one of social obligation. In summary, the palm wine was a labour-intensive, individually produced but socially significant good of ritual pre-eminence. In addition, palm wine was extremely pleasurable to drink and had valued psychotropic effects. This sensory dimension was completely absent from the consumption of coconut copra. The Protestant ethic that gave rise to capitalism does not seem to have theorised sensory experience as a social good (see also Howes 2005b: 296: 'The Marxian theory of value notoriously occludes the sensuous or aesthetic characteristics of the commodity form').

## *Heightened Sensory Events, Co-Produced*

Just how sensuous the palm's fresh produce can be is gleaned from a passage that Edwin Ardener (2018: 145) identified in *The Road to Xanadu: A Study in the Ways of the Imagination* by John Livingstone Lowes (1927). The passage caught Ardener's attention in the course of his research into the explorers' language because of its 'peculiar "stretched" quality'. Admittedly, the quotation that follows concerns the delight of drinking fresh coconut juice rather than palm wine, but even so, it can convey the preciousness of the palm's fresh produce, and how it affects the senses:

> But to proceed further, your Majestie shall understand, that in the place of the stone or coornell, there is in the middest of the said carnositie a void place, which neverthelesse is full of a most cleere and excellent water, in such quantitie as may fill a great Egge shell, or more, or lesse, according to the bignesse of the Cocos, the which water surely, is the most substantiall, excellent and precious to be drunke, that may be found in the World: insomuch that in the moment when it passeth the palate of the mouth, and beginneth to goe downe the throate, it seemeth that from the sole of the foot, to the crowne of the head, there is no part of the bodie but that feeleth great comfort thereby: as it is doubtlesse one of the most excellent things that may be tasted upon earth, and such as I am not able by writing or tongue to expresse. (Cited from Purchas, in Lowes 1927: 314, in Ardener 2018: 145)

'The glory has departed from the coconut', wrote Lowes, 'and a prosaic world has relinquished one delight' (ibid.: 315, as quoted in Ardener 2018: 145). This gets at the nub of capitalist economies, and it pertains to economic worlds both after independence and in late liberalism: it is a prosaic world. The materiality of the cash crop was different from the delicious palm wine, which had a short lifespan, as does most fermented produce, which easily can go off.

Copra was bulkier and involved trading with comparatively larger amounts; it was not primarily for the consumption of locals, nor was its materiality directly linked to an immediate sensory pleasure – for it was through money that pleasures would indirectly be sought and bought, after some delay.

Lowes's quoting of Purchas's description of the delight of drinking coconut juice struck a chord with me when I read it in Ardener (2018), fifteen years after myself having had such a delightful experience. I was waiting in vain at noon for transport along the Mombasa–Malindi highway, and I decided to take a walk to what appeared to be a nearby Giriama village. When I arrived at the several houses of the first hamlet an hour or so later, I was exhausted, parched by the heat, and exceptionally thirsty and tired, as I had underestimated the distance of the village from the road and had not anticipated the sun being so glaring. I was offered a coconut. An elder, sitting in the shade of his thatched house, made a hand gesture and had a young man climb up the thin tree trunk in seconds and bring down several coconuts from on high. The sensuous delight I experienced was no different from that which Lowe described! No field diary entry mentions the occasion (why should the sensory experience of quenching my thirst with fresh coconut juice while waiting for transport matter to a medical anthropological study of Chinese medicine in East Africa?), but it is absolutely unforgettable.

To be sure, I drank coconut juice before and after, fresh and not-so-fresh, but it was that very occasion, that 'sense event', that made the coconut juice so very present as a *pot*, not least due to the hospitality experienced. Certainly, my dehydrated condition demanded it, or afforded it. This affordance or demand was generated through my body's projection into the world, specifically the 'stroll' into what seemed to me to be a nearby village. It was a co-produced sense event all round, as it appeared to be savoured by the elder who had ordered the young man to climb the tree (the young man, as custom required, then walked off), as well as by his female kin and children, sitting in the shade of their home and watching me. My quiet, motionless hosts thereby became part of the sense event. As the fluids visibly revitalised me, pearls of sweat appeared on my face, and I wanted to speak to my hosts. They encouraged me by gestures to wipe my face. Alas, we could not communicate verbally, but it was nevertheless a socially charged sense event, one afforded by the materiality of the delicious *pot* that was the fresh coconut juice.

In summary, as in the case of palm wine, the consumption of a traditional Chinese medical decoction was generally linked to very specific and strong sensuous experiences (often remembered as bitter to very bitter). The sense-perceived odours of the decoctions also filled the kitchen and usually the entire house with a very distinctive smell, such that anyone who entered the premises would know that a household member was ill and demanded extra care. Clearly, Chinese medical treatment of this 'traditional' kind ensured care for the patient through a variety of sensed cues.

In the East Africa of the early 2000s, commerce with formula medicines already had traits of the reformulation regime that Pordié and Gaudillllière (2014) described in South Asia. The Chinese formula medicines were advertised as easy to consume, at any time, quickly and inconspicuously. Their manufacture involved waged labour and happened in spaces that were separated from those of patient care. The ease and speed of their ingestion was an aspect of their efficaciousness and was experienced as being in tune with the pace of modern urban life. In this way, just like the materiality of the fragrant palm wine that was changed into the cash crop copra among the Giriama in the 1960s, the odorific and bitter-tasting Chinese medical decoctions were being replaced by shiny, hygienically packaged formula medicines, which advertised an emergent era of care through commerce.

## Notes

1. On Western medical training in TCM, see Hsu (1999: 241–46). It has since been much intensified (see Karchmer 2005, 2010).
2. These notebooks were filled with his fluent Chinese handwriting and, as used to be custom in the PRC, he put them in the patients' care (fieldwork, 1988–89).
3. Jennings (2005) spent 15–18 June 2004 in this practice, and argues that in East Africa TCM practitioners regularly took the pulse. His publication provides an excellent example of what can go wrong when fieldwork is not long-term, nor conducted with the relevant linguistic competencies.
4. This section elaborates on the contents of the modified and revised Table 1 from Elisabeth Hsu. 2009a. 'Chinese Propriety Medicines: An "Alternative

Modernity?" The Case of the Anti-Malarial Substance Artemisinin in East Africa', *Medical Anthropology* 28(2): 111–40.
5. My fieldwork was thick. Hsu (2009a) consisted of three papers in one, and is thus easily misunderstood: first, it discussed purificatory versus alternative modernity (explained above). Second, it investigated the rationale underlying the industrially produced formula medicines (now Chapter 7's ethnographic focus). Third, it gave a voice to those TCM practitioners who argued that the purified substance *qinghaosu* (artemisinin) was extracted from a Chinese *materia medica*, *qinghao*, which is the case, and that its ethnochemistry was therefore no different from other formula medicines, which is a polemical stance. The latter was a minority viewpoint and is historically inaccurate; see Chapter 9.
6. A notable exception was the AIDS patients treated with Chinese medicine in Muhimbili hospital, Dar es Salaam.
7. On the cultural history of *danggui*, see Li (2017).
8. Cow bezoars, extracted from the bile ducts of cattle, contain deoxycholic acid. This is used as a substitute for bear bile, which contains ursodeoxycholic acid (UDCA).
9. Among the Azande, the now-classic 'poison oracle' arbitrated over 'witchcraft allegations' (Evans-Pritchard 1937) as an institution that was as much about divinatory 'fact-finding' as about making socially visible what everyone already knew (e.g. a case of adultery).
10. Waller (2003: 261) quotes evidence from 1909 that elders used witchcraft to control their juniors, and comments that the colonial law was put in place without the intention of undermining this.

# Chapter 8
# What Makes a *Pot* Efficacious?
## Social Distance, and the Potencies of *Pots*

### Fieldwork: Ethnography Interfacing with History

How were people affected by the new materialities of which Chinese formula medicines were constituted? In order to gain a more intricate understanding of the nexus of communicative technology, materiality and (manual) technique, we will focus on the 'affordances' of the sensory experiences that the medicines' materiality elicited. In other words, rather than treating the formula medicines as medicine 'pots' in a dualist way, that is, as medicines with material contents and immaterial meanings, we will relate to them as *pots* that have a materiality that is sensed and that is constitutive of the relationship between the people involved in making the *pots* 'work' and rendering them, in medical jargon, 'efficacious'. We assume, as emphasised above when discussing the ecology of materials (Chapter 6), an ontological continuum between the sensed *pots* and the people handling and sensuously experiencing them.

No effort is made in this monograph to relate the 'natural' properties to 'cultural' qualities, as a researcher interested in proving that TCM is a science in order to prompt its legitimisation for public health would do. While my research dovetails with that of medical anthropologists studying traditional medicines and their specificities, and the problems involved in modernising and scientising them, I am interested in finding ways to understand anthropologically, rather than just medically, how healing is achieved and how (ritual) dynamics work towards enhancing the self's sense of wholesomeness between self and other. Specifically, I am interested in the ways in which a triadic figuration of patient, practitioner and *pots* that transforms the patient's health status becomes part of the spatial textures in which the transformation takes place. I speak of spatialities rather than socialities to emphasise the material aspects of social relatedness.

## Social Distance and the Efficaciousness of the Exotic Other

Susan Reynolds Whyte, who since the 1960s has worked among the Nyole of Uganda, also discussed foreign medicines and stressed their potency in her classic article 'The Power of Medicines in East Africa' (1988). This chapter too is about the potency of 'exotic substances and techniques':

> One of the most striking characteristics of the Nyole medicine men was that they so frequently had foreign experience and used exotic techniques ... The use of exotic substances and techniques was not only recognized, but emphasized. (Ibid.: 225)

The potency of such 'exotic substances' might be explained, as in the previous chapter, through both their biochemistry and biophysics, as well as in terms of their new materiality, as communicated in culturally recognised ways such as odours or flavours – *wei* in Chinese medicine or *rasa* in Ayurveda.[1]

Whyte (1997, 1988) is grounded in fieldwork undertaken in rural Uganda, in Bunyole, starting in the 1960s. Yet during my fieldwork in the early 2000s it still provided a succinct account of the experiences and choices that partially still affected the patients I examined. Whyte underlined the importance of the social pragmatic perspective when she asked what the choices were that people had for managing misfortune and illness. As she explained, they basically had two. They could make recourse either to 'medicines' – African herbal remedies, talismans, Koranic spells or the ingestion of water that has been spilled over the holy script, and biomedical pharmaceuticals – or they could turn to 'the healing powers of elder kin, ancestors, and spirits'. Whyte observed that there was 'a general trend towards treating suffering by the application of substances rather than the ritual manipulation of relationships' that involved kin, ancestors and spirits (Whyte 1988: 217); the latter choice would lead to public discussions with village elders that would likely be embarrassing for the patients and those responsible for them. This dichotomous view of one's options – of either taking a *dawa* or 'doing otherwise' – I also encountered in the urban settings where I did fieldwork in the early 2000s.[2]

A comparison of the above two choices highlights that a 'medicine', in contrast to other forms of transforming an individual's condition of life, 'is a substance that transforms something – for better or worse' (ibid.: 218). A medicine achieves this through powers that are inherent to it, and it achieves this 'without reference to morality, relationships or intention' (ibid.). In this way, medicines differ from the provision of treatment 'through prayer, ritual and sacrifice' or 'harming through cursing or the power of spirits' (ibid.). The fact that 'the power to transform lies within the substance' makes it possible to apply medicines in private, and often also secretly (ibid.: 219). It allows its consumers to be both discreet (as is possible due to the anonymity of the city) and mobile (or hypermobile).

Whyte (1988: 219) noted that 'misfortune caused by senior relatives or spiritual agents requires negotiation, gift giving and sacrifice in a public ritual'. By contrast, 'the response to sickness caused by medicine was more medicine'. In the first case, 'words had to be spoken so that all, including the agent and the victim, were conscious of the nature of suffering, the relationship involved and the transformation desired'. In the second case, 'open confrontations . . . were extremely rare'; and they would be 'between presumed sorcerers and their victims'. Whyte (ibid.: 220) furthermore stated that 'medicines and ritual were actual alternative choices which Nyole faced in daily life'. Accordingly, 'Choosing medicines . . . might be a way of avoiding ritual obligations and inconveniences'.

In order to understand the choice of taking medicines, one has to account for a variety of factors, among them 'push' and 'pull' factors, or tactics, we might say; one cannot just resort to the concept of the 'pragmatic patient'. Push factors include obviation of ritual inconveniences. Admittedly, ritual obligations in the rural Uganda of the 1960s may not have figured as prominently in the urban East Africa of the early 2000s, where relationships have been described as fragile (Mattes 2019) and precarious (Neumark 2017). In informal settlements, people were neither part of tight kinship-based networks of redistribution nor of state-based economies, or if so, only marginally. Economic hardship among these often first-generation migrants multiplied their come-to-stay marriages or, more precarious still, their come-to-try sexual partnerships (Neumark 2017). Needless to say, fragile and precarious social relations enhanced the push factor towards medicine pots.

What then were the pull factors? Urban textures comprised many different peoples living in a complicated fabric of mutual interdependence to manage the everyday, and in this sense, they were interlaced, but simultaneously they were also drawn into a whirl of constant societal movements. In this ethnically diverse landscape, people consulted diviners, prophets, herbalists and, since the early twentieth century, also biomedical professionals, even if they were from another cultural and ethnic group. As 'strangers', the medical practitioners shared only to a limited extent their ethnic group's sociality and morality. Whyte (1988) noted that the strangers' 'otherness' was experienced as both attractive and repulsive. Ole Bjørn Rekdal (1999) went a step further, arguing that once one left behind a structuralist-functionalist framework, one would see that it was precisely their externality that imbued their medicines with great potency.[3]

Rekdal (1999) noted that medicine men – and in particular so-called female and male herbalists – were in most cases not locals who were embedded in their own culture and spoke the language of their clients. In fact, he made this ethnographic observation into a point with which to criticise the history of anthropological theory: structural-functionalism was interested in seeing the cultural and linguistic, religious and medical institutions of a society reinforce each other in their boundary-making. Meanwhile, the efficaciousness of medicines that motivated observed social practices seemed to be multiplied precisely through structural difference and cultural distance. Rekdal observed with regard to the healers among the Iraqw of Tanzania that:

> Many of these healers did not speak any Iraqw, they often had a very limited knowledge of Iraqw culture, and in their divination and healing procedures most applied techniques and employed paraphernalia from their respective home area. (Rekdal 1999: 459)

Whyte (1988: 226), whose work Rekdal (1999) strangely does not mention, had already signalled earlier that the view of 'the African medicine man as a local resident, embedded in his own tribal culture, serving the needs of his neighbours by manipulating the symbols with which they are familiar' may have applied to some situations, but perhaps not even to a majority of them:

> All medicines, in a sense, come from outside so that it may be misleading to make too strong a contrast between Nyole medicine and foreign medicine, or between African medicine and hospital medicine. (Whyte 1988: 226)

Rekdal (1999) argued that herbalists are usually from another ethnic group, while Whyte (1988: 226) noted that all medicines 'come from outside'. Where Rekdal pointed to a socially relevant observation and suggested that social distance was a culturally constitutive aspect of healing practices (in that it heightened their efficaciousness), Whyte appeared to refer to a cultural definition of medicines: they were by definition externalities that an individual had to appropriate, by ingestion, through skin absorption or otherwise, regardless of whether they would do good or harm. Whyte and Rekdal did not argue along exactly the same lines, but they both independently observed that in East Africa, 'cultural distance' imbued medicines with power. Among these medicines might belong those from the bush – which would be culturally distant in that they were from the wilderness of the forest – or medicines of faraway places, like the island of Pemba in the Indian Ocean where the healers were particularly powerful, as I was also told more than once. Or they came from China, which in a spatial and geographic sense, and also in a cultural and linguistic sense (Wu 2021), was perceived as distant.[4]

People in possession of new, externally acquired medicines often challenge an internally given authority:

> The point should not be missed ... that it is people living and working outside the society or having major external contacts who import medicines; and it is often these same people who challenge established authority within the society. (Parkin 1968: 428–29)

Externally acquired medicines by their mere newness intrinsically challenge established authority. They are 'physical commodities subject to [socio-economic] transaction' (Parkin 1968: 428), and thus are eminently suited to entrepreneurial experimentation and to activities that are not kin-specific (Whyte 1988: 226). The impersonal aspect of the transaction of medicines and their individualistic application surely made people who after independence had the monetary power to acquire them perceive them as liberating. However, as just noted, they simultaneously posed a threat to kin-given, internal authority structures. Among their clientele in the late-liberal early twenty-first century, Chinese medicines were seen as a constitutive aspect of a hyper-modern and interconnnected globality. While their perception as 'natural' and 'traditional' may have made them attractive, their geographic and cultural distance made them powerful and their newness rendered them risky. The new, by definition, is unusual, and therefore cannot be treated as ordinary. It is therefore often treated with ambivalence.

Rekdal (1999) also comments on such ambivalent attitudes to the medicine of the stranger: a much-respected healer among the Iraqw was from the ethnic group of the Maanda Uwa. On the one hand, the Maanda Uwa were disdained because they were considered unclean; they married their cross-cousins, which the Iraqw found incestuous, and they ate donkey meat. On the other hand, the Maanda Uwa had provided the apical ancestor of the Iraqw clan, which possessed the greatest ritual expertise and power. Such ambivalence and ambiguity between the unclean and the powerful is generally inherent to the external and culturally distant. Sometimes, the Chinese formula medicines were met with an ambivalence between diminished medical legitimacy and perceived enhanced potency. They gained much of their potency through the ways that patients and practitioners related to them, and accordingly, handled and perceived them. Their potencies transcended biomedical rationales and evidence-based efficacies. Rather, equivalent to the ground in figure–ground images, the different potencies of a *pot* shaped and were shaped by relations to other *pots* and people.

Naturally, apart from this spatially and structurally given position of the externally acquired, culturally distant and morally ambiguous, there may have been further reasons for which heightened potencies were attributed to the medicines of 'the Chinese'. One reason was, no doubt, medical and empirically verifiable: 'the Chinese antimalarial' was in the early 2000s experienced as an extremely potent drug effecting rapid recovery (see Chapters 4 and 9). Another reason may have had to do with the formula medicines' modernist packaging, glossy appearance and quick consumption routines (as discussed in Chapter 7). In addition, there was the general anti-imperialist inclination to be against anything 'Western'. Apart from this anti-imperialist feeling, which explains much of the principally favorable attitudes of many people towards *dawa ya Kichina*, there was in Tanzania also a historically developed predisposition to imbue the Chinese *pots* with heightened potency, and even with 'magic'.

## *Magic and the Efficaciousness of History*

Some people said that 'the Chinese' understood how to do 'magic' (in English) or *uchawi* (witchcraft, when they spoke Swahili) (Dar es Salaam, March 2002). When engaged in road or construction work, the Chinese typically worked at night (fieldwork, Malindi, January 2006). Others remembered the rapid construction of the TAZARA railway line from 1970 to 1975 (Monson 2013). The speed with which entrepreneurial Chinese clinics 'mushroomed' in Dar es Salaam also made people wonder whether magic was involved.[5] At a time when death from HIV/AIDS was a constant presence in peoples' lives, witchcraft was always a possibility, even if it was not openly discussed.

The rapid increase of Chinese medical practices in the cityscape stirred two sensitive areas of Tanzanian health policies, regarding (1) the private practice of medicine and (2) the government's attitude to traditional medicine. These two issues had been sore points for health professionals since the socialist-oriented period of the 1970s and 1980s (Iliffe 1998: 200–19). Even though during the 1990s, Tanzania had undergone structural reforms towards a more health economics-oriented governance, the ethos of Julius Nyerere's health policies still lingered on. It jarred with the Chinese practitioners' entrepreneurial zeal fostered by Deng Xiaoping's policies in reformist China.

In contrast to neighbouring Kenya, where private clinics were commonplace, Tanzanian salaries for medical professionals had been notoriously low, and prominent politicians would launch attacks on individual doctors who had opened private practices in the past. However, as Iliffe (1998: 218) remarked, the bills to close down private practices were difficult if not impossible to implement, and many private practices were covertly reopened after temporarily being shut.

In the 1990s, when the worldwide waning of the WHO led to World Bank economists becoming influential in health care (Cueto et al. 2019), considerable pressure was put on the Tanzanian Ministry of Health to liberalise the health market. The 'take-off' was in 1996–97, and by March 2001 there were apparently over five hundred privately owned facilities for biomedical health care in Dar es Salaam (personal communications, see also Obrist 2006). Incidentally, the first Chinese medical practice in Dar es Salaam was opened in the period of the 'take-off', in 1996.

The Chinese practitioners baffled their regulators and rivals, as they meddled with the historically developed ways in which Tanzanians negotiated prestige in the medical field. They dispensed 'traditional' medicines, but these were handled like 'modern' ones. They worked in the private sector, but their prices undercut the cost of treatment with free essential drugs in the public sector (which in the patients' calculation included transport costs, consultation fees and the additional medication often prescribed).

Social distance thus imbued the Chinese practitioners and their *pots* with an air of efficaciousness. For the patients who visited Chinese medical clinics, *uchawi* existed, but they explained that this was not what brought them to 'the Chinese'. Indeed, as noted on the opening page of Favret-Saada's (1977) classic, witchcraft exits, but always elsewhere, not here. The more distant a person was to a supposedly bewitched victim, the more likely they were to believe that witchcraft was involved (Lewis 1976).

# The Ethnographic Focus: Potency-Boosters and Their Efficaciousness

The busiest clinic on East Africa's Swahili-speaking coast was air-conditioned, spacious and dominated by a long wall of medicines on display. The formula medicines (*zhongchengyao*) numbered close to one hundred, and they were complemented by around two hundred transparent plastic containers filled with Chinese *materia medica* (*zhongyao*) in powder form. This clinic attracted many male customers, who upon entering the clinic directly moved towards the counter and purchased a red box on which was written in golden script 'The treasure of men/manhood', *Nanbao* 男宝). Why were potency-enhancing Chinese formula medicines so desired, and how were their potency-enhancing effects brought about?[6]

## Beyond the Efficaciousness of Evidence-Based Medicine

For some clients, the purchase of Chinese formula medicines implied a transgression – an opening up to the externally offered, which always poses a challenge to the internally established; a curiosity to investigate, explore, discover and uncover the new, the unknown and the risky that promised to be unusually effective. While in the previous chapter, it was fairly unproblematic to establish the 'objective' properties of Chinese formula medicines as 'pots', explanations for their perceived medical efficaciousness required research into their signature and flavour, and their sensuous and socio-sensory aspects. To understand why formula medicines, among which *Nanbao* belonged, were considered efficacious, an assessment of their 'material quality' was ultimately found to be related to an ontological problem, that of 'multiple efficacies'.

Since most anthropologists, myself included, have been professionally trained to think dualistically, reinterpretations of what comes across as a straightforward cultural constructivist account as a phenomenologically motivated account may seem academic, even irrelevant. However, if we wish to understand why people find certain health care choices attractive, such as the purchase of Chinese formula medicines in urban East Africa, a physiognomic account of the ways in which power, potency and the sensory perception of the *pots'* efficacies were negotiated becomes worthwhile. Where a constructivist account tends to relegate perceived materialities that are contested to the mind of the perceiver, a phenomenological approach considers the Cartesian distinction between mind and matter artificial, a *déformation professionelle* that it aims to overcome.

The efficaciousness of Chinese medical treatment derived from the constellation of a situation in its entirety, as textured by its social and political history (see the preceding section) and with transformative potential due to a combined 'propensity of things', shi 势. The *pots* were not merely the practitioner's paraphernalia, that is, they were not merely inert matter, forming an extension of the practitioner. Rather, they were textured by and had the capacity to texture spatiality. So, a treatment that effected healing was not merely a matter of epistemology, but involved an ecology of matter.

## Beyond the 'Placebo Effect': From Medicine 'Pots' to Handled and Sensed Medicine Pots

So, how was the efficacy of the potency-enhancing formula medicines brought about? Health professionals have an easy answer: it is the 'placebo effect'. However, even though 'the placebo' may be easy to understand for biomedical professionals, it makes little sense to a critical medical anthropologist or to many other social scientists. The placebo effect refers to everything that enhances the efficacy of a treatment other than an identified pharmacologically active substance. Accordingly, the above exploration into the efficaciousness of specific historical developments that increased the social distance of the Chinese practitioners would count as research into the placebo effect. Meanwhile, the spatial texturing instantiated by the handling and sensing of medicines cannot, however, be captured by the concept of the placebo effect.

As Chapters 7, 8 and 9 show, the concept of the placebo is best relegated into the realm from which it comes: debates in biomedicine. Its current existence depends on an ingenious set-up enabling biomedical professionals to produce results that are quantifiable, namely the Randomised Controlled Trial (RCT). However, the principles of the RCT are diametrically opposed to those of any good medical treatment, biomedical or other, as they require treatment for each patient to be standard, identical in relative dosage and carried out systematically. Medical care that attends to personal difference, age, gender, mental and bodily constitution, seasonal variation, weather and other environmental conditions should not be practised, and the physician's learning, personality and experience of delivering artful treatment have to be factored out through additional procedures like double-blinding RCTs. The RCT has been grossly misused as a gold standard for legitimising biomedical treatment vis-à-vis TM/CAM.

Having said this, RCTs on TM/CAM treatment have produced interesting medical anthropological research on social anthroplogical, historical, political, economic, and, in particular, epistemological and ontological questions (see Laplante 2015; Grimley Evans 2010; Barry 2006; Waldram 2000; Hsu 1996). Finally, given the specificities of the medical learning put on trial, they have also spurred the refinement of RCTs in interesting directions, within both epidemiology and CAM research (e.g. Witt et al. 2011; Kaptchuk 2010; MacPherson 2004;).

To repeat, the placebo is a useful concept in the context of designing RCT trials. It is a profession-centric term, developed for the purpose of identifying which brand of a product is more efficacious, but it is far from useful for assessing the complexities of healing, or, more specifically in this case, the social and material lives of people attracted to taking contested medication. In the social sciences, the importance of the placebo effect has been grossly overinflated, and several generations of medical anthropologists have been critiquing this (de Montellano 1975; Sullivan 1993; Kaptchuk 1998; Adams 2002; Moerman 2002; Wahlberg 2008a; Hsu 2011; Csordas 2017; Schwabl and van der Valk 2019).

The term 'placebo' by definition devaluates both the practitioner's and the patient's perception and makes them, so to speak, into 'noise' (Sullivan 1993). Plotting a substance against a placebo, one active, the other supposedly inert, disregards the fact that both have a 'meaning response' (Moerman 2002). Having said this, from a phenomenological perspective, no substance is 'inert' (Csordas 2017); all have a variety of 'affordances' or 'demand characters'. Moreover, chemically speaking, the notion of 'one single pharmacologically active substance' is a social construct and an idealised biomedical model that enables the design of RTCs, while in fact the functionality of poly-natural materials is far more complex (Schwabl and van der Valk 2019). Using the placebo effect as a concept to account for these interdependent biologies working physiologically at different levels, in different strengths and with a variety of probable synergies, which in turn are intricately entwined with a multiplicity of socialities, misses the point.

The question of what made these sexual performance-enhancing formula medicines so desirable and seemingly efficacious in urban areas of East Africa will therefore not be answered in terms of the placebo effect. As Alter (2005b) stressed, Asian medicines are a cultural phenomenon not to be reduced to medicalised TM/CAMs. Accordingly, their efficaciousness should be assessed from a medical anthropological perspective that can do more justice to the complexities at stake.

## Beyond 'Sympathetic Magic': Trans-Species Empowerment and Body Ecological Knowledge That Renders Folk-Medical Meats Effective

In the early days of its appearance on the East African health markets, the Chinese potency-enhancing formula medicine called *Nanbao* had packaging that named thirty-one constituents of the powders contained in its bright red capsules, but the more recent packaging mentioned only five of these thirty-one. They were: donkey's penis (*lüshen* 驴肾), dog's penis (*goushen* 狗肾), seahorse (*haima* 海马), donkey hide (*ejiao* 阿胶) and ginseng (*renshen* 人参). The first three ingredients belonged to what the Chinese medical practitioners I consulted called folk medicines (*caoyao* 草药), and the latter two were recognised as traditional Chinese *materia medica* (*zhongyao* 中药). In order to create an effect, the composite of these and other unnamed 'natural' ingredients had to be ingested. This ethnographic observation coincided with the anthropological finding that, in East Africa, the material appropriation of a medicine into a body or place mattered (e.g. Davis 2000, Fayers-Kerr 2019): a medicine *pot* had to be ingested and incorporated into the body. This procedure of 'empotment' would reaffirm social relatedness (see Chapter 3) as well as directly affect the self's positionality and spatiality (see below).

'Sympathic magic' instantly comes to mind, which in James Frazer's (1890: 12) formulation comprises 'homeopathic magic' that works through likeness and 'contagious magic' that works through tactual contact. Much like the concepts of metaphor and metonymy, the concepts of homeopathic and contagious magic bring into play an interplay of immaterial and material procedures. On the one hand, an immaterial force is made present between entities of, in the case of *Nanbao*, animal and human being, and on the other hand, materials are mixed according to a part–whole rationale where, say, a bit of powder from an animal part empowers the human body as a whole. Anthropologists have long identified the moments at which the metaphorical becomes metonymic as being ritually relevant (e.g. Fernandez 1974), and socially charged (Hsu 2016), and pursuing this structuralist avenue of explanation is in many cases promising indeed.

Meanwhile, I was drawn to the perspectival and ontological discussions that have reconceptualised the issues of 'magic' and 'metaphor' within a multispecies perspective (Viveiros de Castro 1998; Descola 2013a). They inquire into trans-species relationships and ask: how can humans become one with an animal in order to gain mastery over it or even kill it, and how can they, through imitation or by 'eating' it, partake in its strength, intelligence, sensitivity and life force? Where Frazer (1890: 11) noted that like can control or manipulate like at a distance, and Taussig (1993: 252) remarked that mimesis collapses self and other into one, Willerslev (2004a) answers his question of how hunters kill their prey by suggesting that in 'the manipulating power that is present in hunters' imitation of prey rests the dual capacity to incorporate its "Otherness" while in some profound sense remaining the same'. Willerslev then goes on to speak of a 'mirroring of perspectives' and 'mimetic' empathy, of trickery and seduction, of indirect speech and wordplay. He thereby softens and subjunctivises the boundaries between self and other.

Hunters must harness themselves against the danger of falling in love, lovingly giving themselves up and letting metamorphosis happen (e.g. losing their hunting skills, and with them, their humanity as hunters). This mode of understanding the hunter killing their prey as a human being meeting wildlife in a seductive way points in an interesting direction. For one, it keeps us within the realm of the formula medicines' kaleidoscopic hall of mirrors. Rather than viewing the ingestion of animal parts as a metonymic appropriation of the animal's metaphorically given potencies, 'eating' and ingestion would accordingly be a way in which one establishes a relation to the animal that incorporates its Otherness, although there is the threat of thereby losing one's own identity. Notably, it is through seduction and trickery, including wordplay, that one can entertain a very close relation, marked by an intimate tension between self and other, in the face of the danger of giving oneself up entirely (as some hunters are known to have done in the past).

When Willerslev speaks of hunters imitating their animal prey, he speaks of encounters between living beings that bring status and honour, nutrition, and enhancement of the self. Yet here we speak of powders of animal anatomy presented to male clientele in a medical clinic by socially distant Chinese practitioners. Meanwhile, the situation is similarly ambiguous– because these medicines are promising dangerous pleasures (see also Beckmann 2015). They are 'ready to hand' (Willerslev 2004b), on offer to be ingested, and for those who take the risk, potentially powerful. Should we assume that the ontology of trans-species relationships makes no difference between the living and the dead? Or, as in the case of consuming butchered cattle meat, between cutting and connecting (Myhre 2013, 2017)?

As medical anthropological research on organ transplants has demonstrated, even when the organs are harvested from the (brain) dead (Lock 2002), organ recipients often relate to the organs in a way that treats them as living things, suggesting that even among patients living in the enlightened West, a form of animism continues to be cultivated (Sharp 2006). This is all the more so in the case of some living donors whose lives continue with drawn out 'scars of experience' (Lock 1980), reaching from their waist to their thighs, and whose loss of one organ (of which there are only two) is often experienced as the loss of *the* life-engendering organ (the East Asian medical 'kidneys' that comprise the reproductive organs) and a general loss of vitality (Shimazono 2014). Evidently, people's feelings – in North and South, East and West – regarding vital energies and matter are not as clear-cut as the semantics of the English words 'animate' and 'inanimate' might suggest.

Returning to the powders contained in *Nanbao*'s capsules, of the donkey's and dog's reproductive organs and of the seahorse in its entirety, one guesses that they would stir the imagination. The flesh of animals known for their long penises, like donkeys, or of others considered sexually very active, like dogs, is constitutive of this Chinese formula medicine. Seahorses apparently engage in extended courting rituals with just one partner during the mating season. Accordingly, imaginative powers regarding penis size, frequency of sexual contact, and complexity and length of foreplay and intercourse must have motivated the manufacturers' choice of the material composition of *Nanbao*. However, one wonders whether this knowledge about the potent powders affected the practitioners and their clientele, and if so, how.

If metaphor and metonymy were to affect meaning-making, the consumers presumably would have to know what the ingredients were of the material powders they ingested. The ingredients were given in Chinese on the packaging, so were illegible to most clientele. Nevertheless, presumably an oral commentary surrounded them.[7] However, even if the East African clientele knew that donkey, dog and seahorse meats were constitutive of *Nanbao*, would they have understood the above cultural narratives about the sexual conduct of these animals? It is difficult to know. A relativist or cultural-constructivist argument posits that in different cultures the same biological species attracts different myths about it. Consequently, the Chinese cultural meanings attributed to them would likely differ from those of peoples in East Africa – but do they?

In this context, the notion of the 'body ecologic' (Hsu 1999: 78–83, 2007b) may become useful, as it attends to historically evolved biological knowledge constitutive of contemporary cultural practices. An argument that considers 'body ecological' knowledge to inform contemporary 'traditional' medical and 'traditional' scientific knowledge and practice differentiates between different qualities of knowledge. For instance, it may differentiate between 'poetry', 'cunning' and practical 'know-how'.

There is a sort of practical know-how that the Marxist revolutionary Antonio Gramsci recognised and wrote about in his *Prison Notebooks* (1971). He observed that peasants in Sardinia, who were not literate, nevertheless were knowledgeable of the lands they worked on through their agricultural tools and handicraft. Gramsci referred to this practical knowledge as 'common sense' (Crehan 2002, 2016) and sometimes also called it 'good sense' (Robinson 2005).[8] Accordingly, it is to be assumed that much 'traditional' medical knowledge is derived from people's close involvement with the natural environment.

There is thus 'body ecological' knowledge that is closely related to commonsensical knowledge, and 'good sense' in Gramsci's terms belongs in the domain of practical knowledge that arises from a close involvement with the environment (Hsu 2010c). This knowledge is not idiosyncratic, but on a certain level of abstraction, some of the practical insights of 'good sense' can be affirmed by modern science, such as the seasonality of respiratory diseases or malaria (Hsu 2007b).

Observations of 'traditional' medical procedures that fall within the realm of body ecological knowledge often are claimed to belong among knowledge that has 'survived the test of time'. In contemporary Indigenous peoples' movements, activists often combine what I have called 'body ecological knowledge' with 'practical know-how' and a 'good sense', which in creatively combined form they then call 'deep knowledge', about nature and environmental change. It is indeed 'deep knowledge' insofar as it is known to them through the histories of the ecologies they live in.[9]

Body ecological knowledge can also surpass the remit of the local, as in the case of the five *materia medica* mentioned on *Nanbao*'s packaging: dogs and donkeys have spread geographically about as widely as humankind has. Both species speak to a 'conjoined' history of 'trans-species relations', according to Haraway's (2003) biocultural perspective on evolution, and to a 'becoming with'. Dogs became a 'companion species' very early on in human history, and donkeys are already documented as 'working animals' in the ancient civilisations of northern Africa, the Middle East and Europe. So, alongside knowledge of these two animals through folklore and myths (e.g. Kovačič 2015) and poetry (e.g. Galbi 2017), which evidently is culture- or region-specific, the men who purchased *Nanbao* are likely to have had some practical knowledge of these animals' sexual behaviours. Whether or not this was the case before the twentieth century in the case of the seahorse is difficult to know, but the seahorse's appearance has a salient finesse and aesthetics that render it frighteningly fragile, and thus alert one's attention to it. Furthermore, it is not impossible that twenty-first-century consumers of seahorse would have seen video clips on the internet of its ritualised courting (e.g. Castro 2013) and its ability to assume either sex. So, the 'sexual conduct' of dogs and donkeys, more so than of the seahorse, would belong to the 'body ecological' and 'deep' knowledge contained within 'traditional' *materia medica*. This body ecological knowledge need not always just be local, but, as seen with dogs and donkeys, can be transregional and transnational.

The few times I asked patients and practitioners what the above three animals stood for (metaphorically), none spoke of sex or sexual conduct. Instead, they said: 'Fertility' (in English). They said this regardless of whether the animal species itself was particularly fertile (seahorses are, but donkeys apparently are not; see Köhle 2018) or whether it was considered incestuous. Transgender allocation of caring roles (as in the case of male seahorses, who care for their young, kept in a pouch) and trans-species fertilisation (as in the case of the union of donkeys and horses, producing the mule) also seemed to make the animals in question interesting for flexibly enhancing both at once: sexual union and fertility. However, if the clients who ingested *Nanbao* were neither aware nor interested in the animals' sexualities, how could the medicine work through the meaning response, the placebo effect, symbols or metaphor?

Enhanced vitality and fertility were certainly attributes of *Nanbao*'s two other *materia medica*. Ginseng is a traditional Chinese *materia medica*, widely known as an energy-booster, as it enhances *qi* 气 (both *yang qi* 阳气 and *yin qi* 阴气), although it is primarily associated with enhancing longevity (Flitsch 1994) rather than sexual endurance. Finally, the gelatine contained in donkey hide, which is a traditional Chinese *materia medica* known as *ejiao* 阿胶, is well known for its blood-supplementing qualities (*bu xue* 补血) and is a prized lozenge, particularly among teenage Chinese girls coming to terms with their menses (Xin Sun, personal communication, Oxford, 2019). In recent years, a black market surrounding the trade in donkey hide has evolved, as prices have been climbing while stocks of donkeys are dwindling very rapidly, in Africa and elsewhere (Maggs 2021). Today *ejiao* would probably no longer be openly advertised on a formula medicine's packaging, as in recent years it has become a conservation issue (e.g. Köhle 2018).

According to Chinese medical rationales, donkey hide supplemented blood-*yin*. It was thought to enhance women's fertility in particular, while ginseng was valued particularly for its *yangqi* vitality-enhancing effects. Chinese practitioners had ready access to this culture-specific medical rationale, unlike their East African clientele. Donkey hide and ginseng were traditional Chinese *materia medica* treasured for either their *yin*- or *yang*-supplementing affordances.

So, as evidenced by the five ingredients mentioned on the packaging of the potency-boosting 'Treasure of men', its material composition consisted three times of 'folk-medical' (*minjian yixue* 民间医学) meats,[10] namely donkey penis, dog's penis and seahorse, and of two Chinese *materia medica*, namely donkey hide and ginseng, that, according to scholarly Chinese medical rationales and popular non-medical knowledge, boosted *yin* and *yang* energies, To make sense of the powers generated in trans-species relations between human beings and the meats of these three animals remarkable for their species-specific sexual performance, it is necessary to remind ourselves of the body ecological knowledge of the two species that are at the core of human co-evolution – the dog and the donkey – knowledge that for this reason is likely transnational knowledge today.

## Beyond Metaphor: How the Sound of Names and the Materiality of Colours Affect Disposition

If metaphor works exclusively through the powers of the mind (Lévi-Strauss 1963: 186–205) and the imagination (Lambek 2014), the materiality of the potency-boosting Chinese formula medicines would be irrelevant. Nor would changes in the material quality of a formula medicine through substitution matter. We are reminded here of the mind-boggling variation of the material quality of a single formula discussed by Blaikie (2015). However, material variability should not be taken as a sign that the formula's material composition was unrelated to its therapeutic outcomes. Rather, medical anthropologists are required to assess a medicine's efficaciousness as afforded by the interplay of meaning-making on multiple levels of material variability. Metaphor, materiality and (manual) techniques are tightly intertwined.

In the case of the potency-boosters, the principle of substitution was no doubt at play. There is always a tension between what is advertised as being in a 'pot' and the materials in the 'pot'. It is difficult, if not impossible, to know how many ingredients are substituted, and with which substances. Were there adulterations? How many? Were there synergies and incompatibilities? Which aspects of the substances mattered in which respects? Were there good years and bad years, different series of quality production? Personalised treatments are known to attend to the physical constitution of patients, their specific likes and dislikes, so-called compatibilities and incompatibilities, the patient's age and gender, and their spending power (Nichter and Vuckovic 1994; Tan 1994; Whyte et al. 2002; Smith 2018). Furthermore, the composition of a formula has an internal aesthetics and structure that affects which ingredients are included and excluded.

We will now look at other potency-boosting Chinese formula medicines and try to explore how their efficaciousness was configured, having discussed in the previous sections the donkey and dog penis contained in *Nanbao*, which tended to elicit from medics the comment 'placebo effect' and from anthropologists the words 'sympathetic magic' or 'metaphor'. To be sure, the donkey and dog penis were co-constitutive of other formula medines too. One of these, called *huarong weixiong* (the label was in *pinyin* only – no Chinese characters were given), mentioned furthermore the penis of the water buffalo, the goat, the horse and the deer, while the formula medicine called *weigewang* 伟哥王 differentiated between two kinds of dogs, a certain *haigou* 海狗 and a *guanggou* 广狗. The power of metaphor as the main potency-booster was generally invoked as relevant to these cases as well.

From a biomedical viewpoint it is rather inconceivable that penis tissue would contain a pharmacologically relevant substance for the purposes discussed. However, if not merely the penis but also the testicles were considered part of the *materia medica* used, this would contain minute quantitites of bodily substances, namely testosterone and other sexual hormones, that in larger quantities than were contained in the formula medicines could have some of the desired effects. Now, incidentally, the Chinese medical word *shen* 肾, above translated as 'penis', as a technical term in Chinese medicine, has the more general meaning of 'kidneys' or 'kidney system'. The testicles are considered part of this 'kidney system', alongside the head's hair, teeth, ears, bones and the waters (urine, but also other bodily waters). This allows for the possibility that, beyond metaphor, the formula medicine also derived its effects partially and in minute traces from material aspects of its constituents, namely testosterone and other sex hormones. Interestingly, not just in Chinese medicine but also according to East African body ecological knowledge, the meat of the penis tends to be considered part of a larger and more encompassing body part. When Myhre (2013) discusses the dismemberment of a butchered cattle carcass among the Chagga of northern Tanzania, the penis meat is subsumed into the body part called *mrite*, which consists mostly of abdominal subcutaneous fat (which, compared to other tissues, is relatively rich in sex hormones).[11]

In other words, not just the imagination, triggered by metaphor, but also the material aspects of the formula medicine mattered. How did the materiality of the formula medicine come into play? To date, this has remained a mystery to me. From a natural-scientific viewpoint, regarding the properties of the materials in question, even if there were biologically recognisable traces of testosterone in the flesh of the testicles (and in fatty abdominal tissue), the quantities would be too insignificant to 'work' on the body according to biologically comprehensible processes. So, at least, I was told by medical professionals in Europe. Meanwhile, it is important to see, along with Holbraad (2007), that not just immaterial powers of mind and metaphor were at work, but that a material manipulation of some sort of 'power/powders' was also at stake. This is the theme that we will foreground in the following.

Another animal associated with virility was the wolf. A brand of a potency-enhancing medicine produced in the Autonomous Region of Tibet depicted, on the cover of a brass box, several howling wolves. In this case, Tibet was clearly associated with the untamed and the wild, and by extension with unbridled virility, a trope that would be understood at least among a Chinese clientele. Brass was an unusual material, and so was the deep-red plush material on which sat one single capsule. The brass had been welded such that the golden Tibetan and Chinese script stood out and went diagonally across the entire cover. In the right corner, there was some smaller script in Chinese that played on the homophony of *xing* 性, meaning 'nature', 'sex', and *xing* 兴, meaning 'joy'. In this play on the two words' homophony, the material aspect of sound carried meaning.

We note that metaphor played with the imagination and interpretation of the capsule's material ingredients in different ways, and that it was not only the names of the *materia medica* that mattered. For instance, as just seen with *xing* and *xing*, sex and joy, wordplay on homophones and their meanings mattered too. This was not a one-off peculiarity particular to this formula medicine's packaging. It is common in Chinese lexicographic traditions to explain the meaning of words through homophones; this has been so since antiquity (e.g. in the *Erya* 爾雅, in Loewe 1993: 94–99). Furthermore, wishful blessings are often given in terms of words that are homophones, as the above *xing* and *xing* might have been read. Alternatively, foodstuffs and other material culture, as indicated by a homophone, are brought into play. For New Year, for instance, one eats a fish, and the choice of one's menu is explained in terms of a homophone: *yu you yu* 鱼有余, 'fish means there will be leftovers, that is, abundance'. Vice versa, mobile phone numbers that contain the number 4, *si* 四, are avoided, as its homophone means 'to die', *si* 死. Or, more chillingly, in commercial fields of late liberalism, textured by an ever-increasing inequality, these telephone numbers are sold at a discount price.

Wordplay of the kind that relates meaning to the sound of a word can also be seen as a way in which, beyond metaphor, material aspects of words are made to matter, that is, if one considers the sound of a word and the voice of a person to constitute a material aspect of a language event. According to Jakobson and Waugh (1987), who were not unaware of gestalt psychology (Köhler 1929), the sounds of names and words strike the listener in a very material, direct and immediate way. Indeed, in regard to healing technologies, it has been noted that people are unreflectedly affected by the pitch of a sound, which, for instance, if high – as in the case of *xing* and *xing* – is experienced as uplifting (Hsu 2012b).

Not only sound, but also colour has materiality, as demonstrated by Diana Young (2001, see also below). The dark red plush material onto which was planted one single capsule had a soft and soothing tactile quality, which was comforting. Meanwhile, satin had a smooth and cooling quality, reminiscent of cool waters flowing, even if its colour was bright red. Here we are not speaking of colour symbolism, but of atmosphere and affect, attitude and a synaesthetic attuning to the materialities of different tactile textures and colours.

The USA, alongside Tibet, is a place that people in China tend to associate with the powerful. The association is not so much with the unruly and wild, however, as in Chinese, the USA is called the 'beautiful land' (Meiguo 美国). One of the formula medicines on sale in East Africa, called 'Kiss me', came in tablets of light blue colour and rhomboid form that evidently aimed to mimick the efficacy of the American Viagra. It had been 'studied and supervised' by the 'Wisdom Development Co. Ltd.' in the USA and was 'produced' by the Pharon Group Co. Ltd. in Hong Kong and the (north-east Chinese) Shenyang Pharmaceutical Co. Some Chinese doctors also sold Viagra; one sold in addition the Indian brand Venegra, which looked much the same – a blue tablet in rhomboid form. Others sold Chinese formula medicines with that appearance, for instance the above-mentioned *Weigewang* 伟哥王 ('power – elder brother – king'). Imitation of the appearance of successful and well-established brands, like Viagra, was one way in which this formula medicine had sense-perceived material aspects that made meaning. According to the Chinese medical practitioners, however, the medicines that imitated the form and colour of Viagra were not considered the most popular potency-boosters.

Pricing mattered too: heightened prices, and the heightened pain of paying those prices, were thought to increase potency. All potency-boosters, regardless of colour, shape and packaging, were exceedingly expensive; one single pill could cost TZS 3,500–10,000, and sometimes clients would purchase potency-enhancing medicines that cost several times this amount. The price of a service boosts its respectability and the expectation of its efficaciousness. The price certainly has a material aspect to it, particularly when it requires a renouncing of other desires.

Newness mattered, as did the sense of wonder, the feel of freshness, the riskiness of venturing into the unfamiliar, the excitingly uncertain and unknown. For instance, in addition to tablets and capsules, there were sprays. Some came in a lipstick-like packaging, a gold tube with a red top for women and a blue top for men. They were called 'Royal oil for women' (*Nüdiwangyou* 女帝王油) and 'Royal oil for men' (*Nandiwangyou* 男帝王油). Not only was pricing prestigous, the users' status was to be so too. The script on the packaging was in Chinese. It tended to be fine golden script, and as already noted, sometimes it stood out physically. Like a ritual language that is supposed to have a transformative effect in the moment that it is enunciated (e.g. Lévi-Strauss 1963: 186–205), the script clearly had its own aesthetics and sensory efficaciousness, although it mostly was not understood.[12] As in many religious spaces, the potent principle is an inner sanctum that is closed to the public and kept secret. Furthermore, its potency is expected to reveal itself only indirectly. Arguably, knowledge about the masculine performance-enhancing medicines, orally communicated in a low voice, well within the reach of one's breath (Hall 1982: 45–49), endowed these potency-boosters with an additional attribute, that of the secret. The secret, as Simmel ([1908] 1950a) noted, asserts an asymmetrical power relation in an eminently social way, simply by inclusion of you and me and the exclusion of a third party.

Some of these Chinese formula medicines were not derived from animal meats, but contained *chong* 虫, which in Chinese has an extremely wide semantic reach, as it ranges in meaning from insects and worms to tigers and dragons. The *chong* are undomesticated, and like a weed, not wanted, yet are elusive and pregnant with life-bringing energies, as is the wind, which was thought to give birth to insects in antiquity (Sterckx 2002: 169–71). Further potency-boosters thus included the bright red 'Heroic Wind capsules' from a place called Qingyang in Henan province (Xiongfeng Qingyang jiaonang 雄风营养胶囊). They contained, according to the accompanying leaflet, four main ingredients: *Epimedium grandiflorum* (*yinyanghuo* 淫羊藿) and *Astragalus complanatus* (*shayuanzi* 沙苑子), two herbs, alongside male silkworm moth (*xiongcan'e* 雄蚕蛾) and the velvet on the antlers of the deer *Cervus nippon* or *Cervus elaphus* (*lujiaoshuang* 鹿角霜). I could comment on the word *xiong* 雄, meaning male, masculine and heroic, on the materiality of colour and the bright red on the packaging, on the materiality of the sound of *yinyang* 阴阳, or on the soft white velvet of deer antlers and the moth antennae that enable extraordinary sensitivity to pheromones.

The above examples have highlighted how the formula medicine's material ingredients were entwined with the meanings of wordplay, how situational humour played into their appearance and packaging, how the pitch and sound in homophonous words would affect a client's expectations on an unspecific and general level, how colour too had materialities – a warm velvet red differing from a dark red plush material or a bright red flow of silk or satin – how the powerful was implicitly associated with the beautiful, how medicines based on direct mimesis were put on offer yet simultaneously denied efficaciousness, and how virility and heroism were evoked not merely through imagery of untamed wildlife, but also alongside the unwanted yet uncontrollable growth of weeds and winds, on the one hand, and an extraordinary sensitivity towards the other's affective state, on the other.

To reduce to a matter of metaphor the different knowledges indexed by a formula medicine's ingredients, material quality and efficaciousness seems reductionist. The material, sense-perceived and instant-effect-inducing material aspects of the formula medicines and their packaging affected the patients on different levels.

Given that these formula medicines were manufactured to compete in global health markets, it was to be expected that the clients would draw on very different repertoires to make sense of them. Accordingly, the names of these medicines may have appealed to some clients for reasons of their semantics, yet to others they may have been appealing merely due to the materiality of sound. Chinese-speaking customers would read *xing* 性 and *xing* 兴 on the packaging as meaning 'sex' and 'joy', while most of the clients in East Africa were likely primarily affected through the materiality of sound: the high pitched *i* in these two words generally has an uplifting effect (Jakobson and Waugh 1987, Hsu 2012b). That the sound of a name is related to the sense perception of the named has been highlighted by ethnobiologists too, such as Brent Berlin (1992), who drew attention to the phonoaesthetics in folk taxa of living kinds.[13]

As already noted, colour has materiality (Young 2005, 2011, 2018). The texture of the materials, their warmth or coolness to the touch, are part of the experience of colour and modulate people's affective states and attitudes. Skilful healing techniques can effect a synaesthetic 'smell of greenness' (Young 2005) or the high-pitched 'sound of enlivening greenness' (Hsu 2021).

In the course of exploring possible reasons for the perceived efficaciousness of the potency-enhancing formula medicines, we started with metaphor and colour symbolism, but eventually turned to a gestalt-psychologically inspired sensory assessment of medicine *pots*. The sensing and handling of the potency-boosting Chinese medicine *pots*, in the interpretation provided here, worked through modulating the clients' affect, curiosity and sensibilities. The materiality of sound, form, colour or texture, in turn, had an affective dimension (Massumi 2015).

Meanwhile, these potency-boosting formula medicines were sometimes also tied into complex therapeutic procedures. As we will see in the following section, some Chinese medical practitioners made use of the formula medicines in procedures attuned to the timing of different therapeutic interventions. The perceived efficaciousness of the potency-boosters, accordingly, hinged on diagnostic and healing techniques that attended to different temporalities.

## *Technologies of Temporality: Boosting Potency through Complex Chinese Medical Procedures*

Chinese practitioners treated the potency-boosting formula medicines as a rare commodity. In many clinics they were chronically sold out. To prevent this from happening, some practitioners made sure that they sold them only if they were likely to achieve a maximum effect. They therefore stuck to the routine of examining the patient first. Very few knew how to take the pulse; most took the blood pressure instead. This often involved the practitioner leaning over the table towards the patient, and usually also a brief physical contact, although touching bare skin was avoided. The procedure was quick and painless (as is the taking of the pulse that results in the Chinese medical diagnosis of a distinguishing pattern).

The male physicians that I worked with were hesitant to speak to me about the issues discussed here, presumably because I was a woman. Fieldwork in one clinic allowed me to take notes on how the TCM practitioner attended to a patient's common complaints, say, asthma or stomach problems. I also observed treatment for so-called *gesi* (gas) or 'indigestion', which was a frequent complaint. Nothing more was verbalised. It was only when standing by the counter, where patients were asked to pay in cash for both the consultation and the medicines they purchased, that it was impossible to ignore the fact that a box of potency-enhancing formula medicines would be slipped into the large brown bag containing the formula medicines for treating *gesi* or similar. Evidently, asthma or heartburn was a comorbidity that negatively affected sexual performance. Some Chinese medical practitioners thus did not just sell potency-boosters but engaged in a diagnosis that would identify a range of problems that impeded the desired sexual performance.

Patients were often found to have high blood pressure. They were accordingly prescribed antihypertensives, when they had hoped to get one of the famed Chinese potency-boosting formula medicines. We are reminded here of the old *mzee* who visited the clinic in Chake Chake on Pemba island, who had scratched together the money for two *Nanbao* capsules but could have obtained an equivalent antihypertensive for free from the nearby dispensary (Chapter 4, 'Nine Farmers'). When I raised this with the Chinese medical practitioner after the consultation, he shook his head. The antihypertensive drug that he had dispensed was more effective. Other patients who had also suffered from hypertension recounted that the Chinese doctor had treated their 'pressure' in consecutive sessions, often over several weeks, and only after it had been brought under control would the doctor allow them to buy the costly potency-enhancing formula medicine.

Chinese medical learning teaches practitioners to think indirectly, to solve complex problems from multiple perspectives (Scheid 2001, 2007), to get into conversation with the patient and consider social context (Zhang 2007), and to work with a diagnostic toolkit and medical terminology that can account for disorders in a non-invasive way (Farquhar 1992), or at least in a regulatory way (Karchmer 2015), in subtle reintegrative procedures (Zhan 2009) ranging from physiological to psychological balancing acts (e.g. Simons 2015), and avoiding side effects (Lei 2014). Treatment was administered in multiple steps (Pritzker 2014), and initially at low doses, such that the patient could learn how to interpret strange 'sensations' (Sagli 2010, 2017) and the observant practitioner could avert adverse developments (Hsu 2007c). All these considerations may play into the experience of sense events that contribute to the perceived efficaciousness of the above potency-enhancing formula medicines.

Chinese formula medicines were not expected to work on the physiology of men in the same way as Viagra. As already noted, when Chinese doctors prescribed potency-enhancing medicines, like *Nanbao*, they advised their clients not to have intercourse before finishing the prescribed treatment course of about one week. The temporality of this consumption regime of abstinence would in itself likely have a potency-enhancing effect. The Chinese formula drugs were not aphrodisiacs, but were thought to strengthen a man's virility long-term through building up energies, 'slowly, slowly' (*man, man* 慢慢).

Clearly, Chinese medical healing involved techniques of timing, applied with a view to bringing into accord different temporalities and thereby making whole by supplementation and attunement to the social and ecological environment. According to Chinese medical rationales, the potency-boosting formula medicines bolstered *qi* 气, *yang qi* 阳气 or *yin* 阴 waters, or they supplemented the centre by inducing a movement of *qi* 气, that is, *xing qi* 行气, particularly in the digestive system and in the lungs; they were also known to regulate blood circulation.[14] The patients were prescribed different dosages, in different combinations, as the Chinese medical ethos of good practice requires.

Finally, some Chinese doctors commented that their African clients had performance expectations of frequency and duration of intercourse that in their opinion were 'exaggerated' (*guodu* 过度). They explained that according to Chinese medical theory, the frequency of intercourse was age-related; one claimed that it was a common assumption in China that a man over 40 should not have intercourse more than once a week. Evidently, the above techniques were aimed

*What Makes a Pot Efficacious?*

at reconfiguring wholeness through the chiming of different temporalities. *Nanbao* may have appeared a single magic bullet when in fact it was offered as part of a kaleidoscopic choice of different options.

## *It's Not Matter Alone That Matters: Healing and Wholeness*

So, to what extent were the Chinese medical techniques by means of reconfiguring an individual patient's sense of wholeness part of a structurating and culturalising project in East Africa?' Above (in the Introduction and Chapters 3 and 6), I proposed to answer this question by pointing to the triad of Chinese medical practitioners, their medicine pots and their patients, and proposed to investigate their interfacing temporalities. Mauss claimed that the study of techniques, rather than that of cultural representations, would emphasise movement, that is, a toing and froing, and a probing and borrowing, of techniques, in an strife towards self perfection. Medical treatment is then understood as a transformation of people in a way that facilitates their emplacement, which in the case of the fieldwork undertaken, was into new urban spaces. To what extent urban textures, following Lefebvre, would be able to afford the practice of these kaleidoscopically refractured techniques in more than just an ephemeral way, remains to be seen.

At this point let us widen the lens of inquiry and move to a more gender-balanced account. This allows us to notice that in Mombasa's busiest practice, time and again, veiled young women in groups of two or three would enter the clinic and move directly towards the counter in order to purchase 'Guo's slimming capsules' (*Guoshi jianfei jiaonang* 国氏减肥胶囊 or *Guoshou* 国瘦). There was another slimming tea on offer: 'Pellets for moistening the bowels' (*Runchangwan* 润肠丸). According to the accompanying leaflet, this slimming tea consisted in its entirety of traditional Chinese *materia medica*. However, its effects were apparently not sufficiently rapid. Was the relief it provided longterm? Did they know what the capsules contained? During an interview in the middle-class flat nearby, where some of the women lived, I tried to find this out – in vain. The time spent with them was giggly and good fun, but any attempt to speak about the medicines was instantly diverted. Nevertheless, through speaking to other women about this phenomenon, it transpired that young women generally took slimming teas not merely to improve their health, adversely affected by obesity and diabetes, but in particular to enhance their good looks and feminine attractiveness.

So, how did Guo's slimming capsules work? Judging from their observed popularity, one surmises that this fecundity-enhancing formula medicine was perceived as efficacious. Unlike other slimming regimes, it was not considered violent, and was nevertheless said to have rapid effects. The mild sensory events experienced when consuming this slimming tea suited the young women's social status.

According to the leaflet, 'Guo's slimming capsules' contained: (1) '*lingzhi* 灵芝 seed substance', which is a Western medical description for the Chinese *materia medica lingzhi cao* 灵芝草, meaning the 'ensouled mushroom herb' (*Ganoderma Sinense* or *Ganoderma lucidum*); this featured first in Yunnan province's famous *materia medica* (*Diannan bencao* 滇南本草) compiled by Mao Lan 兰茂 (1397–1476), and is not recorded as a Chinese *materia medica* in the textbooks on TCM formulas (*Fangjixue* 1985) and TCM drugs (*Zhongyaoxue* 1984). Furthermore, Guo's slimming capsules were said to contain (2) lactoalbumin, (3) oligosaccharides, (4) the Chinese *materia medica danshen* 丹参 (*Salvia miltiorrhiza*) and (5) the leaves of *Gingko biloba*, *yinxingye* 银杏叶 (rather than its fruits, which are a standard Chinese *materia medica*).[15] It is unlikely that the list of ingredients in Guo's slimming tablets is comprehensive, as it was developed in a field where the mercantile principles of upholding the 'secrets of one's commerce' (*shangye mimi*) reigned.

*Ling zhi cao* 靈芝草 had legendary efficaciousness – it was *the* herb of immortality in Chinese folklore. Already in the *Canon of Mountains and Seas* (*Shan hai jing* 山海經) of the Han dynasty (see Loewe 1993: 357–67) there is an entry on a certain Gu Yao Mountain 姑媱之山, and it is recounted that when the Emperor's daughter died, she 'transformed into the "Yao herb"' (*hua wei yao cao* 化為瑤草) and that 'its fruit was like a *tu qiu* (dodder, *Cuscuta Sinensis* or a rabbit mole). Applying it, was enchanting to men of rank' (*qi shi ru tu qiu, fu zhi mei yu ren* 其實如菟丘 服之眉[媚]於人).

As a commentator notes, it is doubtful that this mountain ever existed. However, as the modern editor Yuan Ke (*Shan hai jing* 1980: 141–42) explains, there is a better-known legend now in circulation that combines two Tang dynasty rhapsodies. It concerns Yao Ji 瑤姬. She was the daughter of Emperor Yan 炎帝, one of the Three Emperors in China's mythic times, who is also known as the Divine Husbandman, Shennong 神農, and celebrated as patron of medicinal plants and pharmacotherapy. When Yao Ji died early, before wedlock, 'her essence and *po*-soul turned into a herb, and its fruit is called the ensouled mushroom' (*jing po wei cao, shi yue ling zhi* 精魄為草，實曰靈芝). This mushroom, *ling zhi*, that is also called the 'ensouled mushroom herb' (*ling zhi cao*), features in many legends, each outdoing one another in spectacle, miracle and prestige.

One of these legends tells of China's first emperor, Qinshi Huangdi 秦始皇帝, who after conquering the warring states in 221 BCE, set the empire's foundations for the next two thousand years (the empire was formally abolished in 1911). In this legend, as documented in the *Records of the Historian* of *c.* 86 BCE (*Shi ji* 史記 1959: Chapter 6, 223; Chapter 158, 3075) of *c.* 86 BCE, the first emperor was consumed by an appetite for fame and power that led him to search for the herb of immortality. This reportedly had disastrous consequences, among them his ordering of Xu Fu 徐福 to sail eastward over the sea in search of the herb, with 780 boys and 780 girls on board, never to return again.[16]

In East Africa, I did not see any practitioner familiarise their clientele with Chinese folklore of this kind. However, in China, despite relentless modernisation efforts, these legends have remained popular knowledge, crossing social strata, as they likely have been for over a millennium. They must have motivated the Ming dynasty scholar-physicians to include this mushroom in the compilation of Yunnan's *materia medica*, and for the professionals who designed the industrialised formula's composition and made it into what looks like the brand marker of Guo's slimming tea, the legends of *ling zhi cao* were no doubt still very alive.

As an aspect of fantastic folklore, these legends infuse everyday life and thereby affect individual health status. During my fieldwork in my ancestral village in Huizhou, southern Anhui province, at the foothills of the Yellow Mountains (in autumn 2009), a local cancer patient who had become a herbalist gave me several *lingzhi* mushrooms on my departure from the field, saying that he had found them high in the mountains. He had been a tea taster by profession and his cancer was of the oral cavity, and he survived his predicted death date by almost a decade. No doubt, legend must have added to his stamina as he climbed the steep rocks on which these mushrooms allegedly grow. Their telling shape suggested, as do the above legends, that longevity – an unspoken desire throughout China, and no doubt many parts of the world – can be achieved through fecundity and fertility, by creating offspring.

In summary, the limitations of reducing the potency-enhancing efficaciousness of Chinese formula medicines to their chemical compounds, which are then assessed in RCTs, are blatantly clear. These items, derived from China's history of material culture, were not actually instantiations of the past, but were newly reconfigured, invented and developed in an era of superdiversity and hypermobility. The ethos was Maoist, namely to integrate Chinese and Western medicine, and in this way, this artefact was an 'alternative modernity', promoted and giving rise to new health regimes. Like other medicines popular within this new health regime, Guo's slimming capsules blurred the boundaries of health, beauty and wealth.

As an aside, we note in this section that even with the broad Maussian definition of 'technique' as 'efficacious action on matter', we cannot capture that which seemed to make the Chinese potency-enhancing formula medicines attractive to their consumers. When it comes to questions of reproduction and fertility, procreation and kinship, issues of attractiveness and seduction, courage and curiosity, inner strength and gendered prowess become particularly salient. Therefore, healing techniques defined in terms of a unidirectional 'action on' [matter] and of 'efficaciousness' reduced to 'medical efficacy' seem insufficient for explaining the above fieldwork experiences. This brings us back to the issues of social relatedness and social distance, institutionalised forms of reciprocity and asymmetry, and also to issues of affect and emotion, honour and self-respect, as discussed in the opening sections of this chapter. To better understand the movements and motivations of the Chinese practitioners' clientele and the transformations they sought in urban spaces, a more comprehensive approach to the dynamic texturing of partially textured spatialities is necessary. Yet to pursue this more comprehensive endeavour, Mauss's definition of matter as acted upon by technology remains an interesting approach, not least – as we will see by the end of the following section – because it allows for an understanding of materiality inclusive of the etymologically related, animate *mater* (mother) and inanimate matrix.

## 'Things of Our Place': The Incorporation of Substance and Its Efficaciousness

Why did the Chinese formula medicines gain significance so quickly in the realm of fertility, procreation and kinship in East Africa? The Chinese appeared to be so alien, so other, so different in so many respects – why should their medicines be used for solving local peoples' reproductive problems, otherwise kept hidden and considered private? In this context, we are reminded that a stranger who is sufficiently different can become a confidant in realms of intimacy (Simmel 1950b). Was it a matter of an 'intimacy with strangers'? Was otherness overcome, as in the case of the eukaryotic cell providing shelter for the prokaryotic holobiont (which eventually morphed into an organelle), by means of engulfment rather than ingestion? It is common practice worldwide that you eat your healer (Schipper 2009)?

If social distance engendered the awe of potency, did it also increase one's attractiveness? How should one handle such attraction that is both risky and rewarding? Was the willingness to be curious about, to buy, to 'try out' and consume these formula medicines one way of getting a handle on the alien and of domesticating the untamed (Simmel [1911] 1950c)? The medicines that the newcomers had on offer demanded incorporation in order to be efficacious (see Chapter 3).

Paradoxically, as will become obvious below, the potency-boosting and fertility-enhancing Chinese formula medicines, above characterised as 'alternatively modern', seem to have appealed to the urbanites in East Africa primarily because they were 'traditional' medicines. 'The traditional' was associated with 'things of our place' (Green 1996) and with the fertility and growth within it ('our place'). Among urbanites, this realm of everyday life that pertained to reproduction was that of *za kienyeji*, 'the traditional'. 'Traditional' medicines were to be used for solving the problems of 'the traditional', *za kienyeji*, 'that out of which we have grown'.

Maia Green's (1996) definition of the 'traditional' as referring to 'things of our place' is very useful for our purposes here. It makes it possible to define the 'traditional' in a positive way, in contrast to the definitions of the WHO and many aid organisations, for whom the term 'traditional medicine' tends to comprise a ragbag of different beliefs and practices that have in common that they are not 'medicine', that is, biomedicine. Green's definition perhaps comes closest to that of *kienyeji* in Stacey Langwick's (2008) gloss on the three terms *dawa za asili*, *dawa za jadi* and *dawa za kienyeji*. As Langwick notes, none of the three Swahili terms refers to an unchanging past. They all imply movement:

> *Kienyeji* implies growth of, and growth out of, a place. *Jadi* captures development through generations. *Asili* suggests derivation – transformation from one state to another. (Langwick 2008: 437, fn. 5)

Langwick's gloss of *kienyeji* as 'growth of, and growth out of, a place' reinforces Green's insights. Green, who has been working long-term with the Pogoro in the region of Morogoro, suggested that the 'traditional' referred to 'things of our place' and contrasted with the 'official', as sanctioned by Christian religion:

> 'Traditional' practice is oriented towards the dead and the spirits associated with territory on whom the fertility of the land and the welfare of its residents depend. It does not so much concern the past directly, as the relation between the people and the spirits. (Green 1996: 488)

However, 'the traditional' is not only linked to place, it is also associated with matter and embodied materialities. Green states that the spirits were disembodied, while the living were entangled in an embodied life.

> Personhood is an attribute of the living, constituted through the performance of appropriate acts and the incorporation of substances classified as medicines. (Green 1996: 488)

A living body was thus expected to incorporate substances in fulfilment of its living. 'Medicines' were not only consumed in the case of an illness or disease, but for the accomplishment of personhood. In this respect, medicines were like food that is eaten together, in commensality. Indeed, a patient's recovery was thought to be effected by 'working together', Green tells us, which meant that healer and patient, and their social entourage, all participated in the eating of the medicines.[17] Furthermore, the incorporation of medicines, just like that of food, could effect the incorporation into a territory.

The sharing of these substances created kinship. Plant medicines incorporated by infants and toddlers, for instance by ingestion of a *shirala* – a medicine made of the ground roots of a tree growing on the paternal kin's land – made the children who ate it part of the land and their paternal kin. Among the Pogoro, this social incorporation of offspring into the father's lineage required an effort. By contrast, the substantial, material relatedness to the mother (*mater*) and maternal kin was given through the feeding of breast milk and maternal care (Green 1996: 491). This material connection to the *mater* was considered a given and required no extra effort. The same logic of making offspring part of the land can also be applied to the more recent ethnography by Geissler and Prince (2010a and 2010b) on the daily procedure of bathing toddlers among the Luo in Kenya. This involved splashing green waters, saturated with fresh plant materials taken from the paternal grandmother's land, onto the toddlers. The playful tone and banter accompanying these bathing techniques affirmed not only tender, loving care, but effected a substantial incorporation of the offspring into the patriline's land. The toddlers absorbed the water through their skin; did this effect a substantial incorporation into the lineage?

Green gives an answer to this question when she notes that the transformative powers of ingested substances 'do not derive from their symbolic properties, but from the specific social conditions governing their manufacture and consumption':

> The mediation of the body's growth and change through the physical incorporation of medicines is integral to the social construction of a personhood premised on a particular experience of the body. (Green 1996: 485)

Green's observations also speak to the anthropology of substances, as discussed for Central Africa by Christopher Davis (2000). Accordingly, the administration and absorption of substances would ultimately be related to a gesturally given but non-verbalised manipulation of ancestral powers. Kate Fayers-Kerr (2013) made this point in respect of the 'eating' of specifically coloured clays, as observed among the Mursi, who collected them from their lineage's ancestral clay pits. As already mentioned in Chapter 3, the 'eating' consisted of applying different hues of colourful clay all over one's body or certain body parts, particularly the face. It indexed, as well as materially consisted of, an absorption and incorporation of ancestral powers from one's patriline's land into one's individual body. A student of

Chinese medicine might speak of the necessity of creating a 'body ecological' ontological continuum to the waters and earths of a place (*shuitu* 水土).[18]

Evidently, the ingestion of potency-enhancing Chinese formula medicines was not merely for therapeutic ends, evaluated in terms of medical efficacies. People were inclined to test the incorporation of these substances, not least for the sake of enhancing and perfectioning their performance as a person; although to procreate, sex need not be enjoyable, procreation is considered more likely if it is.

Paradoxically, the 'alternatively modern' Chinese formula medicines were treated like other 'traditional' medicines. They were sought, paradoxically, as though their 'natural' ingredients had grown on the ancestral land of their consumers. Yet were they indeed consumed for procreation? The social distance to 'the Chinese' engendered exaggerated expectations about the potency of these *pots* (be it the power in the powdered antenna of a male moth or that of an ensouled fungus) which posed a further paradox.

Rather than warding off the foreigners that the Chinese medical practitioners were, patients would disclose their intimate problems of reproductive health and agreed to eat and incorporate the miraculous medicines that they were prescribed and sold. There is a social distance between the genders, which almost everywhere tends to be reinforced through locality-specific gender politics and morality. One has to learn how to take the risk of becoming intimately engaged with the other gender. Ingesting a stranger's strange medicine *pot* may thus be seen as a first step towards the taking of risks before becoming close and intimate. Seen in this way, the consumption of these strange and foreign Chinese formula medicines required a certain courage – the courage to approach and get close to the 'other'. This added a further ironic twist to the purchase and consumption of the enhancement medicines in question. The upwardly mobile urbanites in the East African cityscapes seemed to navigate a hall of mirrors.[19]

Although none of my respondents put it into these words, the ethnographic evidence discussed in this chapter allows us to suggest that, if the issue of procreation was at stake, the Chinese formula medicines were ingested with the aim to make flourishing forests (*silva*) out of dead wood (*hyle*). This latent possibility that *matter* is *mater* (a mother generative of life) may have allowed the Chinese formula medicines to be treated like substances associated with the powers of *za kienyeji*, the 'things of our place'.

To recapitulate, the Chinese formula medicines discussed in this chapter were perceived to be potency- and beauty-enhancing, and as our investigations revealed, due to them being seen as an instantiation of 'the traditional'. Where in Chapter 7, the formula medicines had been treated as an 'alternative *modernity*', this chapter aligned them with techniques that proliferate 'growth in our place', *za kienyeji*. Finally, after providing in Chapter 7 a discussion of the medicine 'pots' in a dualist way, differentiating between their natural scientific 'properties' and Chinese medical 'qualities', this chapter accounted for the *pots* as people handled and sensed them,

## Reflections: Sex in the City and the Leisure Industry

Were the clients of Chinese clinics who purchased the potency-enhancing *Nanbao* and fecundity-enhancing formulas like Guo's slimming tea primarily interested in fecundity and fertility, procreation and longevity? Rachel Spronk did fieldwork in Nairobi in the 2000s, interested in finding out 'how sexuality was embedded in social relations and meanings and therefore how sexuality was related to processes of social transformation' (2009: 500). Interestingly, the people she spoke to and the kinds of dilemmas they experienced, as well as the choices of opinions between which they vacillated (Spronk 2009, 2012), come quite close to the sentiment of some clients I encountered in Kenya's Chinese medical clinics.

It is the case that Chinese practitioners aimed to live in well-established neighbourhoods. Yet as seen in Chapter 3, their clinics were thinly spread across East Africa's urban textures, and several lived in downmarket suburbs and catered to clients from informal settlements. Those patients who said to me that they were 'middle-class' were not as well off as the young professionals Spronk spoke to. The statements they made regarding their searching, their ambitions, their upward mobility and the compromises they made, however, came close to what Spronk said about the 20–30-year-old professionals that she worked with. However, while the Kenyan clientele in Mombasa generally lived in more secure conditions than the Tanzanian clients (see Chapter 4), most of my respondents did not have the spending power of Spronk's professionals in Nairobi, and those who did were very often by chance not available for an interview on the day that I visited them.

Spronk underlined that the young urbanites she worked with were viewed as 'un-African' and 'Westernised', while they were actually very conscious of their Africanness. Sexuality was for them an important aspect of selfhood:

> Sex is a medium for a variety of feelings, emotions and needs; people have sex for fun, to fulfil a desire for intimacy, for a physical thrill, to procreate, to exert power, to humiliate, and much more. Sex is thus a vehicle for powerful feelings that are experienced very subjectively. As an inter-subjective exchange between people, sex is also a symbolic and sensorial interaction between people and this inter-subjective exchange implies intimacy. Last, sexuality is a particularly sensitive conductor of cultural influences and hence of social and political divisions. (Spronk 2009: 501–2)

So-called 'African sexuality', a term promoted in the 1990s, had been at the centre of some research into the prevention of HIV/AIDS. As Spronk (2009: 501) notes, it was discussed mostly in an ahistorical and generalising way, and is best sent into oblivion. To be sure, I did not discuss sex with my interviewees, but this was a topic core to Spronk's research, and indirectly, her findings may throw light on mine. She spoke to about fifty respondents, male and female, characterised as follows:

> They have unlimited access to the internet and hence communicate with friends and relatives abroad. They stay in tune with global trends by surfing the internet, reading magazines, listening to music and watching films. Theirs is a bustling world of 'sophistication' and lifestyle options with its own signifiers and representations of a present-day identity . . . Young professionals are cosmopolitans, not because of a cultural orientation to the West, but because of the convergence of global and local 'cultural compliance' . . . that they embody. They articulate a cosmopolitanism with a particular Kenyan flavour of which they are proud. Fashionable dressing, going out and progressive attitudes are important markers of their modern personality. (Spronk 2009: 505)

Among the young professionals that Spronk worked with, having sex – with contraceptives – was a way of being social and intimate. Sex was casual, an expression of 'fast life', spurred by the consumption of leisure. Interethnic relationships were cultivated and questions of marriage and procreation postponed; ambitions were oriented towards partner choice, companionship, autonomy, self-worth, (female) sexual satisfaction, pleasure and romance. Only a few spoke the language of their parents and grandparents. They took to Westernised dress and music, media and morals. They also mentioned anxieties, uncertainties and ambivalences. They insisted that they were African, but in a modern way. In these debates surrounding Africanness, sexuality was 'at the centre of proper personhood' (ibid.: 516). They were very much concerned with the enhancement of their personal performance and selves, and pleasure-giving sexual performance clearly fell into the realm of an enhanced self.

Meanwhile, as my research showed, Chinese potency-enhancing formulas were generally not purchased by young men, but by the middle-aged, who had the necessary purchasing power and social prestige. Like the sex in the city that Spronk researched, theirs was perhaps not primarily for procreation. Businessmen in their forties and fifties, on business trips and sometimes of another nationality, such as Zambian or South African, were prominent among the clientele who purchased Chinese potency-enhancing drugs.

In the Americas and Europe, the sexual performance perfection industry and the medicalisation of male sexuality have been extensively discussed as aspects of the body as a 'project' (Csordas 1999). In China, not only the expectations of men about their sexual performance (Farquhar 1999; Zhang 2015) but also the medical sciences of male sexuality – in old age, for instance (Wang 2017) – have generated forms of desire previously not openly cultivated. Aspirations for 'good sex', as advertised by an emergent leisure industry in late liberalism, have instilled expectations that are difficult, if not impossible, to satisfy.

Potency-boosters and beauty-enhancing products have been characterised as an enhancement medicine (Edmonds and Sanabria 2014). My fieldwork in East Africa reconfirmed this. In so far they were not actually perceived as pharmaceuticals for treating a sickness. Medical anthropologists have widely demonstrated how energy-boosters, tonics, traditional medicines, hormones, vitamins and other substances are ingested or otherwise incorporated at occasions of commercialised leisure (Rodrigues et al. 2019). Meanwhile, 'impotence' and 'infertility' were borderline phenomena that justified the seeking of medicalised care.

The 'wonders of the exotic' and the 'intimacy with strangers' that potency-boosting formula medicines and beauty-restorative slimming teas enhanced, treated medicine as a substance that had the affordance to transform the person who 'ate' and incorporated it (cf. Parkin 1968; Whyte 1988). Where the 'traditional' was synonymous with 'of our place', 'traditional medicines' have been used to enhance growth and multiply kin derived 'from our place', that is, the ancestral land (Green 1996; Davis 2000; Geissler and Prince 2010a, b). Yet as self and social relatedness have undergone important redefinitions (e.g. Geissler and Prince 2007), reproduction was among some urban professionals no longer a matter of primary concern, nor was the continuation of the patriline through 'blood that is compatible'. Commerce with 'traditional medicines', which ultimately appears to be driven by a rapidly growing global sexual leisure industry, has reconfigured fecundity and fertility concerns, to different degrees, by different sensory means, and in numerous recombinations.

So, in this chapter, rather than providing 'the placebo effect' as a blanket explanation, we discussed how *pots* were sensed and handled, and we threw light on their different potencies and materialities by exploring how people related their efficaciousness to specific sense events. We examined how materialities and manual techniques configured those sense events and enabled different Chinese medical enhancement formulas to be experienced as efficacious. We went beyond colour symbolism, for instance, to investigate the materiality of colour, the phono-aesthetics of colour terms, like the sound 'ee' of the word 'green' and the uplifting synaesthesia it engenders. We also went beyond sound symbolism and attended to pitch and intonation, rhythmicity and the somatic modes of attention it elicited, as in the case of the hope that humorous word play may instil, together with the sheen of gold exuding from free-flowing calligraphy. We touched on legend and folklore, and on the hearsay and imagination of the fantastic growing out of historically motivated attitudes and structuring structures. We pointed to concrete techniques that were meant to affect a change in disposition – at different levels, in many different ways. They were constitutive of the complex technologies of temporarilities that Chinese medical routines can generate and of materially texturing and textured urban space. The social lives of Chinese formula medicines were sensitively affected when handled and sensed as *pots* – *za kienyeji* – in ways that made them become part of social and spatial fields.

## Notes

1. I use the word 'materiality' to signal that I am not speaking of 'inert matter' (as will emerge more clearly at the end of this chapter: the materialities discussed are at the interface of *hyle* and *silva*).
2. 'Doing otherwise' is not easy to package into a single idiom, and turns out to consist of multiple practices deemed empowering and transformative (e.g. Haram and Yamba 2009; Geissler and Prince 2010a; Cooper and Pratten 2015; Myhre 2017).
3. By referring to the concept of externality as a relational one, Rekdal makes possible a change in anthropological discussion from the dualist medicine 'pots' to handled and perceived *pots*.
4. As we will see towards the end of this chapter, these externalities had substance; they were matter that had to be ingested or otherwise absorbed to be efficacious.
5. Some rapid effects of acupuncture were also connected to magic; see Kadetz and Hood (2017: 349–50).
6. This section contains a few excerpts from Elisabeth Hsu. 2009b. 'Wonders of the Exotic: Chinese Formula Medicines on the East African Coast', in Kjersti Larsen (ed.), *Knowledge, Renewal and Religion: Repositioning and Changing Ideological and Material Circumstances among the Swahili on the East African Coast*. Uppsala: Nordiska Afrikainstitutet, pp. 280–99. Used with permission.
7. This certainly heightened the veil of secrecy around them, as secret knowledge is typically orally transmitted (e.g. Simmel [[1908] 1950a).
8. I draw here on common sense and good sense in Gramsci's sense (cf. Robinson 2005), and do not go into the discussion of 'realism' (as did Hsu 2010c).
9. For instance, contemporary Indigenous movements in the southern hemisphere aim to reinstall New Year in June instead of January. This revivalist intention is grounded in their 'deep knowledge', based on the body ecological observation that days are shortest in June and that spring starts in September.
10. The word 'meats' is used here in the sense of Zimmermann ([1982] 1987).
11. The first section [of the butchered carcass] to be removed is called *mrite*, which consists of the subcutaneous fat and tissue on the lower part of the animal's belly. The *mrite* often includes taramea, two tendons that extend down the inside of the hind legs. Genitals are part of a male animal's *mrite*, while the udder is part of a female animal's *mrite* (Myhre 2013: 116).
12. Consider the *hoc est corpus* of Christian ritual that became *hokus pokus*, an idiom that in colloquial German refers to magic (Gabi Alex, personal communication, Oxford, 2007).

13. Freely rolling *r*s and *l*s, for instance, were common in the names of fish and bird folk taxa worldwide, instantiating their swimming and flying sound-wise; see Berlin (1992: 232–59).
14. TCM teachings emphasised dysfunctions between the liver, kidney and *yang* brightness, where *yangming* 阳明 generally referred to the stomach (digestive problems and *gesi*) and sometimes also the heart (anxiety; *Zhongyi neikexue* 1985).
15. The production of leaf extracts is a well-known traditional European and modern German phytotherapeutic procedure, while the Chinese *materia medica* consists of the fruit; see Grimley Evans (2010).
16. The Taiwanese scholar Peng Shuangsong (1984) identified more than twenty landing sites, among them Fukuoka ken 福岡 in Japan, which recently held a celebration with the descendants of this ship's evidently very fecund crew.
17. A medical crisis makes culture by involvement of the entire group (Turner 1968; Lewis 2000; Augé 1986).
18. Incorporating substances of the ancestral land makes the person part of that land – this is well documented. Fayers-Kerr (2018) aims to link these ritual and caring practices of the everyday to the politics of 'autochthony'.
19. Having said that, fertility could be enhanced in other ritual ways too (e.g. van Dijk et al. 1999).

# Chapter 9
# 'The Chinese Antimalarial' as 'Pot' and *Pot*

## Pre-amble

The ethnographic refractions presented in this chapter discuss what people called 'the Chinese antimalarial'. Health professionals and most TCM practitioners considered it not a Chinese formula medicine, but a Western biomedical 'pharmaceutical'. It consisted of one single purified chemical substance and could treat a 'real' disease: malaria. Interestingly, the idiom 'the Chinese antimalarial' referred to several different brands, each made up of a different chemical substance (all artemisinin-derivatives); these multiple manifestations of 'the Chinese antimalarial' changed in chemical composition over time. Importantly, they changed from being a pharmaceutical containing just one purified chemical substance to one consisting of a combination of two to three chemical substances. In what follows, I will first discuss the material aspects of 'the Chinese antimalarial' between 2001 and 2004, that is the different substances that constituted it, and will then discuss how its material composition changed after the World Health Organization published its guidelines regarding ACT (Artemisinin Combination Therapy) in 2005 and 2006.

In regard to fieldwork methods, having so far discussed experiences of siting the field, multisited fieldwork and the inclusion of history in ethnographic considerations, alongside language learning, semi-structured interviewing and working with narrative, let us reflect here on moments in which fieldwork went wrong. In a similar mood, I will reflect on missed opportunities at the end of the chapter. I will specifically ask why fresh plant preparations, as commonly in use among African healers (fieldwork observation), are not considered a viable choice for future public health care in East Africa.

The prevention, management and treatment of malaria is full of success stories for traditional medicine (e.g. Etkin and Ross [1983] 1997; Lei 1999b; Honigsbaum 2001; Willcox et al. 2004; Willcox 2016; Hsu 2014; Laplante 2015; Elliott et al. 2020).[1] This is so in contrast to the missionary's narrative (Comaroff and Comaroff 1992) that the African people lived without medicine until missionary medicine brought salvation to soul and body. Malaria generally is not experienced as the deadly disease in sub-Saharan Africa as it was for the missionaries, and common folk put to use a variety of techniques for treating different forms of malaria.

As is less well known, the preparation of fresh juices against fevers is a widespread phenomenon in 'traditional' medicines (e.g. Laplante 2015; Rutert 2020; Françoise Barbira-Freedman, personal communication, 2014). In this context, it is important to know that fresh herbal antimalarial juices of the Chinese *materia medica* called *qing hao* 青蒿 were recommended in the Chinese formula literature from as early as the fourth century CE onwards. This recommendation was given specifically for treating the acute fever bouts of intermittent fevers (e.g. Hsu 2006a, b; 2009d, 2010b, 2018b; for more detail, see the section of this chapter entitled 'Fieldwork outside the Field'). There is also preliminary ethnoarchaeological evidence to suggest that fresh *qing hao* juices are an effective antimalarial (Wright et al. 2010) and that for whole *qing hao* plant preparations, plasmodial resistance is not a major problem (Elfawal et al. 2012, 2015). Why then is the efficaciousness of this easily prepared, fresh herbal Artemisia-combination therapy, with virtually no side effects, brushed aside by contemporary researchers and ridiculed? Why has so little research been undertaken to investigate the safety and efficaciousness of antimalarial and other fresh-plant preparations for public health alleviation of everyday ailments in sub-Saharan Africa, where many adult patients who are semi-immune? Is it a missed opportunity?

## 'Playing Fields'

Ethnography is entwined with investigations into the history of a place and region, as seen in the previous chapter. Since an herbal antimalarial juice's material aspects are in focus, this chapter takes

*'The Chinese Antimalarial' as 'Pot' and Pot*

inspiration from the 'social lives of things' approach to history (Appadurai 1986). In line with the social life approach that attends to the biography of a commodity in terms of the different values attributed to it (Kopytoff 1986), this chapter will attend to 'playing fields', the changing playing fields in which 'the Chinese antimalarial' featured since its chemical identification in the 1970s. I use the term 'playing field' specifically to refer to the materialities and material constitution of the social fields in which a medicine may feature. By paying attention to the materiality of *pots* (referring both to the vase or pot in the foreground and the stuff in the background in a figure–ground image; see explanations in Chapters 1 and 6), I aim to overcome the decontextualised dualist way of assessing a medicine's material make-up in terms of 'properties' and 'qualities'. Instead, I pay attention to the spatial textures in which it is purchased and used. The ethnographic finding that prompted me to do so was the observation that what people called 'the Chinese antimalarial' changed its chemical profile in accord with the 'playing field' in which it featured.

The notion of 'playing fields' draws on Bourdieu's (1984) notion of the field and the *habitus* as mutually constitutive analytic concepts, a point underlined by Hanks (2005). In my understanding, Bourdieu's 'field' is a non-Euclidean space, much like Lefebvre's (1991) 'textured space', as both the field and the textured space are created by the movements of people. However, just as Bourdieu's *habitus* is strangely disembodied, his social 'field' is disembodied too. Meanwhile, I use the term 'playing fields' not merely as defined by disembodied structuring structures, but also by the textures of the ground, its softness or hardness, the mud or dust that clings to pots and players, their material make-up and its affordances. This requires us to consider the Chinese medicine *pots* as an aspect of the textures, in which their propensity to become co-constitutive of place, comes into play.

## Fieldwork Methods: The Fieldworker at Fault

Styles of conducting fieldwork differ, while the ethical requirement of the fieldworker to be polite and respectful remains unchanged. A fieldworker must respect the mores and customs of the other as other, but this need not mean that the fieldworker must stick to the wall like a fly and extract themselves out of a fieldwork situation. Yes, we are asked to make ourselves 'small' (see Chapter 2, 'Speaking . . . Chinese'), but this need not mean that we cannot raise questions regarding, say, people's clinical practice. I would regularly ask a practitioner why they chose to treat a patient one way rather than another, usually during the brief interval between one patient leaving the consultation room and another entering it. However, this way of doing fieldwork can be experienced as too confrontational.

It felt quite the contrary to me. By attending to the minutiae of their doings and double-checking my recordings with them, I was paying more respect to my respondents than if I were mindlessly copying their information into my notebook and regurgitating it unprobed in publications. So, I had lively discussions with my interviewees, as I was keen to gain a better understanding of Chinese medicine. My intention was not to be patronising, nor to use querying as a technique of surveillance. Even though the moment itself can be embarrassing, and also painful, for both the interviewer and the interviewee, I also do not consider tears something to be avoided at all costs in fieldwork. Fieldwork is always also emotion work.

Having said this, a person who asks direct questions can sometimes come across as insensitive, intrusive and impolite, while the persona that an anthropologist is meant to cultivate shows constant kindness and responsibility towards the interviewee. Our professional ethics require an anthropologist, not only as fieldworker but also as author, to be polite and respectful of other modes of reasoning, manners and customs.

## *Polite Persistence*

Sometimes, a certain polite persistence may be appreciated by your respondents. One day I chanced upon a Chinese medical practice in the late afternoon in the harbour area of Stone Town. As I entered the premises, before even greeting me, the Chinese practitioner ostensibly dialled a number and spoke loudly and for some time into his mobile phone: 'She's arrived here as well', he said in Chinese, and went on chatting in local dialect with his colleague in Moshi. When he finally hung up and turned to me, he let me know that I was known among his friends throughout the country, and that no one liked my snooping around (cf. Braun and Østbø Haugen 2021); I had been doing so, he said, for far too long.

I showed neither shame nor anger at having been told off, even ridiculed. I remained matter of fact, explaining to him that I was a medical anthropologist interested in how Chinese medicine was being practised in East Africa; it was to be expected that my research would not go unnoticed by the handful of practitioners I regularly visited. Then I asked him, politely and in Chinese, for the opportunity to hold an interview with him and the woman practitioner with whom he evidently ran the practice. 'No way', was the answer. Was I allowed to look at such and such a medicine on display behind the counter? Or would he mind if I just stayed put on the chair, as I realised I was tired? He agreed that I looked tired.

The practice was tiny, and I spotted some condoms on display for sale. This was not the only Chinese medical clinic that sold condoms. Although this commodity was Western, it suited Chinese medical rationales, which emphasise preventive health. Sailors were the main customers, he said. Soon thereafter, he and his companion closed the practice. This involved locking the glass door and then pulling an iron gate from both sides, which was held shut by a padlock. Then, during the short period of dusk, the three of us slowly walked down the street, filled with pedestrians in this popular neighbourhood. As we arrived at the door to their flat on the ground floor of a large traditional house, only minutes away from their medical practice, there was a moment of hesitation. 'Come in', they then said. Yet minutes later, my host excused himself, as he was to attend the evening prayer at the mosque. So, I waited for some time alone in their beautifully tiled kitchen.

That evening the two medical practitioners told me that they were relatives. In China their relation was incestuous, but they had both converted to Islam. Among Muslims, cousins of the first degree could get married. This information was thrown at me, unelicited. Love had brought them to East Africa. They did not say so, but it was clear from the conversation that ensued. Later that evening, the couple chaperoned me back to the hotel, again with me walking between them. They were known and greeted by members of the community, moving by in the dark streets or standing as dark silhouettes in the frames of open doors, thereby cooling down house and body in the evening breeze. When we arrived at the starkly illuminated highway leading up to the hotel, I sensed a slight hesitation on their part, as though they did not wish to leave the intimacy of the neighbourhood immersed in darkness that evidently felt safe to them. We parted on good terms, but our encounter did not start so. It required persistent politeness.

## *Listlessness and Lethargy: A Matter of Malaria, Depression or Bewitchment?*

Conflict resolution (say between spouses), mental health problems, soul loss (such as the *dege dege* of infants affected by falciparum malaria convulsions) and cases involving love magic were not brought to Chinese medical practitioners. By contrast, the healer that I worked with in Manzese attended to these sorts of problems. Having said this, there was one episode on Pemba involving a patient who presented with listlessness, lack of energy and the like, having self-diagnosed as suffering from malaria. The Chinese medical practitioner was just about to sell 'the Chinese antimalarial', that is, a course of Artesunate tablets, when I intervened. I did so with good intentions, but I was to experience that my goodwill was misplaced.

I knew that malaria tended to be over-diagnosed (e.g. Chandler et al. 2008), and particularly for depression. After it had become a global burden of disease in sub-Saharan Africa (WHO 1996), it was on everyone's mind. So, patients suffering from depression would be prescribed antimalarials instead of antidepressants. On this occasion I intervened and requested that the TCM practitioner have the young man do a lab test in a private clinic nearby. My educated guess, on the basis of the above psychiatric insights, proved true. The test showed no plasmodial load in support of the patient's self-diagnosis. Given the stigma of mental illness worldwide, and the presence of malaria on everyone's minds, one can easily sympathise with this patient's self-diagnosis. However, although I had read the medical anthropological article on 'fake malaria' (Hausmann Muela et al. 1998), it did not occur to me at the time that I was encountering it. 'Fake malaria' is when patients who consider themselves to suffer from malaria go to the dispensary, have a test done, and if it is negative, doubt the result. In those cases of doubt, suspicions of witchcraft would likely come into play, but witchcraft cannot be blamed for any and everything. True, it works indirectly. According to Hausmann Muela et al. (ibid.), it was, for instance, able to interfere with specific scientific procedures, such as a concealment of the parasites when the patient's blood sample was put under the microscope. Hence, if the self-diagnosed malaria persisted, and the patient went on feeling listless and unwell, it was likely that the patient would suspect the plasmodia had been concealed in the blood sample put under the microscope – by bewitchment. The patient would eventually then consult a healer, their trust in hospital medicine being tenuous anyway, and the healer's treatment of this 'fake malaria', if successful, likely reinforced the train of thought of both patient and healer. Bewitched women seeking refuge in Ashanti shrines in Ghana during the 1950s famously were diagnosed as suffering from a mental disorder, and occasionally depression (Field 1960). Accordingly, malaria and depression both caused listlessness and lethargy, and it is easy to see why this sensed loss of life energies would be attributed to witches, and their notorious greediness.

In general, patients would present Chinese practitioners with complaints that they would bring to hospital medicine, that is, malaria, and not depression. In this particular case, the Chinese medical doctor did not prescribe an antimalarial, and the patient did not walk away with the legendary fast-acting 'Chinese antimalarial' he had hoped to get. He refused to purchase the Chinese formula medicine that the doctor recommended to bring his *qi* into circulation (and thereby lift his spirits).

The understanding that most anthropologists have of malaria is based in that of the Christian missionaries who died within months of arriving in the tropics. As they had no immunity to the disease, it was lethal. This experience of its deadliness for the white man has been reproduced in medical school worldwide to this day. Meanwhile, wherever malaria is endemic, it is not experienced as the deadly fever, but can present in different ways (Beckerleg 1994; Marsland 2007; Kamat 2009; Granado et al. 2011). Due to the anaemia that repeated fever bouts cause, endemic malaria typically presents as listlessness and lethargy.

Had I as the anthropologist not intervened, both the practitioner and the patient would have been satisfied. The practitioner wished to sell his medicine, and the patient had the money to buy it. At the time I thought that I had saved the patient an extra expense, given that, experientially, anaemia from endemic malaria and depression can be experienced as part of a pathological continuum. However, on reflection, one might want to hypothesise that, as shown in Chapter 4 ('The Most Frequent Complaint, Malaria'), artemisinin can clear out a residual load of plasmodia in the blood that would not show up in laboratory tests. A slight betterment of the patient overall sometimes works as a trigger and can kickstart processes that help them to alleviate feelings of depression. In this case, I had better not intervened.

## The Ethnographic Focus: 'The Chinese Antimalarial' as 'Pot' on Different Playing Fields in Multiple Transfigurations, Some Causing Serious Side Effects

There are now three book-length studies on what in East Africa was called 'the Chinese antimalarial', a term in the singular that, as we will see, referred to a plurality of chemically differently constituted drugs. The playing fields on which these three books report involve international organisations, such as the WHO and World Bank, multinational conglomerates, like Novartis, governments (for instance of the PRC and USA) and the research programmes and institutions that they financed. All three monographs are ambitious in remit and cut across the natural sciences, health policy, world history, clinical medicine and, not least, Chinese medical theory and practice, and all not entirely without bias. Of the three, only one is a critical study by a social and medical anthropologist (Meier zu Biesen 2013),[2] and I will draw on it in what follows. This chapter, like the previous ones, focuses on the triad of entrepreneurial practitioners, enterprising patients and medicinal preparations (which in a figure–ground image would make up the foreground, while the playing fields in the background will be shown to have affected the chemical constitution of the antimalarial).[3]

### Artemisinin Monotherapy Brands as OTCs (Medicines Sold Over the Counter)

Research on Chinese medical practices and clinics was charged with an undercurrent of tension, however mildly, throughout my fieldwork. In the early 2000s, local journalists had been vocal about the 'mushrooming' of these clinics, and later the Ministry of Health was restructuring itself and formulating legislation about TM/CAM. The background 'noise' was that of the USA first invading Afghanistan (on 7 October 2001) and then Iraq (on 19 March 2003). In this situation, the local clientele of the practitioners was more welcoming to the anthropologist than were the professionals. During the first two spells of fieldwork in Dar es Salaam, in the 'rainy season' in March 2001 and the 'small rainy season' in December 2001, more than half of over-the-counter transactions in Chinese medical clinics were for the 'Chinese antimalarial', and most of the thirty patients whom I then interviewed in Dar es Salaam considered 'the Chinese antimalarial' *dawa ya Kichina*, where *dawa* referred both to the medicine (*yi* 医) and the medication (*yao* 药). Thus, *dawa ya Kichina* signified both Traditional Chinese Medicine (*zhongyi* 中医) and the biomedical practice (*xiyi* 西医) of Chinese-origin physicians (e.g. those from the Chinese biomedical expert teams, *yiliaodui* 医疗队). As established above, in Chapter 1, *dawa ya Kichina* could also designate just the medications: the Chinese herbal, animal and mineral *materia medica* (*zhongyao* 中药) or biomedical pharmaceuticals produced in China. Among the former belonged a large number of Chinese medical formula medicines (*zhongchengyao* 中成药) and herbal medicines (*caoyao* 草药); among the latter, biomedical pharmaceuticals (*xiyao* 西药). The formula medicines that integrated Chinese and Western medicine (*zhongxiyi jiehe* 中西医结合, e.g. no. 11 in Chapter 7), and in particular 'the Chinese antimalarial', must have shaped some local people's perception that 'Chinese medicine has rapid effects' (see Chapter 4).

Importantly, 'the Chinese antimalarial' was by Western medical standards a 'Western pharmaceutical'. Unlike traditional poly-'natural' pharmaceuticals, it contained one chemical substance only, which, in the 1970s, Professor Tu Youyou 屠呦呦 and her team at the China TCM Academy in Beijing had purified and isolated out of a plant extract. They also identified it almost entirely in chemical structure: this was artemisinin or, in Chinese, *qinghaosu* 青蒿素 (Tu 1977, 2011).[4] Artemisinin and its derivatives had been isolated and developed by modern Chinese scientists in the context of a military task force called 523 (Zhang [2005] 2013). The history of its manufacture was therefore completely different from that of the Chinese formula medicines. Nevertheless, in the early 2000s the patients I interviewed called it a *dawa ya Kichina*.

The alternative antimalarial treatments were with SP/Fansidar (sulfadoxine-pyremethamine) and Nivaquine (chloroquine). However,

SP was known to be harmful for people living with HIV/AIDS, as local newspaper articles, small posters pasted onto the walls in dispensaries and the casual remark of a health worker suggested. Chloroquine was considered basically ineffective but nevertheless was on offer (on this, see also Kamat 2009); traditional healers were allowed to dispense this ineffective medicine as it was thought to cause less harm than good (arguably erroneously). Furthermore, in areas where malaria is endemic, those people who survive into adulthood generally experience reinfections as episodes similar to the flu, marked by headaches and joint aches (e.g. Granado et al. 2011: 108). It was common practice in the early 2000s to treat these with painkillers. Some patients preferred painkillers, explaining that antimalarials adversely affected their gut. Unlike the expatriates, who were interested in taking prophylactic antimalarials – Malarone (atovaquone and proguanil hydrochloride), Lariam (mefloquine) and various brands of doxycycline, which is a tetracycline antibiotic, the locals took antimalarials only in cases of acute infection. Given this range of choice, 'the Chinese antimalarial' was praised for both (1) effecting a rapid clearance from fevers and (2) having absolutely no side effects. Scientists and professionals are rightly sceptical of laypersons' perceptions that produce the gossip of the day, but in this case, local perceptions have been validated by biomedical research as accurate (e.g. Hien and White 1993: Table 1; Ribeiro and Olliaro 1998).

However, even for government employees with a regular income, 'the Chinese antimalarial' was fairly expensive. A Fansidar tablet cost TZS 75, and a treatment cycle was made up of three of these, while a box of 'the Chinese antimalarial' required a five-day treatment cycle and cost TZS 4,500. One government clerk on the lowest salary grade, who lived in the far outskirts of the city, explained that he did not take any antimalarials at all, as they all were very bitter and adversely affected his stomach ulcers. After spending TZS 7,000 in vain on a comorbidity that he tried to have treated, first in the Chinese medical clinic and then, for double the price, in the Aga Khan hospital, he felt that he no longer had any money for treating his malaria and reverted to taking Panadol instead when he felt flu-like. Another government employee, however, who lived in a well-established neighbourhood, declared that 'the Chinese antimalarial' was relatively inexpensive. He explained that he would go to the local dispensary to get a blood test done, as it cost only a few shillings there, and then buy a full treatment course of 'the Chinese antimalarial' from the nearby Chinese medical clinic. He was one of the few people who knew that there were different brands and that none was a prophylactic. He said that the Chinese doctor had requested that he return to test the efficacy of the treatment, but he refused to do so as it was an extra expense. When asked whether he would take an entire treatment cycle after the fever had abated on the first day, he claimed that he did so. He responded to this question as almost all of my interviewees did. Patients also showed compliance with other Chinese medical treatments, even if they had to take tablets for an entire week. They may of course have said this to please the interviewer, but a variety of other observations (the readiness with which they showed me their packages of medication and the tablets that were left in them, the certainty and speed with which they told me the prescribed dosage, etc.) suggested that the local public health personnel had done well in impressing on them how important it was to adhere to one's prescriptions and dosage. The few exceptions seemed to prove the rule.

The chemical substances that made up 'the Chinese antimalarial' were multiple. In 2001 three main brands were on offer. These included Artesunate, which contained artesunate (dihydroartemisinin hemisuccinate) and was produced by Guilin Pharma; Artemedine,[5] which contained artemether (artemisinin with a methyl-group) and was produced by the Kunming Pharmaceutical Corporation; and Cotecsin (or Co-texin), which contained dihydroartemisinin and was produced by the Beijing COTEC New Technology Corporation; Cotecsin was particularly valued among expatriates in Kenya. Each package contained 40 mg for the first day and 20 mg for the subsequent four days (the WHO recommended a seven-day treatment with precisely these dosages; see Phillips-Howard 2002: 320).

Licensed pharmacists sold the Belgian Arinate and the French Artesumax at a price of about TZS 6,500 in 2002. The Chinese and European brands both used Chinese plant materials, but only the latter produced tablets to GMP standards. In the following years two Tanzanian brands became available, Malather and Thaitanzunate, which both sold for less, c. TZS 3,500. Both contained artemisinin for a treatment course, but the latter contained only 100 mg instead of 120 mg. In Kenya, by contrast, the Belgian brand was aggressively advertised on television. The audiences targeted were not the sufferers, who typically are poverty-stricken (WHO 2012), but enterprising, fairly educated (Form 4) middle-class men. In the mid-2000s, the prize that the year's four most successful Kenyan distributors of Arinate received was a spanking new BMW sports car.

Most locals were not aware that 'the Chinese antimalarial' could not be used as a prophylactic – but who, apart from the foreign tourist or expatriate, would take them prophylactically anyway? Locals did, however, know that it was unusual for an 'antimalarial' to have no side effects, but they did not understand why. Expatriates occasionally talked chemistry. I got the clearest scientific explanation of the pharmacokinetics of artemisinin from a researcher at NIMR (National Institute for Medical Research) on one of my first days in the field in Dar es Salaam. He had offered to give me a lift back to my hotel when we were caught in a traffic jam that lasted over an hour. 'Prophylactic antimalarials interrupt the life cycle of the vector in the liver', he explained. 'In the hepatic schizont stage?', I asked (vaguely remembering bits of my undergraduate lectures on the well-known four *Plasmodium* species that cause malaria). 'Yes', he said, and continued that the side effects accordingly arose primarily from damage to the liver. Artemisinin and its derivatives, by contrast, worked on the red blood cells in the bloodstream that were infected by the parasites (in the life stage of haploid merozoites). The molecule artemisinin had a highly labile, heat-sensitive but highly efficacious peroxide bridge (Hien and White 1993). It effected, so to speak, an 'explosion' of the infected red blood cells. This explained the speed with which it cleared high fevers. However, even though over 99.9 per cent of the parasites causing a bout of fever were killed by a few artemisinin tablets, it was easy for the remaining 0.1 per cent to proliferate and multiply, causing a new fever bout. This was called 'recrudescence', he said. Recrudescence itself did not cause resistance to the molecule artemisinin, but it heightened the possibility of the parasite developing resistance to it over time.

'Recrudescence' was evidently a concept that caused concern, but even though I repeatedly brought up the theme at conferences in Africa, Europe and East Asia, most scientists were rather vague about it. It was again during a serendipitous off-record moment that I was competently informed by an expert expatriate, this time the director of KEMRI (Kenya Medical Research Institute). While conducting fieldwork in Mombasa, I had been invited to spend Christmas 2005 with his family in Kilifi, and as he was seeing me off, we stood by the road for over an hour, waiting for a *matatu* bus.[6] In 2005, the WHO recommendation had been issued for artemisinin monotherapies as the treatment of choice for severe *P. falciparum* malaria, but 'recrudescence' (and the heightened risk it posed of the parasite developing resistance against the purified substance artemisinin) was the main reason that they were discouraged in 2006, when the WHO made a firm recommendation for ACT (Artemisinin Combination Therapy) instead.[7] In ACTs, artemisinin is combined with a conventional antimalarial synthetic substance that attacks the schizonts in the liver. The addition of this synthetic substance also made it possible to reduce the period of a treatment cycle to three days only. However, it might be precisely due to this change in the drug's chemical composition that anthropologists would now note hesitations in local people's perception of 'the Chinese antimalarial'.

## *Import-Export Bulk Trade with ACTs (Artemisinin Combination Therapy)*

By winter 2007–8, when I was doing fieldwork in Kampala, Uganda, the playing fields of 'the Chinese antimalarial' had changed. It was no longer sold in the grey zone of legality in Chinese medical clinics, in which it had made up over 50 per cent of over-the-counter transactions in the early 2000s. The reason was obvious. The Chinese medical practitioners had the permission to sell 'traditional', 'natural', 'herbal' treatment only, but not purified chemical substances, as those classified as Western medications. Paradoxically, as some Chinese practitioners remarked, 'the Chinese antimalarial' was now on offer exclusively in licensed Western medical pharmacies. Coartem (a combination of artemether and lumefantrine) was now the main product on sale. However, the price of a treatment course had tripled (it was the equivalent of TZS 14,000), as to be expected of a brand by a Swiss firm, Novartis. Furthermore, 'the Chinese antimalarial' was no longer the wonder drug that miraculously cleared malarial fever bouts within hours and had no side effects. Despite scientific articles to the contrary, rumours abounded of its severe side effects (e.g. Meier zu Biesen 2013: 332–60).

Evidently, both the substances in 'the Chinese antimalarial' and the 'playing fields' in which it was sold had changed. It no longer consisted of a single purified substance – artemisinin or one of its derivatives, among them dihydroartemisinin – nor was it sold any longer in Chinese medical clinics. It was now produced by 'the Swiss', was exorbitantly expensive and had multiple side effects. 'Are you sure it is a wonder drug?', one of my respondents queried. Furthermore, as I was to discover in my fieldwork, within fewer than ten years the term *dawa ya Kichina* had acquired yet another shade of meaning, which superseded some of the others.

When I explained to locals in Kampala that I was studying *dawa ya Kichina*, people would guide me to young men involved in the competitive selling of *Tianshui* 天水 or simply, 'Tiens' natural products (Wan 2011). These young men, in turn, led me into rooms in multistorey supermarkets, jammed up with chairs and large cardboard boxes – vestiges from a previous meeting. *Tianshui*, which traced its roots to Southeast Asia, struck me as a commerce-oriented movement in the name of health. This health enterprise was an entirely different social phenomenon from the one I was studying, as it involved the organisation of large group meetings, not unlike those of the Pentecostals, during which herbal health products, mostly in pill, tablet, capsule, granule and cream form, were advertised and sold *en masse* to individuals. This happened, importantly, on credit, as patients were tasked with selling these health products on to others in a snowball effect. This as-yet-understudied social movement was directed at people suffering from undefined chronic health problems who through a combination of intense group experiences and personal redefinition were led not only into better health, but also into total bankruptcy and, sometimes, complete social rupture with their families.

Had the Chinese medical clinics disappeared from the health field? No – they were there, as elsewhere in urban East Africa, thinly spread out throughout the city, advertising themselves to the entire spectrum of patients as they always had, ranging from the upper-middle-class population in the fairly well-to-do neighbourhoods to the crowds at loud and busy bus stations. 'The Chinese antimalarial' had once provided the Chinese doctors with a steady flow of income, but they evidently did not depend on it. Their services had been diverse from the start.

However, 'the Chinese' appeared to be more numerous than ever before, and businesspeople were populating an emergent field of state-subsidised medical commerce with high-tech biotechnology. These businesspeople were not medical doctors. They imported in bulk Chinese ACT brands alongside Chinese-manufactured surgical instruments and hospital furniture into Uganda. These brands included Artequin (a combination of artesunate and mefloquine), Duo-cotecsin (a combination of dihydroartemisinin and piperaquine phosphate) and Arco (a combination of artemisinin and naphthoquine). Arco, in particular, heralded this new era of pharmacoengineering. Importantly, Arco could be administered in a single dose, as advertised by a glossy brochure containing very high-quality graphics and colour photography. As in the case of the material aspects of the formula medicines' packaging discussed at length in Chapter 8, the main biotechnological effort seemed to have been spent on easing the consumption of the new product as a commercial commodity, and thereby heightening sales and profit margins, in place of improving the quality of its production or distribution.

In summary, through the study of 'the Chinese antimalarial' we have been able to discern within the late-liberal global health market two distinctive playing fields, related to different economies. In the early 2000s, Traditional Chinese Medical doctors had been involved in the dispensation of a variety of different artemisinin monotherapies, but by 2008 Chinese import-export traders, with Chinese brands of ACTs, had become the main players in the antimalarial health economies. The former had offered health provision as individualistic petty entrepreneurs, working with unregulated medicines in unregulated health markets within a grey zone of legality, while the latter were proponents of a growing, aggressively lucrative health commerce fed by international and national subsidies.[8] In these playing fields, the reputation of 'the Chinese antimalarial' had changed. Locals were generally not aware that this had to do with a change in the chemistry of the drug, that is, the thinginess of the thing.

Meanwhile, the organisation Tiens offered as a yearly prize an intercontinental trip (e.g. one week in Brazil) to those who had been able to sell the most drugs in bulk. They were almost exclusively young men. Ostensibly, they were not selling crack (Bourgois 1996) but 'doing good' by selling health products. There was an air of vibrant competition, out of which came increasingly visible winners and losers. The winners' aggressive selling strategies were likely matched, within the very same organisation, by the losers' acquisition of drugs in bulk on credit during the emotional high of a therapeutic group meeting and their subsequent failure to find an outlet for selling them on. As the prizes in this health economy involved fast cars and travel afar for enterprising, male individuals, these Tiens 'natural herbs' advertised the mobility and cultural diversity, even superdiversity, of late liberalism. To what extent the crowds they worked with experienced healing in the long run as well would be worth further study.

## Reflections: What Happened to the Fresh Plant Preparations as 'Pots'? Missed Opportunities for Handling Herbal *Pots* with Good Sense

The 'active man-in-the-mass' was engaged in a practical activity, according to Gramsci (1979), and 'revolutionary potential' could be found in such practical activities, guided by 'common sense'. Although overall, Gramsci's attitude to common sense is ambivalent (Crehan 2016), two of his comments are relevant here.

First, as already noted, Gramsci considered common sense to have revolutionary potential. Accordingly, there is political potential in the recognition of the commonsensical efficaciousness of herbal preparations, even if they are made from a weed-like sweet wormwood (*Artemisia annua* L.). Any claim that a potentially serious disease can be managed at the grassroots with practical know-how ultimately amounts to a political statement.

Second, Gramsci treated 'common sense' as a specific domain of knowledge.[9] He discussed 'common sense' in the context of: a) the connections between common sense, religion and philosophy, b) the relation between science, religion and common sense and c) language, 'languages' and common sense. We are familiar with the idea of differentiating between the 'logics' of different knowledges and domains of knowledge.[10] In other words, those three domains of knowledge, which intersect with the knowledge domains of 'traditional' medicines, at one level involve craftsmanship. Good sense arises from a craftsman's practical engagement with the world.

A missed opportunity would be, for health carers, not to consider practices pursued at the grassroots as manifestations of knowledge, namely practical knowledge and good sense.

After returning from the field, I was motivated to do extensive reading on ethnographies of East Africa, on the Chinese medical teams (*yiliaodui* 医疗队), on Chinese *materia medica* (*zhongyao*) and in particular, on *Artemisia annua*. I searched for studies on the traditional Chinese medical *qinghao* 青蒿 (*Artemisia annua* L.), rather than on the purified chemical substance that this plant produces, *qinghaosu* 青蒿素 (artemisinin). Not a single paper had been written on its history (despite several misleading titles). This contrasted with the articles in their thousands on the molecular structure, biochemistry, pharmacokinetics and clinical efficacy of *qinghaosu*. Likewise, protagonists of *qinghao* as a herbal antimalarial had shown little curiosity to learn from premodern Chinese medical practice and writings. The founder of the organisation Anamed, for instance, developed what in my fieldwork people called 'antimalarial herbal teas', although in the early 2000s only a few urbanites had had direct experience of these. Anamed's 'natural herb' method involved the drying of leaves, the boiling of water and the ingestion of infusions (e.g. Willcox et al. 2004), which to a student of Chinese medicine has more affinity with German phytotherapy involving infusions (pouring boiling water over the dried *materia medica*) than with Chinese medical decoctions (simmering the dried *materia medica* over a small fire and decanting the liquid that is then ingested). It appeared as though scientists and NGO activists considered premodern Chinese scientific knowledge completely irrelevant. Or was it that they lacked the necessary linguistic and ethnobiological knowledge to make sense of the texts in which this body ecological knowledge is contained? Had they failed to recognise an opportunity to make whole and heal when you have the flu-like symptoms of stomach aches and headaches, dizziness, listlessness and joint pains that the malaria causes that is perceived as a 'nuisance' rather than lethal disease by adults in sub-Saharan Africa? Just like drinking water is offered at every street corner in urban spaces for revitalising the dehydrated, would drinking the 'fresh weed juice', made of the herbal antimalarial *Artemisia annua*, revitalise the anaemic? Which spatial textures would most likely afford Chinese medical juice therapies of the kind and turn them into spatial practices of East Africa in the longterm?

## *Fieldwork outside the Field*

In preparation for fieldwork outside the field, I ventured into unknown textual territories. I had been trained in acupuncture during fieldwork in 1988/89, but was unfamiliar with both the *materia medica* texts and the formula literature, recognised today as two different genres: the Chinese *bencao* 本草 and *fangji* 方剂 literatures. I began a translation project in 2001 on all *qinghao* entries in the *bencao* up to 1596 (see Hsu 2010b) and another one in 2011 on all *qinghao* entries in the *fangji* up to 1911, in five volumes (Hsu et al. forthcoming). It was a small workshop at Green Templeton College, University of Oxford, that led to a collaboration between the pharmacognosist Dr Colin Wright and myself in 2006. The scientific results of this 'ethno-archaeological' research have been published in Wright et al. (2010) in a special issue of *Molecules*, honouring Professor Tu Youyou. Meanwhile, the experiential aspects of this ethno-archaeological project have interesting implications for future textual and medical anthropological research.

The fieldwork outside the field concerned a project that was 'ethno-archaeological' insofar as it consisted of re-enacting a *qinghao* recipe recorded by the alchemist-physician Ge Hong 葛洪 (340 CE) in the *Emergency Recipes Kept in One's Sleeve* (*Zhou hou bei ji fang*) 肘後備急方, Chapter 3.16.

> Another recipe: *qing hao*, one bunch, take two *sheng* [2 x 0.2 litres] of water for soaking it, wring it out for taking the juice, ingest it in its entirety (又方 青蒿一握 以水二升漬 絞取汁 盡服之).[11]

In 2006, the *A. annua* seeds germinated well and grew into bushy plants at Hailey House in Oxfordshire, easily reaching 2.5 to 3 metres in height in early June, when they were harvested. After a several-hour-long drive up the M1, they were prepared in a laboratory at the School of Pharmacy, University of Bradford. Two *sheng* in the Jin dynasty (fourth century) were four decilitres of water (not two litres, as one of my respondents working in Ethiopia suggested!); this is general knowledge, recorded in the standard dictionary *Hanyu dacidian* 汉语大词典. Yet the branches of the fresh plants were a metre long. The only way to soak 'a bunch of *qinghao*' in water was by

'The Chinese Antimalarial' as 'Pot' and Pot

detaching the fine foliage from the stems. The fresh foliage, stripped off the long branch-stems of a single plant, usually weighed about 70 g, and this foliage could be crammed into 4 dl of water, such that all leafy material was just about covered with water.

While I was busy carrying out the instructions of Ge Hong's text, Dr Colin Wright tinkered around without any textual instructions in front of him, aiming to extract juice out of the fresh plant leaves without soaking them in water. Within less than an hour he found a way of first pounding the leaves with a pestle in a small mortar, and then pressing out little drops of green juice from the pulp with index finger and thumb. He explained that the dosage for conducting a test on mice was in millilitres. Such practice-based tinkering had evidently also happened in premodern China. Li Shizhen 李时珍, incorporated the above formula by Ge Hong into his *Classified Materia Medica*, *Bencao gangmu* 本草綱目, posthumously published in 1596, but Li did not quote it verbatim, as that would have been pedantic and no scholar with self-respect would have done so. He came up with a recommendation, which was to pound the fresh plant materials: 'Use one bunch of *qing hao*, two *sheng* of water, pound with a pestle to juice and ingest it' (用青蒿一握 水二升 搗汁 服之). Alongside other minor changes, he replaced Ge Hong's recommendation to 'wring it out' – that is, wring out the plant after soaking it in water – with the wording 'pestle it'. This was exactly what Dr Wright had done! He had pestled fresh leaf into a pulp, out of which he pressed fresh juice in very small quantities.

In the Bradford pharmacognosy laboratory, we soon found that situational practicalities were key to the procedure of preparing the medicine. In the meantime the question regarding Ge Hong's formula was: for how long should we soak the leaves? The text was not explicit about this. I had tried to wring out the fresh leaves to no avail. My efforts only destroyed some epithelial cells such that the fresh plant's pleasant but penetrating scent filled the entire lab.

The text was vague, but the practice required a decision. I proposed to address the question in a systematic manner and find out how long one should soak the plant for through a string of trial and error experiments, say, every two hours. Colin, however, appealed to common sense, saying: 'It is 6 p.m. now; you are welcome to stay in the lab and do your systematic trial and error experimentation, but I am going home. I have family and I am hungry. Dinner will be served at 7 p.m. You have had a busy day, you got up at the crack of dawn, you drove far on the motorway, you only had a bite for lunch, you must be tired and hungry too. We can continue our experiment tomorrow.' And so we did. Colin had what Antonio Gramsci called 'good sense'. We were guided in a commonsensical way, not by the text, but by practical knowledge regarding our bodies. This afforded us a good night's sleep. This Gramscian good sense about one's own body was presumably not unlike that which the bodies of Chinese physicians have afforded since medieval times.

The following morning it was possible to wring out the plant. The foliage was soft and dark green. It was what in a Chinese text is called *lan* 爛, generally translated as 'rotten'. However, after soaking overnight, the foliage was not rotten, just soft. It was as soft, perhaps, as overcooked boiled vegetables, which in colloquial Chinese are also *lan*. Interestingly, after 2006, I continued to translate the word *lan* as 'rotten' because this was its standard translation, despite this practical experience. However, rotten plant materials have a different biochemistry, and I now translate *lan* as 'soft', as I had experienced it in my own hands.

If *lan* refers to the state in which the leaves are soft enough to be handled, it refers to a change in biophysics. Had I adopted a more physiognomic approach to word meaning, I would have taken more seriously the phenomena that I dealt with hands-on. For instance, when the *Bencao mengquan* 本草蒙荃 (quoted in Hsu 2010b: 103) says 生搗 爛絞汁, I would have revised my translation to the following: 'When they are fresh, pound them; when they are soft, wring out the juice.' Evidently, this reading of the word *lan* 爛 arose from a practical engagement with the world. The perception of the soft plant materials was inextricably linked to their handling.

Fifteen hours had passed between going for dinner and returning to the lab, whereas in the culture of a premodern physician the night may have been shorter, and this cultural difference may have affected the thinginess of the thing and its efficacy. Moreover, my skills at wringing out the plant were rather imperfect. The malariological tests, undertaken at the Swiss Tropical Institute in Basel on the following day, demonstrated that Li Shizhen's rendering of Ge Hong's recipe and the herbal antimalarial juice made from pounding fresh plant materials effected a 96 per cent recovery of malarial mice infected with *P. berghei* (Wright at al. 2010); however, my unskilled wringing out of the softened plant materials produced too watery an emulsion to have antimalarial effects.

Several attempts to continue this research project within academia failed. We encountered problems with getting the right seed, its growing, its harvesting and transport, and with funding. Businesspeople operating in today's commercialised fields of 'natural herbs' saw little profit in it: 'Why make a juice, it poses problems for distribution.' Colleagues in phytochemistry were inclined to believe that the efficaciousness of a fresh juice was greater than that of an infusion, but the problem of dosage when working with fresh plants was a consistently raised objection to the viability of a project for developing an antimalarial juice. Indeed, the variability in chemical composition of fresh plant materials is a well-known problem in ethnomedicine, and is also acknowledged in the Chinese *materia medica* (when, for instance, exact information is provided regarding when to harvest which plant parts). Public health regimes require research into dosage, also in juicing practices. The empowerment of health care at the grassroots that fresh *qinghao* juice affords has not been instantiated in the playing fields of tight biomedical malarial control, but the coronavirus crisis has spurred scientific research, if not into juices, into 'natural' teas (Nair 2021; Nie 2021), as all whole plant preparations prevent rapid generation of resistant strains (Elfawal et al. 2015).

## A Missed Opportunity?

In summary, Chinese medical formula medicines treated a wide range of disorders, and once a patient felt healed, they attracted patients with similar ailments. These practices, sometimes considered self-medication routines, were found to be best explained in terms of a reformulation regime (Pordié and Gaudillière 2014) in an early stage. Meanwhile, as seen in Chapter 7, disproportionate efforts by health professionals to maintain the notorious asymmetries between purified biomedicine and marginalised forms of TM/CAM were observed.

Interestingly, locals brought their reproductive issues to strangers, as Chinese medicine practitioners were often perceived to be, and regionally mobile clientele appeared to perceive the performance of good sex as a form of self-enhancement. Medicalised reproductive medicine has seen a rapid expansion in late liberalism, alongside a rapid increase, globally, of the leisure industries advertising sex for pleasure rather than for procreation.

Paradoxically, perhaps, in this context, the 'alternatively modern' Chinese formula medicines were sought, not merely because they were packaged as modern, but because they were considered traditional medicines, and traditional medicines had a well-known use. They enhanced the fecundity of the ancestral lands, the multiplication of kin and infant growth (Green 1996; Geissler and Prince 2010a; Fayers-Kerr 2013), and the hyper-ironic twists of post-postmodernity seemed to imbue the potency-boosting Chinese formula medicines with the affordances of local traditional medicines.

Finally, this chapter demonstrated how a succession of different 'playing fields' affected changes in the material make-up of what people called 'the Chinese antimalarial'. People in urban East Africa generally spoke of 'the Chinese antimalarial' as though it was one single thing. However, as demonstrated above, its chemical constitution was modified hand in hand with the transformations of the playing fields in which it was enacted. In the early 2000s, in the unregulated health markets of urban East Africa, various unregulated brands of artemisinin monotherapy flourished as over-the-counter antimalarials dispensed by Chinese medical practitioners. After the WHO recommendation of 2006, however, ACTs belonged among the bulk wares of Chinese import-export traders in heavily subsidised antimalarial donor economies.

Meanwhile, what Kopytoff (1986: 213) asked of doing the biography of a thing still applies: 'What, sociologically, are the possibilities inherent in its "status" and in the period and culture, and how are these possibilities realised?' Commodities are not merely transacted in a monetary economy, but form part of a moral economy. The playing fields of 'the Chinese antimalarial' that I described were both highly commercialised, but they were part of different moral economies. Artemisinin monotherapy was dispensed in the informal sector in urban East Africa in the early 2000s, while Artemisinin Combination Therapy (ACT) was part of a subsidised and richly endowed global health economy after 2006. Both the fairly affordable artemisinin monotherapy and the expensive ACTs were co-constitutive of the playing fields that enabled their use and of the patients that ingested them. Artemisinin monotherapy brands had barely any side effects, while the chemistry of the ACTs caused many side effects, some very serious.

Meanwhile, only pre-twentieth-century health fields have afforded fresh herbal antimalarial *qinghao* juice. The juice was a home remedy, easily made, easily dispensed, at low cost, yet probably rather high risk; one guesses that dosage affected its usage. Yet current public health regimes rely on RCTs for the legitimised usage of any medicine, and the chemistry of fresh plant materials is too complex for current research routines. The investigation into playing fields underlined that the materiality of the thing, in this case a fresh plant preparation, is co-constitutive of the sociality that makes its existence possible, or impossible. Is this a missed opportunity?

# Notes

1. This list is embarrassingly short, mentioning merely a few landmark publications.
2. The other two books, written in the orbit of either the Wellcome Trust or USAID, are by Zhang Jianfang ([2005] 2013), on Professor Li Guoqiao 李國橋 at the Guangzhou TCM University, and by Dana G. Dalrymple (2013).
3. This section elaborates on excerpts of Elisabeth Hsu. 2015. 'From Social Lives to Playing Fields: "The Chinese Antimalarial" as Artemisinin Monotherapy, Artemisinin Combination Therapy and *Qinghao* Juice', in Laurent Pordié and Anita Hardon (eds), 'Stories and Itineraries on the Making of Asian Industrial Medicines', special issue, *Anthropology & Medicine* 22(1): 75–86.
4. Much later in her life, Professor Tu was honoured with the Lasker and Nobel prizes in 2012 and 2015.
5. At the time, it did not actually have a brand name, and was known by its generic name, artemether.
6. At the time, hardly any articles had reported resistance to artemisinin *in vivo*, and if they had, they were controversial. For a more recent account of the situation in Kilifi, see Ndungu (2013). The IC50 remains exceedingly low *in vitro*.
7. The exact wording has been difficult to locate, but see WHO (2005: 28, under paragraph 3.4.2): 'Intramuscular artemether is included in the WHO complementary model list of Essential Drugs as a reserve antimalarial . . . Artesunate suppositories have now been produced according to Good Manufacturing Practice. Experience with these products is limited but their use may be appropriate for emergency treatment prior to referral at health facility and community levels in severely ill patients who are unable to swallow oral medication when im artemether (or iv quinine) is not available.'

For the change in policy in the following year, see WHO ([2006] 2011: 21, paragraph 7.1]; identical to WHO 2010): 'Artemisinin should not be used as monotherapy, as this will promote resistance to this critically important class of antimalarials. . . . In endemic regions, some semi-immune malaria patients could be cured using an incomplete dose or treatment regimens that would be unsatisfactory in patients with no immunity. In the past, this had led to different recommendations for patients considered as semi-immune and those considered as non-immune. This practice is no longer recommended.'

8. This field-based observation was reinforced in the news, e.g. 'Malaria and the Politics of Disease', *The Economist*, 8 April 2008. See also Meier zu Biesen (2013: 301 ff.).

9. For example, domain specificity may pertain to the theme of study, e.g. whether the 'object' engaged with is 'inanimate' or 'animate', different registers of speech and their truth claims, or situations, e.g. mathematics in the classroom versus daily life householding (Lave 1988; Lave and Wenger 1991).

10. For instance, the Ngaju Dayak in Katingan, Borneo, have been found to engage three different ways of knowing when engaging with the environment, called *pengatawa* (lexical and conceptual knowledge), *kaji* (arcane and esoteric knowledge) and *katau* (practical knowledge), where *tau* means 'to be able to do something' or 'knowing how to do something', like weaving, harvesting rattan or telling a story (Bizard 2014).

11. For a comprehensive translation of the Chinese *materia medica* texts on *qing hao* until 1596, see Hsu (2010b).

# Conclusion
# Kaleidoscopic Refractions

## Thinking beyond the Ethnic Lens

The notion of economic 'emplacement' has existed for a good decade in migration studies. It is an analytic concept that arose from the same aversion to research that – without further reflection – assumes that there are 'ethnic entrepreneurs' whose activities are best explained in terms of cultural traditions, engrained behavioural patterns and given moral frameworks (Glick Schiller and Çağlar 2013: 495). Such assumptions about 'ethnic entrepreneurs' preclude research into the multiple and nuanced processes by which people 'emplace' – or tangibly 'empot' (as suggested in Chapter 3) – themselves into new surroundings, regardless of whether they are mobile, migrant or sedentary. These assumptions also facilitate research that homogenises a wide range of observed tensions into 'culture clashes', where 'culture' appears to be the problem that has to be overcome. Unfortunately, this 'methodological nationalism' (Wimmer and Glick Schiller 2003) still today unduly affects not only migration studies, but any anthropological study on the foreigner, the stranger, the migrant and the mobile entrepreneur.

Glick Schiller and Çağlar (2013), whose article I found amid stacks of my photocopied 'to read' literature in the course of clearing my desk as this book project was coming to an end, have long expressed the issues at its core.

> By rejecting the ethnic lens scholars can explore the ways in which all people, including people of migrant background, deploy multiple frames of action and forms of belonging. (Ibid.: 495)

This is to treat people as people and not have them 'boxified' before one's study even begins. Just as we have done in this monograph,

Glick Schiller and Çağlar (ibid.) proposed to 'approach the study of migrant businesses by exploring urban-based entrepreneurial activities as a mode of emplacement', whereby 'emplacement' was understood to focus 'analytic attention on the conjuncture of time and place'. More specifically, economic emplacement has been defined as 'a relationship between the continuing restricting of a city within networks of power and migrants' efforts to settle and build networks of connection within the constraints and opportunities of a specific locality'.

To be sure, an assessment of economic emplacement goes beyond a 'view from below' that also focuses on the everyday, but remains 'confined by description'. Economic emplacement arises in a negotiated sphere of 'structures and narratives, as they emerge in particular moments in the historical trajectory and multiscalar positioning of specific cities' (Glick Schiller and Çağlar 2013: 495). In their study of migrant entrepreneurs in Halle/Saale, eastern Germany, at a time when the city was shrinking, Glick Schiller and Çağlar (2013) observed how the migrant entrepreneurs diversified their goods for different groups of customers, how their repertoire increasingly comprised inexpensive commodities catering to an expanding, poorly paid and unemployed clientele, and how they invaded empty spaces as they moved away from the city centre due to shrinking business opportunities, thereby newly enlivening the periphery.

'Empotment', as discussed in Chapter 3, and as presented as a process relevant to all themes discussed throughout the book, can be defined exactly along the same lines, as part of a multiscalar process specific to certain, often historically given constellations. It additionally emphasises that substances, materials and matter are involved in this process, conceived as one that affects and involves the body handling materials.

The East African contexts in which this happened were declining economies, yet the migrant entrepreneurs I studied were not destitute. They all had more than one option to play with; there was irony, and irony about this irony. At the beginning of my fieldwork, Chinese commodities were seen as providing value for money and being super-effective, but towards the end, many started to be seen as cheap. Glick Schiller and Çağlar (2013) remain path-breaking for our purposes here. Issues discussed in migration studies should not be treated differently from mainstream social anthropology.

## *Wanderung* and *Wandlung*

As noted already in pre-Second World War studies, *Wanderung* and *Wandlung* are cognates. People on the move instigate culture change. Specifically, Marcel Mauss pointed to the three great principles relevant to the study of 'civilisation', as undertaken in his days, which in Adolf Bastian's formulation pertained to: 1) the *Elementargedanke* (the basic idea), 2) the *geographische Provinz* (the geographic sector) and 3) *Wanderung und Wandlung*. While these formulations never had much traction, Mauss found the third worth commenting on. He emphasised their intrinsic relatedness:

> *Wanderung* – migration, travel, and the vicissitudes of civilisation – and with it, as in the case of autonomous evolution, the *Wandlung* of civilization, the transformation of civilisation by the borrowing of elements, by migrations, by mixtures of the peoples bearing these elements, or by *autonomous* activity on the part of these peoples. (Mauss [1927/30] 2006b: 59, italics added)

Today, migration studies are often treated as a domain of the (applied) social sciences, separate from that of general sociology and anthropology, as though there were an 'autonomous evolution' of a civilisation, on the one hand – the normal sort of phenomenon a social anthropologist would study – and *Wanderung* effecting cultural change, on the other. Interestingly, even today, when migration and mobility have increased in visibility and importance for the social sciences and humanities, they are nevertheless still studied in separate institutes or research groups. Yet Mauss flatly contradicted this dichotomising habit of thinking; *Wanderung* and *Wandlung* were cognates, he said, and 'autonomous evolution' would always involve 'borrowing' from elsewhere and from whoever is perceived as 'other'. Chinese medicine in East Africa is a curious phenomenon of migration, and specifically of so-called 'lifestyle migration', in the domain of the rapidly emergent area studies field CA/AC. Yet as this monograph aims to underline, its study also permits interesting reflections on the figuration of sociality more generally (that is, if one disposes of the ethnic lens). The social changes over time in a space, *Wandlung*, as instigated by *Wanderung*, are in this monograph not by definition treated as a specialist theme of creolisation, hybridity or superdiversity. Rather, this book aims to speak to questions of culturalising efforts in general.

For Mauss, 'economic pressure', as discussed in the context of the quotation below, was only a recent development. For him, the more important issue for understanding the evolution and developments of so-called 'civilisation' was 'exchanges of techniques'. So, if an aspiration to health and healing was involved, as in our case, its practices could be interpreted as activities of self-improvement in a way that involves sociality and affects social relatedness. For the study of such efforts towards self-perfection, Mauss proposes to focus on techniques and the arts.

> Yet all this commercial aspect is less important than the phenomenon of borrowing and the spread of techniques. In normal circumstances . . . a society will strive to acquire and make its own the techniques it recognises as superior. . . . Most of the time . . . borrowing is a matter of self-interest, a quest for a better and easier life. (Mauss 2006b: 47)

Accordingly, *Wandlung* as instigated through *Wanderung* would involve the borrowing of elements and the mixing of people bearing these elements, and, as Mauss underlined in the previous quotation, also an 'autonomous activity' on the part of these people (Mauss 2006b: 59). We are told to focus on the technique, the arts, the handicraft and the technologies. For the fieldworker, this implies an attentiveness to given specificities: 'It is essential to move from the concrete to the abstract and not the other way round' (Mauss [1935] 2006a: 78).

## The One, Two, Three of the Phenomenology of the Body

In focus have been fieldwork experiences involving efforts to effect in one's own self, and in the other, a transformation that would lead to a sense of wholeness and wholesomeness among the participants involved in a medical procedure, whether human or non-human.[1] I have not provided, and have no intention to produce, a list of the spaces in which specific techniques became constitutive of the sense of wholeness that they induced. Here, I merely wish to recapitulate some general points.

The first point pertains to Merleau-Ponty's (1945) definition of the body as being at the intersection of the self moving through space. So, a body in search of health is one that is moving. This may be movement as effected by muscular locomotion or by an affective movement in the sense of turning one's attention towards the other. It may also imply being moved in a more interiorised way – say, in common parlance, on an emotional level. Movement can also refer to bodies and people whose mobility involves long distances. The wholeness towards which healing activities are oriented would accordingly be generated only if someone is willing to move or be moved in one or more of the above senses. The self must want to move or be moved before any healing can happen.

The second point regards techniques that instigated a sense of wholeness; it is that movements always have an orientation, a directionality. Phenomenologists have demonstrated in multiple ways that the self's movements are oriented towards a *Thou*, and happen within an already given *Thou*-relation. Contra solipsism, which posits that ultimately, the self is locked into itself, phenomenologists each in their different ways emphasise that the movement of the self is a movement towards the other, away from itself. This self tends to comprehend itself as part of a *Thou*-relation, and healing thus involves techniques that affect the self as part of the *Thou*. There are 'propensities in things', and organisms have (pre)dispositions, so to speak, which facilitate learning sophisticated techniques in order to create polyphonically attuned temporalities. The orientation is outward, towards the other, who is usually already understood to be mingling with the self. This may be so, for instance, when providing comfort by sitting next to a person, holding hands, or if not, feeling their warmth, while emphasising the tactile aspects of speaking – the mingling of breath, for instance, rather than the meanings of what is being said.

Third, these movements do not happen in a spatial vacuum, but arise in response to given textures. As so often said, assemblages are re-assemblages, and figurations are reconfigured. However, not everything goes. Things have a propensity to fracture along certain lines and not others. Some bits remain clunky, and their associations with others may be sticky and enduring. We are dealing with heterogeneous materials in an unevenly textured space.

## What Makes Whole? Reflections on Reflections

The ethnographic core of the monograph has now been recast so as to elaborate on Merleau-Ponty's *Phenomenology of Perception*. This just happened, almost effortlessly. The process first involved finding a language that can account both for social and material, epistemological and ontological aspects of healing. This language was found in Henri Lefebvre's (1991) *The Production of Space*. By making space, place and emplacement (or rather, as I argue in this book, 'empotment' alongside 'emplotment') part of a dynamic that mobilises patients and practitioners into probing and eventually incorporating foreign, strange and exotic medicines into their daily life routines, I hope to have opened up new ways to think anthropologically about healing, namely as a technique of transformation, a becoming part of a place, and also an orientation towards the world.

How might people at risk find modes of living together, to be configured such that they comprehend themselves as forming a whole? The argument of this book works with the rendering of 'autopoiesis' as an 'autonomous figuration' or 'spontaneous (re-)configuration' – of the self, of self-*and*-other in a *Thou*-relation, of things and fields (and not as a 'self-making'). For sure, there are propensities in things and organisms to trigger this process, but this ethnography highlights that the triggering into becoming transformed can happen, regardless of size and scale, autonomously, but not unaffected by the textures of the space of which it is part. Part I started with the movement through space that enables a medical encounter, Part II was about the people – patients, practitioners and paramedical professionals – and Part III engaged with the ontologies of the medicine *pots*. Specifically, the final three chapters discussed the composition of hybrid modern-traditional formula medicines, the efficaciousness of enhancement procedures and the ontological changes that 'the Chinese antimalarial' underwent, from *qinghao* to *qinghaosu* and beyond.

Each chapter was introduced with an ethnographic section on 'fieldwork methods'. These methods sections were written in such a way as to be relevant to any reader interested in 'the ethnographic method'. The sections on siting the field, language-learning, semi-structured interviewing, working with narrative, tackling prickly issues, integrating the historical into the ethnographic and finding fault with oneself as a fieldworker discussed actual field experiences.

Furthermore, since anthropological theory has evolved since the ethnographic core of the book was first composed two de-

## Conclusion

cades ago, each chapter was rounded off with a section on a 'reflection', ruminating on 'theory' – specifically Alfred Schütz's foregrounding of the *Thou*-relation and Paul Grice's cooperative principle in Part I; Marcel Mauss's insistence on studying concrete techniques for understanding cultural evolution and de Certeau's (1984) tactics, echoing the Chinese 'propensity of things' (Jullien 1995), in Part II; and Ingold's (2000) sensory anthropology and Davis's (2000) anthropology of substances in Part III. We pointed to the wide range of different micro-skills and substances that can, in indirect ways, enable patients and practitioners to reconfigure their relations to each other and the places that they seek to inhabit.

## Note

1. This is not because I was unaware of the misunderstandings, conflicts and deceit happening in East African health fields between Chinese businesspeople and their local and regional competitors for clientele. Furthermore, it was impossible to turn a blind eye to the geopolitical perspective and the Belt and Road Initiative, as the Chinese medical entrepreneurs were perceived as part of the BRI's texturing of urban spaces.

# References

The references are in six separate sections: 1. academic publications, inclusive of dissertations and doctoral theses, 2. premodern texts, 3. TCM textbooks, 4. unpublished seminar presentations, 5. investigative journalism and grey literature, and 6. my own publications. Too many colleagues and friends to be mentioned here have contributed through joint discussions to this bibliography, but I wish to acknowledge Ms Yuxin Peng, University of Oxford, for her invaluable assistance with compiling it. Larry D. Sweazy is acknowledged for his work on the index.

## Academic Publications

Adams, Vincanne. 2002. 'Randomized Controlled Crime: Post-Colonial Sciences in Alternative Medicine Research', *Studies of Social Science* 32(5–6): 659–90.

Adams, Vincanne, et al. 2005. 'The Challenge of Cross-Cultural Clinical Trials Research: Case Report from the Tibetan Autonomous Region, People's Republic of China', *Medical Anthropology Quarterly* 9(3): 267–89.

Adams, Vincanne, Nancy J. Burke and Ian Whitmarsh. 2014. 'Slow Research: Thoughts for a Movement in Global Health', *Medical Anthropology* 33(3): 179–97.

Ahern, Emily M. 1975. 'Sacred and Secular Medicine in a Taiwan Village: A Study of Cosmological Disorders', in Arthur Kleinman, Peter Kunstadter, E. Russell Alexander and James L. Gale (eds), *Medicine in Chinese Cultures: Comparative Studies of Healthcare in Chinese and Other Societies*. Bethesda, MD: Geographic Health Studies, John E. Fogarty International Center for Advanced Study in the Health Sciences, pp. 91–113.

Alden, Chris, Daniel Large and Ricardo de Oliveira (eds). 2008. *China Returns to Africa: A Rising Power and a Continent Embrace*. London: Hurst.

Alter, Joseph S. (ed.). 2005a. *Asian Medicine and Globalization*. Philadelphia, PA: University of Pennsylvania Press.

———. 2005b. 'Introduction: The Politics of Culture and Medicine', in Joseph S. Alter (ed.), *Asian Medicine and Globalization*. Philadelphia, PA: University of Pennsylvania Press, pp. 1–20.

Andrews, Bridie. 2014. *The Making of Modern Chinese Medicine, 1850–1960*. Vancouver: University of British Columbia Press.

Appadurai, Arjun. (ed.). *The Social Life of Things: Commodities in Cultural Perspective*. Cambridge: Cambridge University Press.

Ardener, Edwin. 2007. 'Some Outstanding Problems in the Analysis of Events', in *The Voice of Prophecy and Other Essays*, ed. Malcolm Chapman. Oxford: Berghahn, pp. 86–104.

———. [2007] 2018. 'The Voice of Prophecy: Further Problems in the Analysis of Events', in *The Voice of Prophecy and Other Essays*, ed. Malcolm Chapman, 2$^{nd}$ expanded edn. Oxford: Berghahn, pp. 134–54.

Augé, Marc. 1986. 'L'Anthropologie de la maladie', *L'Homme* 26(97/98): 81–90.

Austin, John Langshaw. [1955] 1962. *How To Do Things With Words*. Cambridge, MA: Harvard University Press.

Banks, Marcus, and André Gingrich. 2006. 'Introduction: Neo-Nationalism in Europe and Beyond', in André Gingrich and Marcus Banks (eds), *Neo-Nationalism in Europe and Beyond: Perspectives from Social Anthropology*. Oxford: Berghahn, pp. 1–26.

Barnes, Linda L. 1998. 'The Psychologizing of Chinese Healing Practices in the United States', *Culture, Medicine and Psychiatry* 22(4): 413–43.

———. 2009. 'Practitioner Decisions to Engage in Chinese Medicine: Cultural Messages under the Skin', in Gunnar Stollberg and Elisabeth Hsu (eds), 'Globalizing Chinese Medicine', special issue, *Medical Anthropology* 28(2): 141–65.

Barry, Christine Ann. 2006. 'The Role of Evidence in Alternative Medicine: Contrasting Biomedical and Anthropological Approaches', *Social Science & Medicine* 62(11): 2646–57.

Bates, Donald G. (ed.). 1995. *Knowledge and the Scholarly Medical Traditions*. Cambridge: Cambridge University Press.

Bateson, Gregory. [1955] [1972] 1973a. 'A Theory of Play and Fantasy', in *Steps to an Ecology of Mind: Collected Essays in Anthropology, Psychiatry, Evolution and Epistemology*, 2$^{nd}$ edn. Frogmore: Paladin, 150–66.

———. 1973b. 'Redundancy and Coding', in *Steps to an Ecology of Mind: Collected Essays in Anthropology, Psychiatry, Evolution and Epistemology*, 2$^{nd}$ edn. Frogmore: Paladin, pp. 387–401.

Beckerleg, Susan. 1994. 'Medical Pluralism and Islam in Swahili Communities in Kenya', *Medical Anthropology Quarterly* 8(3): 299–313.

Beckmann, Nadine. 2012. 'Medicines of Hope? The Tough Decision for Anti-Retroviral Use for HIV in Zanzibar, Tanzania', *Journal of Eastern African Studies* 6(4): 690–708.

———. 2015a. 'The Quest for Trust in the Face of Uncertainty: Managing Pregnancy Outcomes in Zanzibar', in Elizabeth Cooper and David Pratten (eds), *Ethnographies of Uncertainty in Africa*. London: Palgrave Macmillan, pp. 59–83.

———. 2015b. 'Pleasure and Danger: Muslim Views on Sex and Gender in Zanzibar', in Erin Stiles and Katrina Daly-Thompson (eds), *Gendered Lives in the Western Indian Ocean: Islam, Marriage, and Sexuality on the Swahili Coast*. Columbus, OH: Ohio State University Press, pp. 117–40.

Benson, Michaela, and Karen O'Reilly. 2015. 'From Lifestyle Migration to Lifestyle in Migration: Categories, Concepts and Ways of Thinking', *Migration Studies* 4(1): 20–37.

# References

Bensky, Dan, Steven Clavey and Erich Stoeger, with Andrew Gamble. 2004. *Chinese Herbal Medicine: Materia Medica*, 3rd edn. Seattle, WA: Eastland Press.

Berlin, Brent. 1992. 'Manchung and Bikua: The Non-Arbitrariness of Ethnobiological Nomenclature', in *Ethnobiological Classification: Principles of Categorization of Plants and Animals in Traditional Societies*. Princeton, NJ: Princeton University Press, pp. 232–59.

Bernard, Harvey Russell. 1994. *Research Methods in Anthropology: Qualitative and Quantitative Approaches*, 2nd edn. London: Sage.

Biao, Xiang. 2013. *Making Order from Transnational Migration: Labor, Recruitment Agents and the State in Northeast China*. Princeton, NJ: Princeton University Press.

Biao, Xiang, 2011. 'A Ritual Economy of "Talent": China and Overseas Chinese Professionals', Brenda S.A. Yeoh and Shirlena Huang (eds), 'In and Out of Asia: The Cultural Politics of Talent Migration', special issue, *Journal of Ethnic and Migration Studies* 37 (5): 821–38. Reprinted as book in 2012, London: Routledge.

Bibeau, Gilles. 1985. 'From China to Africa: The Same Impossible Synthesis between Traditional and Western Medicines', *Social Science & Medicine* 21(8): 937–43.

Bierlich, Bernhard M. 2007. *The Problem of Money: African Agency and Western Medicine in Northern Ghana*. Oxford: Berghahn.

Blacking, John. 1977a. 'Towards an Anthropology of the Body', in John Blacking (ed.), *The Anthropology of the Body*. London: Academic Press, pp. 1–28.

——— (ed.). 1977b. *The Anthropology of the Body*. London: Academic Press.

Blaikie, Calum. 2015. 'Wish-fulfilling Jewel Pills: Tibetan Medicines from Exclusivity to Ubiquity', *Anthropology & Medicine* 22(1): 7–22.

Blaikie, Calum, Sienna Craig, Barbara Gerke and Theresia Hofer. 2015. 'Co-producing Efficacious Medicines: Collaborative Event Ethnography with Himalayan and Tibetan *Sowa Rigpa* Practitioners', *Current Anthropology* 56(2): 178–204.

Blommaert, Jan. 2013. *Ethnography, Superdiversity and Linguistic Landscapes: Chronicles of Complexity*. Bristol: Multilingual Matters.

Boas, Franz. 1911. 'Introduction', in *Handbook of American Indian Languages*, vol. 1. Washington, DC: Government Printing Office, pp. 1–83. Retrieved 9 January 2022 from http://biblio.wdfiles.com/local--files/boas-1911-introduction/boas_1911_introduction.pdf.

Boddy, Janice Patricia. 1989. *Wombs and Alien Spirits: Women, Men, and the Zar Cult in Northern Sudan*. Madison, WI: University of Wisconsin Press.

Bode, Maarten. 2004. 'Ayurvedic and Unani Health and Beauty Products: Reworking India's Medical Traditions', PhD thesis. Amsterdam: Faculty of Social and Behavioural Sciences, University of Amsterdam.

———. 2008. *Taking Traditional Knowledge to the Market: The Modern Image of the Ayurvedic and Unani Industry, 1980–2000*. Hyderabad: Orient Longman.

Booth, Karen. 2004. *Local Women, Global Science: Fighting AIDS in Kenya*. Bloomington, IN: Indiana University Press.

Bourdieu, Pierre. [1958] 1979. 'The Kabyle House or the World Reversed', in *Algeria 1960*, Cambridge: Cambridge University Press, pp. 133–55.
———. [1972] 1977. *Outline of a Theory of Practice*. Cambridge: Cambridge University Press.
———. [1979] 1984. *Distinction: A Social Critique of the Judgement of Taste*. London: Routledge.
Bourgois, Philippe. 1996. 'In Search of Masculinity: Violence, Respect and Sexuality among Puerto Rican Crack Dealers in East Harlem', *British Journal of Criminology* 36(3): 412–27.
Bram, Barclay. 2020. 'Help-Seekers, Callers and Clients: Embodied History in China's Psy-Boom', *Medical Anthropology Quarterly* 34(2): 286–300.
Bräutigam, Deborah. 2009. *The Dragon's Gift: The Real Story of China in Africa*. Oxford: Oxford University Press.
———. 2011. 'Chinese Development Aid in Africa: What, Where, Why, and How Much?', in Jane Golley and Song Ligang (eds), *Rising China: Global Challenges and Opportunities*. Canberra: ANU Press, pp. 203–22.
Bray, Francesca. 1995. 'A Deathly Disorder: Understanding Women's Health in Late Imperial China', in Donald Bates (ed.), *Knowledge and the Scholarly Medical Traditions*. Cambridge: Cambridge University Press, pp. 235–50.
Braun, Lesley Nicole, and Heidi Østbø Haugen. 2021. 'The Weight Women Carry: Research on the Visible and Invisible Baggage in Suitcase Trade between China and Africa', *The Professional Geographer* [online first]. https://doi.org/10.1080/00330124.2021.1950554.
Brown, Theodore, Marcos Cueto and Elizabeth Fee. 2006. 'The World Health Organization and the Transition from "International" to "Global" Public Health', *American Journal of Public Health* 96(1): 62–72.
Bruchhausen, Walter. 2006. *Medizin zwischen den Welten: Vergangenheit und Gegenwart des medizinischen Pluralismus im südöstlichen Tansania*. Göttingen: V&R University Press/Bonn: Bonn University Press.
Callon, Michel. 1986. 'Some Elements for a Sociology of Translation: Domestication of the Scallops and the Fishermen of St-Brieuc Bay', in John Law (ed.), *Power, Action and Belief: A New Sociology of Knowledge?* London: Routledge & Kegan Paul, pp. 196–233.
Campinas, Manuel. 2020. 'Stones, Demons, Medicinal Herbs, and the Market: Ethnic Medicine and Industrial Aspirations among the Qiang of Western Sichuan', PhD thesis. London: London School of Hygiene & Tropical Medicine.
Candelise, Lucia. 2008. 'La médecine Chinoise dans la pratique médicale en France et en Italie, de 1930 à nos jours: Représentations, reception, tentatives d'intégration', PhD thesis, 2 vols. Paris: École des Hautes Études en Sciences Sociales, with the Univeristy of Milano-Bicocca.
———. 2011. 'Chinese Medicine Outside of China: The Encounter between Chinese Medical Practices and Conventional Medicine in France and Italy', *China Perspectives* 3: 43–50.
Caplan, Patricia. 2004. 'Struggling to be Modern: Recent Letters from Mafia Island', in Patricia Caplan and Farouk Topan (eds), *Swahili Modernities*:

*Culture, Politics, and Identity on the East Coast of Africa*. Trenton, NJ: Africa World Press, pp. 43–60.

Ceuppens, Bambi, and Peter Geschiere. 2005. 'Autochthony: Local or Global? New Modes in the Struggle over Citizenship and Belonging in Africa and Europe', *Annual Review of Anthropology* 34(1): 385–407.

Chandler, Clare IR, Caroline Jones, Gloria Boniface, Kaseem Juma, Hugh Reyburn and Christopher JM Whitty 2008. 'Guidelines and Mindlines: Why Do Clinical Staff Over-Diagnose Malaria in Tanzania? A Qualitative Study', *Malaria Journal* 7: 53. https://doi.org/10.1186/1475-2875-7-53.

Chatelard, Solange. 2018. 'From Imperialism to Intimacy: An Ethnography of the First Chinese Migrants to Zambia 1980–Today', PhD thesis. Paris: Sciences Po.

Chen, Meixuan, Paul Kadetz, Christie Cabral and Helen Lambert. 2020. 'Prescribing Antibiotics in Rural China: The Influence of Capital on Clinical Realities', *Frontiers in Sociology* 5: Article 66.

Chiang, Howard. 2015. *Historical Epistemology and the Making of Modern Chinese Medicine*. Manchester: Manchester University Press.

Clarke, Bruce. 2012. 'Autopoiesis and the Planet', in Henry Sussman (ed.), *Impasses of the Post-Global: Theory in the Era of Climate Change*, vol. 2. Ann Arbor, MI: Open Humanities Press, pp. 58–75.

Cochran, Sherman. 2006. *Chinese Medicine Men: Consumer Culture in China and Southeast Asia*. Cambridge, MA: Harvard University Press.

Coderey, Céline, and Laurent Pordié (eds). 2019. *Circulation and Governance of Asian Medicine*. London: Routledge.

Cohen, Emma, et al. 2010. 'Rowers' High: Behavioural Synchrony is Correlated with Elevated Pain Thresholds', *Biology Letters* 6(1): 106–08.

Coleman, Simon, and Peter Collins. 2006. 'Introduction: "Being . . . Where?" Performing Fields on Shifting Grounds', in Simon Coleman and Peter Collins (eds), *Locating the Field: Space, Place and Context in Anthropology*. Oxford: Berg, pp. 1–22.

Comaroff, Jean, and John L. Comaroff. 1992. *Ethnography and the Historical Imagination*. Boulder, CO: Westview Press.

——— . 2009. *Ethnicity, Inc.* Chicago: University of Chicago Press.

Comaroff, Jean, and John Comaroff (eds). 1993. *Modernity and its Malcontents: Ritual and Power in Postcolonial Africa*. Chicago: University of Chicago Press.

Cooper, Elizabeth, and David Pratten (eds). 2015. *Ethnographies of Uncertainty in Africa*. London: Palgrave Macmillan.

Craig, Sienna R. 2012. *Healing Elements: Efficacies and the Social Ecologies of Tibetan Medicine*. Berkeley, CA: California University Press.

Craig, Sienna R., and Denise M. Glover 2009. 'Conservation, Cultivation and Commodification of Medicinal Plants in the Greater Himalayan-Tibetan Plateau', Sienna R. Craig and Denise M. Glover (eds) 'Medicinal Plant Cultivation, Conservation and Commoditization in the Himalaya and Tibet', special issue, *Asian Medicine* 5(2): 219–42.

Crehan, Kate. 2002. *Gramsci, Culture, and Anthropology*. Berkeley, CA: University of California Press.

———. 2016. *Gramsci's Common Sense: Inequality and Its Narratives*. Durham, NC: Duke University Press.
Croizier, Ralph C. 1968. *Traditional Medicine in Modern China: Science, Nationalism, and the Tensions of Cultural Change*. Cambridge, MA: Harvard University Press.
———. 1976. 'The Ideology of Medical Revivalism in Modern China', in Charles Leslie (ed.), *Asian Medical Systems: A Comparative Study*. Berkeley, CA: University of California Press, pp. 341–55.
Crossley, Nick. 2005. 'Mapping Reflexive Body Techniques: On Body Modification and Mapping', *Body and Society* 1(1): 1–35.
Csordas, Thomas J. [1988] 1990. 'Embodiment as a Paradigm for Anthropology', *Ethos* 18(1): 5–47.
———. 1993. 'Somatic Modes of Attention', *Cultural Anthropology* 8(2): 135–56.
———. 1994a. *The Sacred Self: A Cultural Phenomenology of Charismatic Healing*. Berkeley, CA: University of California Press.
———. 1994b. 'Introduction: The Body as Presentation and Being-in-the-World', in Thomas J. Csordas (ed.), *Embodiment and Experience: The Existential Ground of Culture and Self*. Cambridge: Cambridge University Press, pp. 1–24.
———. (ed.). 1994c. *Embodiment and Experience: The Existential Ground of Culture and Self*. Cambridge: Cambridge University Press.
———. 1999. 'The Body's Career in Anthropology', in Henrietta L. Moore (ed.), *Anthropological Theory Today*. London: Polity Press, pp. 172–233.
———. 2002. *Body/Meaning/Healing*. Basingstoke: Palgrave Macmillan.
———. 2008. 'Intersubjectivity and Intercorporeality', *Subjectivity* 22(1): 110–21.
———. 2011. 'Subjectivity: Ethnographic Investigations', *Subjectivity* 4(2): 204–6.
———. 2017. 'The Impossibility of the Inert: Placebo and the Essence of Healing', Somatosphere, June 23. Retrieved 9 January 2022 from http://somatosphere.net/2017/the-impossibility-of-the-inert-placebo-and-the-essence-of-healing.html/.
Cueto, Marcos, Theodore M. Brown and Elizabeth Fee. 2019. *The World Health Organization: A History*. Cambridge: Cambridge University Press.
Cushing, Frank H. 1892. 'Manual Concepts: A Study of the Influence of Hand-Usage on Culture-Growth', *American Anthropologist* 5(4): 289–318.
Daniel, E. Valentine. 1984. 'The Pulse as an Icon in Siddha Medicine', in E. Valentine Daniel and Judy F. Pugh (eds), *South Asian Systems of Healing*. Leiden: Brill, pp. 115–26. Reprinted in David Howes (ed.) 1991, *The Varieties of Sensory Experience: A Sourcebook in the Anthropology of the Senses*. Toronto: University of Toromnto Press, pp. 100–10.
Das, Veena, and Ranendra K. Das. 2005. 'Urban Health and Pharmaceutical Consumption in Delhi, India', *Journal of Biosocial Science* 38(1): 69–82.
Davies, James, and Dimitrina Spencer (eds). 2010. *Emotions in the Field: The Psychology and Anthropology of Fieldwork Experience*. Stanford, CA: Stanford University Press.

# References

Davies, Janette. 2007. 'Necessary In-Betweens: Auxiliary Workers in a Nursing-Home Hierarchy', in Kent Maynard (ed.), *Medical Identities: Health, Wellbeing and Personhood*. Oxford: Berghahn, pp. 117–33.

Davis, Christopher. 2000. *Death in Abeyance: Illness and Therapy among the Tabwa in Central Africa*. Edinburgh: Edinburgh University Press.

Davis, Dona Lee (ed.). 1988. 'Historical and Cross-Cultural Perspectives on Nerves', special issue, *Social Science & Medicine* 26(12): 1197–1259.

Dawkins, Richard. 1976. *The Selfish Gene*. Oxford: Oxford University Press.

De Certeau, Michel. 1984. *The Practice of Everyday Life*. Berkeley, CA: University of California Press.

De Montellano, Ortiz B. 1975. 'Empirical Aztec Medicine: Aztec Medicinal Plants Seem to Be Effective If They Are Judged by Aztec Standards', *Science* 188(4185): 215–20.

De Saussure, Ferdinand. 1916. *Cours de linguistique générale*, ed. Charles Bally and Albert Sechehaye, assisted by Albert Riedlinger. Lausanne: Payot.

Descola, Philippe. [2005] 2013a. *Beyond Nature and Culture*, trans. J. Lloyd. Chicago: University of Chicago Press.

———. [2011] 2013b. *The Ecology of Others*, trans. G. Godbout and B. P. Luley. Chicago: Prickly Paradigm Press.

Desjarlais, Robert. 1996. 'Presence', in Carol Laderman and Marina Roseman (eds), *The Performance of Healing*. London: Routledge, pp. 143–64.

Despeux, Catherine. 1996. 'Le corps, champ spatio-temporel, souche d'identité', *L'Homme* 137: 87–118.

Despret, Vinciane. 2004. 'The Body We Care for: Figures of Anthropo-zoogenesis'. *Body and Society* 10(2–3): 111–34.

Devisch, Renaat. 1993. *Weaving the Threads of Life: The Khita Gyn-Ecological Healing Cult among the Yaka*. Chicago: University of Chicago Press.

Dilger, Hansjörg. 2007. 'Healing the Wounds of Modernity: Salvation, Community and Care in a Neo-Pentecostal Church in Dar Es Salaam, Tanzania', *Journal of Religion in Africa* 37(1): 59–83.

Dilger, Hansjörg, and Dominik Mattes. 2018. 'Im/mobilities and Dis/connectivities in Medical Globalisation: How Global is Global Health?' *Global Public Health* 13(3): 265–75.

Dilger, Hansjörg, and Ute Luig (eds). 2010. *Morality, Hope and Grief: Anthropologies of AIDS in Africa*. Oxford: Berghahn.

Dobler, Gregor. 2008. 'Solidarity, Xenophobia and the Regulation of Chinese Businesses in Namibia', in Chris Alden, Daniel Large and Ricardo Soares de Oliveira (eds), *China Returns to Africa: A Rising Power and a Continent Embrace*. London: Hurst, pp. 237–55.

———. 2017. 'China and Namibia, 1990 to 2015: How a New Actor Changes the Dynamics of Political Economy', *Review of African Political Economy* 44(153): 449–65.

Douglas, Mary. 1966. *Purity and Danger: An Analysis of Concepts of Pollution and Taboo*. London: Routledge & Kegan Paul.

Duden, Barbara. [1987] 1991. *The Woman Beneath the Skin: A Doctor's Patients* in *Eighteenth-Century Germany*, trans. T. Dunlap. Cambridge, MA: Harvard University Press.

Dunk, Pamela. 1989. 'Greek Women and Broken Nerves in Montreal', in L. S. Greene (ed.), 'Health, Culture and the Nature of Nerves', special issue, *Medical Anthropology* 11(1): 29–45.

Durkheim, Émile. [1912] 1915. *The Elementary Forms of the Religious Life*, trans. J. W. Swain. London: Allen and Unwin.

Edmonds, Alexander, and Emilia Sanabria. 2014. 'Medical Borderlands: Engineering the Body with Plastic Surgery and Hormonal Therapies in Brazil', *Anthropology & Medicine* 21(2): 202–16.

Elfawal, Mostafa A., Melissa J. Towler, Nicholas G. Reich, Douglas Golenbock, Pamela J. Weathers and Stephen M. Rich. 2012. 'Dried Whole Plant *Artemisia annua* as an Antimalarial Therapy', *PloS one* 7(12): e52746.

Elfawal, Mostafa A., et al. 2015. 'Dried Whole-Plant *Artemisia annua* Slows Evolution of Malaria Drug Resistance and Overcomes Resistance to Artemisinin', *PNAS* 112(3): 821–26.

Elias, Norbert. [1939] 1969. *The Civilizing Process, vol. 1: The History of Manners*. Oxford: Blackwell.

———. 1978. *What is Sociology?* New York: Columbia University Press.

Elliot, Alice, Roger Norum and Noel B. Salazar (eds). 2017. *Methodologies of Mobility: Ethnography and Experiment*. Oxford: Berghahn.

Elliott, Elizabeth, Robin Ejsmond-Frey, Nicola Knight, and R.I.M. Dunbar. 2020. 'Forest Fevers: Traditional Treatment of Malaria in the Southern Lowlands of Laos', *Journal of Ethnopharmacology* 249: 112187.

Etkin, Nina L., and Paul J. Ross. [1983] 1997. 'Malaria, Medicine and Meals: A Biobehavioral Perspective', in L. Romanucci-Ross, Daniel E. Moerman and Laurence R. Tancredi (eds), *The Anthropology of Medicine: From Culture to Method*, 3rd edn. New York: Praeger, pp.169–209.

Evans-Pritchard, Edward Evan. 1937. *Witchcraft, Oracles and Magic among the Azande*. Oxford: Clarendon Press.

Farnell, Brenda. 2000. 'Getting Out of the Habitus: An Alternative Model of Dynamically Embodied Social Action', *Journal of the Royal Anthropological Institute* 6(3): 397–418.

Farquhar, Judith B. 1992. 'Time and Text: Approaching Chinese Medical Practice through Analysis of a Published Case', in Charles Leslie and Allan Young (eds), *Paths to Asian Medical Knowledge*. Berkeley, CA: University of California Press, pp. 62–73.

———. 1994. *Knowing Practice: The Clinical Encounter of Chinese Medicine*. Boulder, CO: Westview.

———. 1999. 'Technologies of Everyday Life: The Economy of Impotence in Reform China', *Cultural Anthropology* 14(2): 155–79.

Favret-Saada, Jeanne. 1977. *Les mots, la mort, les sorts. La sorcellerie dans le Bocage* [Deadly Words: Witchcraft in the Bocage], Paris: Gallimard.

Fayers-Kerr, Kate Nialla. 2013. 'Beyond the Social Skin: Healing Arts and Sacred Clays among the Mun (Mursi) of Southwest Ethiopia', DPhil thesis. Oxford: University of Oxford.

# References

———. 2018. 'Clay, Cosmology, and Healing', in Timothy Clack and Marcus Brittain (eds), *The River: Peoples and Histories of the Omo-Turkana Area*. Oxford: Archaeopress, pp. 71–75.

———. 2019. 'Becoming a Community of Substance: The Mun, the Mud and the Therapeutic Art of Body Painting', in Louise Attala and Luci Steel (eds), *Body Matters: Exploring the Materiality of the Human Body*. Chicago: University of Chicago Press, pp. 109–34.

Feierman, Steven. 1981. 'Therapy as a System-in-Action in Northeastern Tanzania', *Social Science & Medicine* 15B(3): 353–60.

Ferguson, James. 2015. *Give a Man a Fish: Reflections on the New Politics of Distribution*. Durham, NC: Duke University Press.

Fernandez, James. 1974. 'The Mission of Metaphor in Expressive Culture [and Comments and Reply]', *Current Anthropology* 15(2): 119–45.

Ferzacca, Steve. 2002. 'Governing Bodies in New Order Indonesia', in Mark Nichter and Margaret Lock (eds), *New Horizons in Medical Anthropology*. London: Routledge, pp. 35–57.

———. 2004. 'Lived Food and Judgments of Taste at a Time of Disease', *Medical Anthropology* 23(1): 41–67.

Field, Margaret. 1960. *Search for Security: An Ethno-Psychiatric Study of Rural Ghana*. London: Faber and Faber.

Flitsch, Mareile. 1994. *Der Ginsengkomplex in den Han-chinesischen Erzähltraditionen des Jiliner Changbai-Gebietes: Erfassung, Darstellung und Analyse der Jiliner Ginsengerzählungen unter Verwendung selbst gesammelten Materials und unter besonderer Berücksichtigung der Volksliteratur- und Volkskundeforschung Jilins 1949–1988*. Frankfurt: Peter Lang.

Frank, Robert. 2004. *Globalisierung 'Alternativer' Medizin: Homöopathie und Ayurveda in Deutschland und Indien*. Bielefeld: Transcript.

Frank, Robert, and Gunnar Stollberg. 2004. 'Conceptualizing Hybridization: On the Diffusion of Asian Medical Knowledge to Germany', *International Sociology* 19(1): 71–88.

Frazer, James George. 1890 [1981]. *The Golden Bough*. New York: Gramercy Books.

Friedson, Steven Michael. 1996. *Dancing Prophets: Musical Experience in Tumbuka Healing*. Chicago: University of Chicago Press.

Furth, Charlotte. 1999. *A Flourishing Yin: Gender in China's Medical History, 960–1665*. Berkeley, CA: University of California Press.

Gaonkar, Dilip P. 1999. 'On Alternative Modernities', *Public Culture* 11(1): 1–18.

Garfield, Richard, and Eugenio Taboada. 1984. 'Health Services Reforms in Revolutionary Nicaragua', *American Journal of Public Health* 74(10): 1138–44.

Geissler, Wenzel, and Ruth Jane Prince. 2007. 'Life Seen: Touch and Vision in the Making of Sex in Western Kenya', *Journal of Eastern African Studies* 1(1): 123–49.

———. 2010a. *The Land is Dying: Contingency, Creativity and Conflict in Western Kenya*. Oxford: Berghahn.

———. 2010b. 'Persons, Plants and Relations: Treating Childhood Illness in a Western Kenyan Village', in Elisabeth Hsu and Stephen Harris (eds), *Plants, Health and Healing: On the Interface of Ethnobotany and Medical Anthropology*. Oxford: Berghahn, pp. 179–223.

Gerke, Barbara (ed.). 2013. 'Mercury in Ayurveda and Tibetan Medicine', special issue, *Asian Medicine* 8(1): 1–239.

———. 2021. *Taming the Poisonous: Mercury, Toxicity, and Safety in Tibetan Medical Practice*. Heidelberg: Heidelberg University Publishing.

Geurts, Kathryn Linn. 2002. *Culture and the Senses: Bodily Ways of Knowing in an African Community*. Berkeley, CA: University of California Press

Gibson, James J. 1979. *The Ecological Approach to Visual Perception*. Boston: Houghton Mifflin.

Gilbertson, Adam Lloyd. 2013. 'The Ecology of Risk in an Informal Settlement: Interpersonal Conflict, Social Networks, and Household Food Security', DPhil thesis. Oxford: University of Oxford.

———. 2015. 'Food Security, Conjugal Conflict, and Uncertainty in "Bangladesh", Mombasa, Kenya', in Elizabeth Cooper and David Pratten (eds), *Ethnographies of Uncertainty in Africa*. London: Palgrave Macmillan, pp. 84–108.

Glick Schiller, Nina. 2005. 'Transnational Urbanism as a Way of Life: A Research Topic not a Metaphor', *City & Society* 17(1): 49–64.

Glick Schiller, Nina, Linda Basch and Cristina Szanton Blanc. 1995. 'From Immigrant to Transmigrant – Theorizing Transnational Migration', *Anthropological Quarterly* 68(1): 48–63.

Glick Schiller, Nina, Ayse Çağlar and Thaddeus C. Guldbrandsen. 2006. 'Beyond the Ethnic Lens: Locality, Globality, and Born-Again Incorporation', *American Ethnologist* 33(4): 612–33.

Glick Schiller, Nina, and Ayse Çağlar. 2008. 'Migrant Incorporation and City Scale: Towards a Theory of Locality in Migration Theories', in M. Povrzanovic Frykman (ed.), *Willy Brandt Series of Working Papers in International Migration and Ethnic Relations*. Malmö: Malmö University. Reprinted in 2009, *Journal of Ethnic and Migration Studies* 35(2): 177–202.

———. 2013. 'Locating Migrant Pathways of Economic Emplacement: Thinking beyond the Ethnic Lens', *Ethnicities* 13(4): 494–514.

———. 2015. 'Displacement, Emplacement, and Migrant Newcomers: Rethinking Urban Sociabilities within Multiscalar Power', *Identities: Global Studies in Culture and Power* 23(1): 17–34.

Gonçalves Martín, Johanna. 2016. 'The Path of Health and the Elusiveness of Fertility: Partial Translations between Yanomami People and Doctors in the Venezuelan Amazon', PhD thesis. Cambridge: University of Cambridge.

Good, Byron J. 1994. *Medicine, Rationality, and Experience: An Anthropological Perspective*. Cambridge: Cambridge University Press.

Good, Byron. J., and Mary-Jo DelVecchio Good. 1994. 'In the Subjunctive Mode: Epilepsy Narratives in Turkey', *Social Science & Medicine* 38(6): 835–42.

Good, Mary-Jo DelVecchio, Esther Mwaikambo, Erastus Amayo and James Machoki. 1999. 'Clinical Realities and Moral Dilemmas: Contrasting Perspec-

tives from Academic Medicine in Kenya, Tanzania, and America', *Daedalus* 128(4): 167–96.
Gramsci, Antonio. 1971. *Selections from the Prison Notebooks of Antonio Gramsci*, ed. Quintin Hoare and Geoffrey Nowell-Smith. London: Lawrence and Wishart.
Granado, Stefanie, Lenore Manderson, Brigit Obrist and Marcel Tanner. 2011. 'Appropriating Malaria: Local Responses to Malaria Treatment and Prevention in Abidjan, Cote d'Ivoire', *Medical Anthropology* 30(1): 102–21.
Grasseni, Cristina (ed.). 2007. *Skilled Visions: Between Apprenticeship and Standards*. Oxford: Berghahn Books.
Green, Maia. 1996. 'Medicines and the Embodiment of Substances among Pogoro Catholics, Southern Tanzania', *Journal of the Royal Anthropological Institute* 2(3): 485–98.
Green, Paul. 2014. 'Contested Realities and Economic Circumstances: British Later-Life Migrants in Malaysia', in Michael Janoschka and Heiko Haas (eds), *Contested Spatialities, Lifestyle Migration and Residential Tourism*. London: Routledge, pp. 145–57.
Grice, Paul. [1967] 1989. 'Logic and Conversation', in *Studies in the Way of Words*. Cambridge, MA: Harvard University Press, pp. 22–40.
Grillo, Ralph D. 1973. *African Railwaymen: Solidarity and Opposition in an East African Labour Force*. Cambridge: Cambridge University Press.
Grimley Evans, John. 2010. 'East goes West, *Ginkgo biloba* and Dementia', in Elisabeth Hsu and Stephen Harris (eds), *Plants, Health and Healing: On the Interface of Ethnobotany and Medical Anthropology*. Oxford: Berghahn, pp. 229–61.
Guenzi, Caterina. 2021. *Words of Destiny: Practicing Astrology in North India*. Albany, NY: SUNY Press.
Günel, Gökçe, Saiba Varma and Chika Watanabe. 2020. 'A Manifesto for Patchwork Ethnography', Society for Cultural Anthropology, 9 June. Retrieved 10 January 2022 from https://culanth.org/fieldsights/a-manifesto-for-patchwork-ethnography.
Hall, Edward T. [1966] 1982. *The Hidden Dimension*. New York: Anchor Books.
Hallowell, Irving A. [1954] 2017. 'The Self and Its Behavioral Environment', in *Culture and Experience*. Philadelphia: University of Pennsylvania, pp. 75–111.
Hanks, William F. 2005. 'Pierre Bourdieu and the Practices of Language', *Annual Review of Anthropology* 34(1): 67–83.
Hannerz, Ulf. 1987. 'The World in Creolisation', *Africa* 57: 546–59.
Haram, Liv, and C. Bawa Yamba (eds). 2009. *Dealing with Uncertainty in Contemporary African Lives*. Uppsala: Nordika Afrikainstitutet.
Haraway, Donna Jeanne 1988. 'Situated Knowledges: The Science Question in Feminism and the Privilege of Partial Perspective', *Feminist Studies* 14(3): 575–99.
———. 2003. *The Companion Species Manifesto: Dogs, People, and Significant Otherness*. Chicago: Prickly Paradigm Press.
———. 2016. *Staying with the Trouble: Making Kin in the Chthulucene*. Durham, NC: Duke University Press.

Hardiman, David, and Projit Bihari Mukharji (eds). 2013. *Medical Marginality in South Asia: Situating Subaltern Therapeutics*. London: Routledge.

Hardon, Anita, and Nurul Ilmi Idrus. 2015. 'Magic Power: Changing Gender Dynamics and Sex-Enhancement Practices among Youths in Makassar, Indonesia', in Laurent Pordié and Anita Hardon (eds), 'Drugs' Stories and Itineraries: On the Making of Asian Industrial Medicines', special issue, *Anthropology & Medicine* 22(1): 49–63.

Harré, Roy, and Ben Rampton. 2002. 'Creole Metaphors in Cultural Analysis: On the Limits and Possibilities of (Socio-) Linguistics', *Critique of Anthropology* 22(1): 31–51.

Haudricourt, André-Georges. 1987. *La Technologie, science humaine: Recherche d'histoire et d'ethnologie des techniques*. Paris: Éditions de la Maison des Sciences de l'Homme.

———. 2010. *Des gestes aux techniques: Essai sur les techniques dans les sociétés pré-machinistes*. Paris: Éditions de la Maison des Sciences de l'Homme.

Haugen, Heidi, and Jørgen Carling. 2005. 'On the Edge of the Chinese Diaspora: The Surge of Baihuo Business in an African City', *Ethnic and Racial Studies* 28(4): 639–62.

Hausmann Muela, Susanna, Joan Muela Ribera and Marcel Tanner. 1998. 'Fake Malaria and Hidden Parasites – The Ambiguity of Malaria', *Anthropology & Medicine* 5(1): 43–61.

Hicks, Dan. 2010. 'The Material-Cultural Turn: Event and Effect', in Dan Hicks and Mary C. Beaudry (eds), *The Oxford Handbook of Material Culture Studies*. Oxford: Oxford University Press, pp. 26–99.

Hien, Tran, and Nicholas J. White. 1993. 'Qinghaosu', *The Lancet* 341 (8845): 603–8.

Hinde, Robert A. 2015. *Our Culture of Greed: When is Enough Enough?* London: Spokesman.

Ho, Ming-jung. 2001. 'Discourses on Immigrant Tuberculosis: A Case Study of New York City's Chinese Labourers', DPhil thesis. Oxford: University of Oxford.

———. 2003. 'Migratory Journeys and Tuberculosis Risk', *Medical Anthropology Quarterly* 17(4): 442–58.

Hoey, Brian A. 2005. 'From Pi to Pie: Moral Narratives of Noneconomic Migration and Starting Over in the Postindustrial Midwest', *Journal of Contemporary Ethnography* 34(5): 586–624.

———. 2014. *Opting for Elsewhere: Lifestyle Migration in the American Middle Class*. Nashville, TN: Vanderbilt University Press.

Holbraad, Martin. 2007. 'The Power of Powder: Multiplicity and Motion in the Divinatory Cosmology of Cuban Ifá (or Mana, Again)', in Amiria Henare, Martin Holbraad and Sari Wastell (eds), *Thinking Through Things: Theorising Artefacts Ethnographically*. London: Routledge, pp. 189–225.

Holbraad, Martin, and Morten Axel Pedersen. 2017. *The Ontological Turn: An Anthropological Exposition*. Cambridge: Cambridge University Press.

Horden, Peregrine, and Elisabeth Hsu (eds). 2013. *The Body in Balance: Humoral Medicines in Practice*. Oxford: Berghahn.

Howes, David (ed.). 1991. *The Varieties of Sensory Experience: A Sourcebook in the Anthropology of the Senses*. Toronto: University of Toronto Press.

———. 2005a. 'Introduction', in David Howes (ed.), *Empire of the Senses: The Sensual Culture Reader*. Oxford: Berg, pp. 1–17.

———. 2005b. 'HYPERESTHESIA, or, The Sensual Logic of Late Capitalism', in David Howes (ed.), *Empire of the Senses: The Sensual Culture Reader*. Oxford: Berg, pp. 281–303.

Huang, Hsuan-Ying. 2014. 'The Emergence of the Psycho-Boom in Contemporary Urban China', in Howard Chiang (ed.), *Psychiatry and Chinese History*. London: Pickering and Chatto, pp. 183–284.

Huizinga, Johan. [1938] 1980. *Homo Ludens: A Study of the Play-Element in Culture*. London: Routledge & Kegan Paul.

Hunter, Kathryn M. 1993. *Doctors' Stories: The Narrative Structure of Medical Knowledge*. Princeton, NJ: Princeton University Press.

Iliffe, John. 1998. *East African Doctors: A History of the Modern Profession*. Cambridge: Cambridge University Press.

Ingold, Tim. 2000. *The Perception of the Environment: Essays on Livelihood, Dwelling and Skill*. London: Routledge.

———. 2007a. *Lines: A Brief History*. London: Routledge.

———. 2007b. 'Earth, Sky, Wind, and Weather', in Elisabeth Hsu and Chris Low (eds), 'Wind, Life, Health: Anthropological and Historical Perspectives', special issue no. 2, *Journal of the Royal Anthropological Institute*: S19–S38.

———. 2008. 'When ANT Meets SPIDER: Social Theory for Arthropods', in Carl Knappett and Lambros Malafouris (eds), *Material Agency: Towards a Non-Anthropocentric Approach*. Boston: Springer. pp. 209–16.

———. 2009. 'Against Space: Place, Movement, Knowledge', in Peter Kirby (ed.), *Boundless Worlds: An Anthropological Approach to Movement*. Oxford: Berghahn, pp. 29–43.

———. 2011. *Being Alive: Essays on Movement, Knowledge and Description*. London: Routledge.

———. 2012. 'Toward an Ecology of Materials', *Annual Review of Anthropology* 41: 427–42.

———. 2013. *Making: Anthropology, Archaeology, Art and Architecture*. London: Routledge.

———. 2014. 'Making and Growing: An Introduction', in Elizabeth Hallam and Tim Ingold (eds), *Making and Growing: Anthropological Studies of Organisms and Artefacts*. Farnham: Ashgate, pp. 1–24.

Jackson, Michael. 1983a. 'Knowledge of the Body', *Man* 18(2): 327–45.

———. 1983b. 'Thinking through the Body: An Essay on Understanding Metaphor', *Social Analysis* 14: 127–48.

Jakobson, Roman, and Linda R. Waugh [1979] 1987. *The Sound Shape of Language*. Berlin: Mouton de Gruyter.

James, Wendy. 1998. '"One of Us": Marcel Mauss and "English" Anthropology', in Wendy James and Nick J. Allen (eds), *Marcel Mauss: A Centenary Tribute*. Oxford: Berghahn, pp. 3–26.

James, Wendy, and David Mills (eds). 2005. *The Qualities of Time: Anthropological Approaches*. Oxford: Berg.

Janzen, John. 1978. *The Quest for Therapy: Medical Pluralism in Lower Zaire*. Berkeley, CA: University of California Press.

———. 1992. *Ngoma: Discourses of Healing in Central and Southern Africa*. Berkeley, CA: University of California Press.

Janzen, John, and Gwyn Prins (eds). 1981. 'Causality and Classification in African Medicine and Health', special issue, *Social Science & Medicine* 15B(3): 169–437.

Jenkins, Richard. 2002. *Pierre Bourdieu*, 2nd edn. London: Routledge.

Jennings, Michael. 2005. 'Chinese Medicine and Medical Pluralism in Dar es Salaam: Globalisation or Glocalisation?' *International Relations* 19(4): 457–74.

Jiangsu Xinyi Xueyuan 江苏新医学院 (eds). [1977] 1986. *Zhongyao dacidian* 中药大辞典 [Great dictionary of Chinese medical drugs]. Shanghai: Shanghai keji chubanshe.

Jullien, François. [1992] 1995. *The Propensity of Things: Toward a History of Efficacy in China*. New York: Zone Books.

Jung, Carl. G. 1968. 'Foreword', in *The I Ching or Book of Changes*, trans. R. Wilhelm. London: Routledge, pp. 33–62.

Kadetz, Paul. 2014. 'Unpacking Sino-African Health Diplomacy: Problematizing a Hegemonic Construction', *St. Antony's International Review* 8(2): 149–72.

Kadetz, Paul, and Johanna Hood. 2017. 'Outsourcing China's Welfare: Unpacking the Outcomes of "Sustainable" Self-Development in Sino-African Health Diplomacy', in Beatriz Carrillo, Johanna Hood and Paul Kadetz (eds), *Handbook of Welfare in China*. Cheltenham: Edward Elgar, pp. 338–60.

Kamat, Vinay R. 2009. 'Cultural Interpretations of the Efficacy and Side Effects of Antimalarials in Tanzania', *Anthropology & Medicine* 16(3): 293–305.

Kapferer, Bruce. 1984. 'The Ritual Process and the Problem of Reflexivity in Sinhalese Demon Exorcisms', in John J. MacAloon (ed.), *Rite, Drama, Festival, Spectacle*. Philadelphia, PA: Institute for Human Issues, pp. 179–207.

———. [1987] 1991. *A Celebration of Demons Exorcism and the Aesthetics of Healing in Sri Lanka*. 2nd. edn. Bloomington: Indiana University Press.

———. 2004. 'Ritual Dynamics and Virtual Practice: Beyond Presentation and Meaning', in Don Handelman and Galina Lindquist (eds), 'Ritual in Its Own Right: Exploring the Dynamics of Transformation', special issue, *Social Analysis* 48(2): 33–54.

Kaptchuk, Ted J. 1998. 'Intentional Ignorance: A History of Blind Assessment and Placebo Controls in Medicine', *Bulletin of the History of Medicine* 72: 389–433.

Kaptchuk, Ted J., et al. 2010. 'Placebos without Deception: A Randomized Controlled Trial in Irritable Bowel Syndrome'. *PLOS ONE* 5(12): e15591. https://doi.org/10.1371/journal.pone.0015591.

Karchmer, Eric I. 2005. 'Orientalizing the Body: Postcolonial Transformations in Chinese Medicine', PhD dissertation. Chapel Hill, NC: University of North Caroline at Chapel Hill.

———. 2010. 'Chinese Medicine in Action: On the Postcoloniality of Medical Practice in China', *Medical Anthropology* 29(3): 226–52.

———. 2015. 'Slow Medicine: How Chinese Medicine Became Efficacious Only for Chronic Conditions', in Howard Chiang (ed.), *Historical Epistemology and the Making of Modern Chinese Medicine*. Manchester: Manchester University Press, pp. 188–216.

Katz, Pearl. 1985. 'How Surgeons Make Decisions', in Robert A. Hahn and Atwood D. Gaines (eds), *Physicians of Western Medicine: Anthropological Approaches to Theory and Practice*. Dordrecht: Reidel, pp. 155–75.

Kelly, Tara. 2014. 'Plants, Power, Possibility: Maneuvering the Medical Landscape in Response to Uncertainty', DPhil thesis. Oxford: University of Oxford.

Kielmann, Karina. 1998. 'Barren Ground: Contesting Identities of Infertile Women in Pemba, Tanzania', in Margaret M. Lock and Patricia A. Kaufert (eds), *Pragmatic Women and Body Politics*. Cambridge: Cambridge University Press, pp. 127–63.

Kieschnick, John. 2003. *The Impact of Buddhism on Chinese Material Culture*. Princeton, NJ: Princeton University Press.

King, Helen. 2013. 'Female Fluids in the Hippocratic Corpus: How Solid was the Humoral Body?', in Peregrine Horden and Elisabeth Hsu (eds), *The Body in Balance: Humoral Medicines in Practice*. Oxford: Berghahn, pp. 25–52.

Kirmayer, Laurence J. 1992. 'The Body Insistence on Meaning: Metaphor as Presentation and Representation in Illness Experience', *Medical Anthropology Quarterly* 6(4): 323–46.

———. 2003. 'Reflections on Embodiment', in James MacLynn Wilce (ed.), *Social and Cultural Lives of Immune Systems*. London: Routledge, pp. 282–302.

Kleinman, Arthur. 1980. *Patients and Healers in the Context of Culture: An Exploration of the Borderland between Anthropology, Medicine, and Psychiatry*. Berkeley, CA: University of California Press.

———. 1986. *Social Origins of Distress and Disease: Depression, Neurasthenia, and Pain in Modern China*. New Haven, CT: Yale University Press.

———. 1988. *The Illness Narratives: Suffering, Healing, and the Human Condition*. New York: Basic Books.

——— (ed.). 2011. *Deep China: The Moral Life of the Person, What Anthropology and Psychiatry Tell us about China Today*. Berkeley, CA: University of California Press.

Kloos, Stephan. 2010. 'Tibetan Medicine in Exile: The Ethics, Politics and Science of Cultural Survival', PhD dissertation. San Francisco and Berkeley, CA: Universities of California at San Francisco and Berkeley.

———. 2017. 'The Pharmaceutical Assemblage: Rethinking Sowa Rigpa and the Herbal Pharmaceutical Industry in Asia', *Current Anthropology* 58(6): 693–717.

Knauft, Bruce. 2002a. 'Critically Modern: An Introduction', in Bruce Knauft (ed.), *Critically Modern: Alternatives, Alterities, Anthropologies*. Bloomington, IN: Indiana University Press, pp. 1–56.

——— (ed.). 2002b. *Critically Modern: Alternatives, Alterities, Anthropologies*. Bloomington, IN: Indiana University Press.

Köhle, Natalie, and Shigehisa Kuriyama (eds). 2018. *Fluid Matter(s): Flow and Transformation in the History of the Body*. Canberra: ANU Press.
Köhler, Wolfgang G. 1929. *Gestalt Psychology*. New York: Liveright.
Kohrt, Brandon, and Ian Harper. 2008. 'Navigating Diagnoses: Understanding Mind–Body Relations, Mental Health, and Stigma in Nepal', *Culture, Medicine and Psychiatry* 32(4): 462–91.
Kopytoff, Igor. 1986. 'The Cultural Biography of Things: Commoditization as Process', in Arjun Appadurai (ed.), *The Social Life of Things: Commodities in Cultural Perspective*. Cambridge: Cambridge University Press, pp. 64–91.
Kovačič, Tanja. 2015. 'How to Know Whether a Dog is Dangerous: Myth, Superstition and Its Influence on the Human–Dog Relationship', *Ars et Humanitas* 9(1): 227–43.
Krause, Kristine. 2011. 'Sickness, Migration and Social Relations: Therapeutic Practices and Medical Subjectivities among Ghanaian Migrants in London', DPhil thesis. Oxford: University of Oxford.
Krause, Kristine, David Parkin and Gabi Alex (eds). 2014. 'Turning Therapies: Placing Medical Diversity', special issue, *Medical Anthropology* 33(1): 1–84.
Kuper, Adam. [1977] 2015. *Anthropology and Anthropologists: The British School in the Twentieth Century*, 4th edn. London: Routledge.
Kuriyama, Shigehisa. 1999. *The Expressiveness of the Body and the Divergence of Greek and Chinese Medicine*. New York: Zone Books.
Lambek, Michael. 2014. 'The Interpretation of Lives or Life as Interpretation: Cohabiting with Spirits in the Malagasy World', *American Ethnologist* 41(3): 491–503.
Lampton, David M. 1977. *The Politics of Medicine in China: The Policy Process, 1949–1977*. Boulder, CO: Westview.
Landy, David (ed.). 1977. *Culture, Disease and Healing*. New York: Macmillan.
Langer, Susanne Katherina. 1953. *Feeling and Form: A Theory of Art*. London: Routledge & Kegan Paul.
Langford, Jean M. 2002. *Fluent Bodies: Ayurvedic Remedies for Postcolonial Imbalance*. Durham, NC: Duke University Press.
Langwick, Stacy Ann. 2006. 'Geographies of Medicine: Interrogating the Boundary between "Traditional" and "Modern" Medicine in Colonial Tanganyika', in Tracy J. Luedke and Harry G. West (eds), *Borders and Healers: Brokering Therapeutic Resources in Southeast Africa*. Bloomington, IN: Indiana University Press, pp. 143–65.
———. 2008. 'Articulate(d) Bodies: Traditional Medicine in a Tanzanian Hospital', *American Ethnologist* 35(3): 428–39.
———. 2010. 'From Non-Aligned Medicines to Market-Based Herbals: China's Relationship to the Shifting Politics of Traditional Medicine in Tanzania', *Medical Anthropology* 29(1): 15–43.
———. 2011. *Bodies, Politics, and African Healing: The Matter of Maladies in Tanzania*. Bloomington, IN: Indiana University Press.
———. 2018. 'A Politics of Habitability: Plants, Healing, and Sovereignty in a Toxic World', *Cultural Anthropology* 33(3): 415–43.

Laplante, Julie. 2015. *Healing Roots: Anthropology in Life and Medicine*. Oxford: Berghahn.
———. 2016. 'Becoming Plant: Jamu in Java, Indonesia', in Elizabeth Anne Olson and John R. Stepp (eds), *Plants and Health: New Perspectives on the Health–Environment–Plant Nexus*. Cham: Springer, pp. 17–65.
Laplante, Julie, Ari Gandsman and Willow Scobie (eds). 2020. *Search after Method: Sensing, Moving, and Imagining in Anthropological Fieldwork*. Oxford: Berghahn.
Large, Daniel. 2008. 'Beyond "Dragon in the Bush": The Study of China–Africa Relations', *African Affairs* 107(426): 45–61.
Larkin, Bruce D. 1971. *China and Africa, 1949–1970: The Foreign Policy of the People's Republic of China*. Berkeley, CA: Center for Chinese Studies.
Larsen, Kjersti. 2008. *Where Humans and Spirits Meet: The Politics of Rituals and Identified Spirits in Zanzibar*. Oxford: Berghahn.
———. 2019. 'By Way of the Qur`an: Appeasing Spirits, Easing Emotions and Everyday Matters in Zanzibar', in Zulfikar Hirji (ed.), *Approaches to the Qur`an in Sub-Saharan Africa*. Oxford: Oxford University Press, pp. 317–40.
Larsen, Kjersti, Françoise Le Guennec-Coppens and Sophie Mery. 2001. 'Knowledge, Astrology and the Power of Healing in Zanzibar', *Journal des Africanistes* 72(2): 175–86.
Last, Murray. 1981. 'The Importance of Knowing about not Knowing: Observations from Hausaland', in John Janzen and Gwyn Prins (eds), 'Causality and Classification in African Medicine and Health', special issue, *Social Science & Medicine* 15B(3): 387–92.
———. 1986. 'Introduction', in Murray Last and G. L. Chavunduka (eds), *The Professionalisation of African Medicine*. Manchester: Manchester University Press, pp. 1–19.
Last, Murray, and G. L. Chavunduka (eds). 1986. *The Professionalisation of African Medicine*. Manchester: Manchester University Press.
Latour, Bruno. [1984] 1988. *The Pasteurization of France*, trans. Alan Sheridan and John Law. Cambridge, MA: Harvard University Press.
———. 1993. *We Have Never Been Modern*. Cambridge, MA: Harvard University Press.
———. [1993] 2000a. 'The Berlin Key or How to Do Words with Things', trans. L. Davis, in Paul M. Graves-Brown (ed.), *Matter, Materiality and Modern Culture*. London: Routledge, pp. 10–21.
———. 2000b. 'When Things Strike Back: A Possible Contribution of "Science Studies" to the Social Sciences', *The British Journal of Sociology* 51(1): 107–23.
———. 2004. 'How to Talk about the Body? The Normative Dimension of Science Studies', *Body and Society* 10 (2–3): 205–29.
Lave, Jean. 1988. *Cognition in Practice: Mind, Mathematics and Culture in Everyday Life*. Cambridge: Cambridge University Press.
Lave, Jean, and Etienne Wenger. 1991. *Situated Learning: Legitimate Peripheral Participation*. Cambridge: Cambridge University Press.

Law, John, and Lin Wen-Yuan. 2018. 'Tidescapes: Notes on a *shi*-Inflected Social Science', *Journal of World Philosophies* 3(1): 1–16.

Laws, Megan. 2019. '"You're a Trickster": Mockery, Egalitarianism, and Uncertainty in Northeastern Namibia', *Social Analysis* 63(1): 1–21.

Leder, Drew. 1990. *The Absent Body*. Chicago: University of Chicago Press.

Lee, Jo, and Tim Ingold. 2006. 'Fieldwork on Foot: Perceiving, Routing, Socializing', in Simon Coleman and Peter Collins (eds), *Locating the Field: Space, Place and Context in Anthropology*. Oxford: Berg, pp. 67–86.

Lefebvre, Henri. 1974. *La production de l'éspace*. Paris: Anthropos.

———. [1974] 1991. *The Production of Space*, trans. D. Nicholson-Smith. Oxford: Blackwell.

Lei, Sean Hsiang-lin. 1999a. 'When Chinese Medicine Encountered the State: 1910–1949', PhD dissertation. Chicago: University of Chicago.

———. 1999b. 'From Changshan to a New Anti-Malarial Drug: Re-Networking Chinese Drugs and Excluding Chinese Doctors', *Social Studies of Science* 29(3): 323–58.

———. 2014. *Neither Donkey nor Horse: Medicine in the Struggle Over China's Modernity*. Chicago: University of Chicago Press.

Leroi-Gourhan, André. [1964] 1993. *Gesture and Speech*, trans. A. B. Berger. Cambridge, MA: MIT Press.

Leslie, Charles (ed.). 1976. *Asian Medical Systems: A Comparative Study*. Berkeley, CA: University of California Press.

———. 1980. 'Medical Pluralism in World Perspective', in Charles Leslie (ed.), 'Medical Pluralism', special issue, *Social Science & Medicine* 14B(4): 190–96.

Leslie, Charles, and Allan Young (eds). 1992. *Paths to Asian Medical Knowledge*. Berkeley, CA: University of California Press.

Leung, Angela Ki Che, and Charlotte Furth (eds). 2010. *Health and Hygiene in Chinese East Asia: Policies and Publics in the Long Twentieth Century*. Durham, NC: Duke University Press.

Levinson, Stephen C. 1983. *Pragmatics*. Cambridge: Cambridge University Press.

Lévi-Strauss, Claude. [1958] 1963. 'The Effectiveness of Symbols', in *Structural Anthropology*, trans. C. Jacobson and B. G. Schoepf. London: Basic Books, pp. 186–205.

Levitt, Peggy, and Nina Glick-Schiller. 2004. 'Conceptualizing Simultaneity: A Transnational Social Field Perspective on Society', *International Migration Review* 38(3): 1002–39.

Lewis, Gilbert A. 1975. *Knowledge of Illness in a Sepik Society: A Study of the Gnau, New Guinea*. London: Athlone Press.

———. 1976. 'Fear of Sorcery and the Problem of Death by Suggestion', in J. B. Loudon (ed.), *Social Anthropology & Medicine*. London: London Academic Press, pp. 111–43.

———. 1995. 'The Articulation of Circumstance and Causal Understandings', in Dan Sperber, David Premack and Ann James Premack (eds), *Causal Cognition: A Multidisciplinary Debate*. Oxford: Oxford University Press, pp. 558–77.

———. 2000. *A Failure of Treatment*. Oxford: Oxford University Press.

———. [1979] 2021. *Pandora's Box: Ethnography and the Comparison of Medical Beliefs*. Chicago: Hau Books/University of Chicago Press.

Li, Anshan. 2006. 'On the Adjustment and Transformation of China's African Policy', *West Asia and Africa* (CASS, China Academy of the Social Sciences) 8.

———. 2009. 'Zhongguo yuanwai yiliaodui de lishi, guimo ji qi yingxiang' 中国院外医疗队的规模及其影响 [Chinese medical teams abroad: History, scale and impact], *Waijiao pinglun* 外交评论 [Foreign affairs review] 1: 25–45.

———. 2011. 'Chinese Medical Cooperation in Africa: With Special Emphasis on the Medical Teams and Anti-Malaria Campaign'. Discussion paper 52. Uppsala: Nordiska Afrikainstitutet.

———. 2021. *China and Africa in Global Context: Encounters, Policy, Cooperation and Migration*. London: Routledge.

Li, Jen-der 李貞德. 2017. 'Nüren yaoyao kao – dangguide yiliao wenhuashi shitan' 女人要藥考—當歸的醫療文化史試探 ['The essential medicine for women': A cultural history of danggui *Angelica sinensis* L. in China], *Zhongyang yanjiuyuan lishi yuyan yanjiusuo jikan* 中央研究院歷史語言研究所集刊 88(3): 521–88.

Lindquist, Galina. 2005. *Conjuring Hope: Magic and Healing in Contemporary Russia*. Oxford: Berghahn.

Littlewood, Roland, and Maurice Lipsedge. 1982. *Aliens and Alienists: Ethnic Minorities and Psychiatry*. Harmondsworth: Penguin.

Livingstone, Julie. 2012. *Improvising Medicine: An African Oncology Ward in an Emerging Cancer Epidemic*. Durham, NC: Duke University Press.

Lloyd, Geoffrey Ernest Richard. 1983. *Science, Folklore and Ideology: Studies in the Life Sciences in Ancient Greece*. Cambridge: Cambridge University Press.

Lock, Margaret. 1978. 'Scars of Experience: The Art of Moxibustion in Japanese Medicine and Society', *Culture, Medicine and Psychiatry* 2(2): 151–75.

———. 1980. *East Asian Medicine in Urban Japan: Varieties of Medical Experience*. Berkeley, CA: University of California Press.

———. 1991. 'Nerves and Nostalgia: Greek-Canadian Immigrants and Medical Care in Québec', in Beatrix Pfleiderer and Gilles Bibeau (eds), 'Anthropologies of Medicine: A Colloquium on West European and North American Perspectives', special issue, *Curare* 91(7): 87–103.

———. 1993. *Encounters with Aging: Mythologies of Menopause in Japan and North America*. Berkeley, CA: University of California Press.

———. 2002. *Twice Dead: Organ Transplants and the Reinvention of Death*. Berkeley, CA: University of California Press.

Loewe, Michael (ed.). 1993. *Early Chinese Texts: A Bibliographical Guide*. Berkeley, CA: Society for the Study of Early China and the Institute of East Asian Studies.

Löffler, Lorenz G. 2012. *Ethnographic Notes on the Mru and Khumi of the Chittagong and Arakan Hill Tracts: A Contribution to our Knowledge of South and Southeast Asian Indigenous Peoples Mainly Based on Field Research in the Southern Chittagong Hill Tracts*. Cambridge, MA: Harvard University Press.

*References*

Loizos, Peter, and Costas Constantinou. 2007. 'Hearts, as well as Minds: Well-being and Illness among Greek Cypriot Refugees', *Journal of Refugee Studies* 20(1): 86–107.

Loudon, Joseph Buist (ed.). 1976. *Social Anthropology & Medicine*. London: Academic Press.

Low, Setha M. 1994. 'Embodied Metaphors: Nerves as Lived Experience', in Thomas J. Csordas (ed.), *Embodiment and Experience: The Existential Ground of Culture and Self*. Cambridge: Cambridge University Press, pp. 139–62.

Lowes, John Livingston. 1927. *The Road to Xanadu: A Study in the Ways of the Imagination*. Boston: Houghton Mifflin.

Luedke, Tracy J., and Harry G. West (eds). 2006. *Borders and Healers: Brokering Therapeutic Resources in Southeast Africa*. Bloomington, IN: Indiana University Press.

Luhmann, Niklas. 1986. 'The Autopoiesis of Social Systems', in R. Felix Geyer and Johannes van der Zouwen (eds), *Sociocybernetic Systems: Observation, Control and Evolution of Self-Steering Systems*, vol. 2. London: Sage, pp. 95–112.

Luisi, Pier Luigi. 2006. 'Autopoiesis: The Logic of Cellular Life', in *The Emergence of Life: From Chemical Origins to Synthetic Biology*. Cambridge: Cambridge University Press, pp. 155–81.

Lupton, Deborah. 1997. 'Consumerism, Reflexivity and the Medical Encounter', *Social Science & Medicine* 45(3): 373–81.

Ma, Eun-Jeong. 2008. 'Medicine in the Making of Post-Colonial Korea, 1948–2006', PhD dissertation. Ithaca, NY: Cornell University.

———. 2015. 'Join or be Excluded from Biomedicine? JOINS and Post-Colonial Korea', *Anthropology & Medicine* 22(1): 64–74.

MacPherson, Hugh. 2004. 'Pragmatic Clinical Trials', *Complementary Therapies in Medicine* 12(2): 136–40.

Maggs, Heather C., Andrew Ainslie and Richard M. Bennett, 2021. 'Donkey Ownership Provides a Range of Income Benefits to the Livelihoods of Rural Households in Northern Ghana'. *Animals* 11(3154). https://doi.org/10.3390/ani11113154.

Mamdani, Mahmood. 2007. *Scholars in the Marketplace: The Dilemmas of Neo-Liberal Reform at Makerere University, 1989–2005*. Kampala: Fountain Publishers.

Mandelbrot, Benoit B. 1983. *The Fractal Geometry of Nature*, revised edn. New York: W.H. Freeman.

Margulis, Lynn. 1991. 'Symbiogenesis and Symbiontism', in Lynn Margulis and René Fester (eds) *Symbiosis as a Source of Evolutionary Innovation: Speciation and Morphogenesis*. Cambridge, MA: MIT Press, pp. 1–14.

———. 1997. 'Big Trouble in Biology: Physiological Autopoiesis versus Mechanistic Neo-Darwinism', in Lynn Margulis and Dorion Sagan (eds), *Slanted Truths: Essays on Gaia, Symbiosis, and Evolution*. New York: Springer, pp. 265–82.

———. 1998. *Symbiotic Planet. A New Look at Evolution*, New York, NY: Basic Books.

## References

Marsland, Rebecca. 2007. 'The Modern Traditional Healer: Locating "Hybridity" in Modern Traditional Medicine, Southern Tanzania', *Journal of Southern African Studies* 33(4): 751–65.
Martin, Emily. 1987. *The Woman in the Body: A Cultural Analysis of Reproduction*. Boston: Beacon Press.
Massey, Doreen. 2005. *For Space*. London: Sage.
Massumi, Brain. 2015. *Politics of Affect*. Cambridge: Polity Press.
Mattes, Dominik. 2019. *Fierce Medicines, Fragile Socialities: Grounding Global HIV Treatment in Tanzania*. Oxford: Berghahn.
Mattes, Dominik, Bernhard Hadolt and Brigit Obrist. 2020. 'Introduction', in 'Rethinking Sociality and Health through Transfiguration', special papers, *Medicine Anthropology Theory (MAT)* 7(1): 66–86.
Mattingly, Cheryl. 1998. *Healing Dramas and Clinical Plots: The Narrative Structure of Experience*. Cambridge: Cambridge University Press.
———. 2010. *The Paradox of Hope: Journeys through a Clinical Borderland*. Berkeley, CA: University of California Press.
Mauss, Marcel. [1906] 1979a. *Seasonal Variations of the Eskimo: A Study of Social Morphology*, trans. J. J. Fox. London: Routledge & Kegan Paul.
———. [1925] 1954. *The Gift: Forms and Functions of Exchange in Archaic Societies*. London: Cohen & West.
———. [1920/1953] 2006b. 'The Nation', in *Techniques, Technology and Civilisation*, ed. Nathan Schlanger. Oxford: Berghahn, pp. 41–48.
———. [1927] 2006b. 'The Divisions of Sociology', in *Techniques, Technology and Civilisation*, ed. Nathan Schlanger. Oxford: Berghahn, pp. 49–54.
———. [1929] 2006b. 'Debate on the Origins of Human Technology', in *Techniques, Technology and Civilisation*, ed. Nathan Schlanger. Oxford: Berghahn, pp. 55–56.
———. [1929/30] 2006b. 'Civilisations, Their Elements and Forms', in *Techniques, Technology and Civilisation*, ed. Nathan Schlanger. Oxford: Berghahn, pp. 57–74.
———. [1935] 1973. 'Techniques of the Body', trans. B. Brewster, *Economy and Society* 2(1): 70–88.
———. [1935] 1979b. 'Body Techniques', trans. B. Brewster, in *Sociology and Psychology: Essays*. London: Routledge & Kegan Paul, pp. 95–123.
———. [1935] 2006a. 'Techniques of the Body', trans. B. Brewster, in *Techniques, Technology and Civilisation*, ed. Nathan Schlanger. Oxford: Berghahn, pp. 77–96.
———. [1936] 1950. 'Les techniques du corps', in *Sociologie et anthropologie*. Paris: PUF, pp. 365–86.
———. [1913–53] 2006b. *Techniques, Technology and Civilisation*, ed. Nathan Schlanger. Oxford: Berghahn.
———. [1967] 2007. *Manual of Ethnography*, trans. D. Lussler, ed. Nick J. Allen. Oxford: Berghahn.
Meier zu Biesen, Caroline. 2013. *Globale Epidemien – Lokale Antworten: Eine Ethnographie der Heil-pflanze Artemisia annua in Tansania*. Frankfurt: Campus.

———. 2018. 'From Coastal to Global: The Transnational Flow of Ayurveda and its Relevance for Indo-African Linkages', *Global Public Health* 13(3): 339–54.
Merleau-Ponty, Maurice. 1945. *Phénoménologie de la perception*. Paris: Gallimard.
———. [1945] 1962. *Phenomenology of Perception*, trans. C. Smith. London: Routledge.
———. [1945] 2012. *Phenomenology of Perception*, trans. D. A. Landes. London: Routledge.
Mesaki, Simeon. 2009a. 'Witchcraft and the Law in Tanzania', *International Journal of Sociology and Anthropology* 1(8): 132–38.
———. 2009b. 'The Tragedy of Ageing: Witch Killings and Poor Governance among the Sukuma', in Liv Haram and C. Bawa Yamba (eds), *Dealing with Uncertainty in Contemporary African Lives*. Uppsala: Nordika Afrikainstitutet, pp. 72–90.
Migliore, Sam. 1994. 'Gender, Emotion, and Physical Distress: The Sicilian-Canadian "Nerves" Complex', *Culture, Medicine and Psychiatry* 18(3): 271–97.
Moerman, Daniel E. 2002. *Meaning, Medicine and the 'Placebo Effect'*. Cambridge: Cambridge University Press.
Mol, Annemarie. 2002. *The Body Multiple: Ontology in Medical Practice*. Durham, NC: Duke University Press.
Monson, Jamie. 2009. *Africa's Freedom Railway: How a Chinese Development Project Changed Lives and Livelihoods in Tanzania*. Bloomington, IN: Indiana University Press.
———. 2013. 'Remembering Work on the Tazara Railway in Africa and China, 1965–2011: When "New Men" Grow Old', *African Studies Review* 56(1): 45–64.
Morris, Katherine. 2012. *Starting with Merleau-Ponty*. London: Continuum.
Mosko, Mark S. 2005. 'Introduction: A (Re)turn to Chaos: Chaos Theory, The Sciences, and Social Anthropological Theory', in Mark S. Mosko and Frederick H. Damon (eds), *On the Order of Chaos: Social Anthropology and the Science of Chaos*. Oxford: Berghahn, pp. 1–46.
Mosko, Mark S., and Frederick H. Damon (eds). 2005. *On the Order of Chaos: Social Anthropology and the Science of Chaos*. Oxford: Berghahn.
Myhre, Knut Christian. 2013. 'Membering and Dismembering: The Poetry and Relationality of Animal Bodies in Kilimanjaro', *Social Analysis* 57(3): 114–31.
———. 2017. *Returning Life: Language, Life Force, and History in Kilimanjaro*. Oxford: Berghahn.
Nair, Manoj, Y. Huang, D. A. Fidock, S. J. Polyak, J. Wagoner, M. J. Towler and P. J. Weathers 2021. '*Artemisia annua* L. Extracts Inhibit the *In Vitro* Replication of SARS-CoV-2 and Two of Its Variants', *Journal of Ethnopharmacology* 274(2): 114016.
Ndungu, Duncan Ndegwa. 2013. 'Study of Resistance to Artemisinins in Plasmodium Falciparum Isolates from Kilifi County', master's thesis. Njoro: Egerton University.

# References

Neumark, Tom. 2017. 'A Good Neighbour is Not One That Gives: Detachment, Ethics and the Relational Self in Kenya', *Journal of the Royal Anthropological Institute* 23(4): 748–64.

Newton, Paul N., Arjen Dondorp, Michael Green, Mayfong Mayxay, Nicholas J. White. 2003. 'Counterfeit Artesunate Antimalarials in Southeast Asia', *The Lancet* 362(9378): 169.

Nichols-Belo, Amy. 2018. '"Witchdoctors" in White Coats: Politics and Healing Knowledge in Tanzania', *Medical Anthropology* 37(8): 722–36.

Nichter, Mark. 1980. 'The Layperson's Perception of Medicine as Perspective into the Utilization of Multiple Therapy Systems in the Indian Context', *Social Science & Medicine* 14B(4): 225–33. Reprinted in M. Nichter. 1996. *Anthropology and International Health: Asian Case Studies*. Amsterdam: Gordon and Breach, pp. 203–37.

———. 2008. 'Coming to Our Senses: Appreciating the Sensorial in Medical Anthropology', in Devon E. Hinton, David Howes and Laurence J. Kirmayer (eds), 'Medical Anthropology of Sensations', special issue, *Transcultural Psychiatry* 45(2): 163–97.

Nichter, Mark, and Nancy Vuckovic. 1994. 'Agenda for an Anthropology of Pharmaceutical Practice', *Social Science & Medicine* 39(11): 1509–25.

Nichter, Mark, and Margaret Lock (eds). 2002. *New Horizons in Medical Anthropology: Essays in Honour of Charles Leslie*. London: Routledge.

Nie, Chuanxiong, Jakob Trimpert, Sooyeon Moon, Rainer Haag, Kerry Gilmore, Benedikt B. Kaufer and Peter H. Seeberger. 2021. 'In Vitro Efficacy of Artemisia Extracts Against SARS-CoV-2', *Virology Journal* 18(1): 182.

Niewöhner, Jörg, and Margaret Lock. 2018. 'Situating Local Biologies: Anthropological Perspectives on Environment/Human Entanglements', *BioSocieties* 13(4): 681–97.

Ngubane, Harriet. 1977. *Body and Mind in Zulu Medicine: An Ethnography of Health and Disease in Nyuswa-Zulu Thought and Practice*. London: Academic Press.

Obeyesekere, Gananath. 1985. 'Depression, Buddhism, and the Work of Culture in Sri Lanka', in Arthur Kleinman and Byron Good (eds), *Culture and Depression: Studies in the Anthropology and Cross-Cultural Psychiatry of Affect and Disorder*. Berkeley, CA: University of California Press, pp. 134–52.

Obrist, Brigit. 2003. 'Urban Health in Daily Practice: Livelihood, Vulnerability and Resilience in Dar es Salaam, Tanzania', *Anthropology & Medicine* 10(3): 275–90.

———. 2004. 'Medicalization and Morality in a Weak State: Health, Hygiene and Water in Dar Es Salaam, Tanzania', in Helle Samuelsen and Vibeke Steffen (eds), 'The Relevance of Foucault and Bourdieu for Medical Anthropology: Exploring New Sites', special issue, *Anthropology & Medicine* 11(1): 43–57.

———. 2006. *Struggling for Health in the City: An Anthropological Inquiry of Health, Vulnerability and Resilience in Dar es Salaam, Tanzania*. Bern: Peter Lang.

Ohnuki-Tierney, Emiko. 1993. *Rice as Self*. Princeton, NJ: Princeton University Press.

Ong, Aihwa. 1999. *Flexible Citizenship: The Cultural Logic of Transnationality*. Durham, NC: Duke University Press.

Onori, Luciano, and Guido Visconti. 2012. The *Gaia* Theory: from Lovelock to Margulis. From a Homeostatic to a Cognitive Autopoietic Worldview. *Rendiconti Lincei* 23: 375–386. https://doi.org/10.1007/s12210-012-0187-z.

Ots, Thomas. 1990a. *Medizin und Heilung in China: Annäherungen an die traditionelle chinesische Medizin*, 2nd revised edn. Berlin: Reimer.

———. 1990b. 'The Angry Liver, the Anxious Heart and the Melancholy Spleen', *Culture, Medicine and Psychiatry* 14(1): 21–58.

Panofsky, Erwin. 1951. *Gothic Architecture and Scholasticism*. Latrobe, PA: Archabbey Press.

Parkin, David. 1968. 'Medicines and Men of Influence', *Man* 3: 428–39.

———. 1969. *Neighbours and Nationals in an African City Ward*. London: Routledge & Kegan Paul.

———. 1972. *Palms, Wine and Witnesses: Public Spirit and Private Gain in an African Farm Community*. London: Chandler.

———. 1990. 'East Africa: The View from the Office and the Voice from the Field', in Richard Fardon (ed.), *Localizing Strategies: Regional Traditions of Ethnographic Writing*. Edinburgh: Scottish Academic Press, pp. 182–203.

———. 1991a. 'Simultaneity and Sequencing in the Oracular Speech of Kenyan Diviners', in Philip M. Peek (ed.), *African Divination Systems: Ways of Knowing*. Bloomington, IN: Indiana University Press, pp. 173–89. See also revised version in Parkin 2021, Chapter 17, 343–60.

———. 1999. 'Mementoes as Transitional Objects in Human Displacement', *Journal of Material Culture* 4(3): 303–20.

———. 2000. 'Islam among the Humours: Destiny and Agency among the Swahili', in Ivan Karp and D. A. Masolo (eds), *African Philosophy as Cultural Inquiry*. Bloomington, IN: Indiana University Press, pp. 50–65.

———. 2007. 'Wafting on the Wind: Smell and the Cycle of Spirit and Matter', in Elisabeth Hsu and Chris Low (eds), 'Wind, Life, Health: Anthropological and Historical Perspectives', special issue no. 2, *Journal of the Royal Anthropological Institute*: S39–S53.

———. 2011. 'Trust Talk and Alienable Talk in Healing: A Problem of Medical Diversity'. *MMG Working Paper* 11. Göttingen: Max Planck Institute for the Study of Religious and Ethnic Diversity.

———. 2013. 'Balancing Diversity and Well-Being: Words, Concepts and Practice in Eastern Africa', in Peregrine Horden and Elisabeth Hsu (eds), *The Body in Balance: Humoral Medicines in Practice*. Oxford: Berghahn, pp. 171–96.

———. 2016. 'From Multilingual Classification to Translingual Ontology: A Turning Point', in Karel Arnaut, Jan Blommaert, Ben Rampton and Massimiliano Spotti (eds), *Language and Superdiversity*. London: Routledge, pp. 71–88.

———. 2021. *The Transformative Materiality of Meaning Making*. Bristol/Blue Ridge Summit, PA: Multilingual Matters.

Parkin, David, Kristine Krause and Gabi Alex (eds). 2013. 'Therapeutic Crises, Diversification and Mainstreaming', special issue, *Anthropology & Medicine* 20(2): 117–202.

# References

Peng, Shuangsong 彭雙松. 1984. *Xufu yanjiu* [The study of Xufu]. Taibei: Fuhui tushu chubanshe.
Phillips, John. 2006. 'Agencement/Assemblage', *Theory, Culture & Society* 23(2–3): 108–9.
Phillips-Howard, Penelope. 2002. 'Regulation of the Quality and Use of Artemisinin and Its Derivatives', in Colin W. Wright (ed.), *Artemisia*. London: Taylor & Francis, pp. 248–59.
Pieke, Frank N., Pál Nyíri, Mette Thunø and Antonella Ceccagno. 2004. *Transnational Chinese: Fujianese Migrants in Europe*. Stanford, CA: Stanford University Press.
Pieke, Frank N., and Janet Salaff (eds). 2007. 'New Chinese Diasporas', special issue, *Population, Space and Place* 13(2): 81–156.
Pieterse, Jan Nederveen. 1994. 'Globalization as Hybridization', *International Sociology* 9(2): 161–84.
———. 1995. 'Globalization as Hybridization', in Mike Featherstone, Scott Lash and Roland Robertson (eds), *Global Modernities*. London: Sage, pp. 54–77.
Pike, Kenneth L. [1954] 1967. 'Etic and Emic Standpoints for the Description of Behaviour', in *Language in Relation to a Unified Theory of the Structure of Human Behavior*, 2nd edn. The Hague: Mouton, pp. 37–72.
Pink, Sarah. 2011. 'From Embodiment to Emplacement: Re-Thinking Competing Bodies, Senses and Spatialities', *Sport, Education and Society* 16(3): 343–55.
Polanyi, Michael. 1966. *The Tacit Dimension*. Chicago: University of Chicago Press.
Pool, Robert. 1994. *Dialogue and the Interpretation of Illness: Conversations in a Cameroon Village*. Oxford: Berg.
Pordié, Laurent. 2008. *Tibetan Medicine in the Contemporary World: Global Politics of Medical Knowledge and Practice*. London: Routledge.
———. 2010. 'The Politics of Therapeutic Evaluation in Asian Medicine', *Economic and Political Weekly* 45(18): 57–64.
———. 2015. 'Hangover Free! The Social and Material Trajectories of Party-Smart', in Laurent Pordié and Anita Hardon (eds), 'Drugs' Stories and Itineraries: On the Making of Asian Industrial Medicines', special issue, *Anthropology & Medicine* 22(1): 34–48.
Pordié, Laurent, and Anita Hardon (eds). 2015. 'Drugs' Stories and Itineraries: On the Making of Asian Industrial Medicines', special issue, *Anthropology & Medicine* 22(1): 1–96.
Pordié, Laurent, and Jean-Paul Gaudillière. 2014. 'The Reformulation Regime in Drug Discovery: Revisiting Polyherbals and Property Rights in the Ayurvedic Industry', in Volker Scheid and Sean Hsiang-lin Lei (eds), 'Beyond Tradition: Asian Medicines and STS', special issue, *East Asian Science, Technology and Society* 8(1): 57–79.
Porkert, Manfred. 1974. *The Theoretical Foundations of Chinese Medicine: Systems of Correspondence*. Cambridge, MA: MIT Press.
Prince, Ruth Jane, and Rebecca Marsland. 2013. *Making and Unmaking Public Health in Africa: Ethnographic and Historical Perspectives*. Athens, OH: Ohio University Press.

Pritzker, Sonya. 2014. *Living Translation: Language and the Search for Resonance in U.S. Chinese Medicine*. Oxford: Berghahn.
Pye, David. 1968. *The Nature and Art of Workmanship*. London: Cambridge, at the University Press.
Quet, Mathieu, et al. 2018. 'Regulation Multiple: Pharmaceutical Trajectories and Modes of Control in the ASEAN', *Science, Technology and Society* 23(3): 485–503.
Raviola, Giuseppe, M'Imunya Machoki, Esther Mwaikambo and Mary-Jo DelVechhio Good. 2002. 'HIV, Disease Plague, Demoralization, and "Burnout": Resident Experience of the Medical Profession in Nairobi, Kenya', *Culture, Medicine and Psychiatry* 26(1): 55–86.
Rekdal, Ole Bjørn. 1999. 'Cross-Cultural Healing in East African Ethnography', *Medical Anthropology Quarterly* 13(4): 458–82.
Rhodes, Lorna Amarasingham. 1980. 'Movement among Healers in Sri Lanka: A Case Study of a Sinhalese Patient', *Culture, Medicine and Psychiatry* 4: 71–92.
———. 1984. 'Time and the Process of Diagnosis in Sinhalese Ritual Treatment', in E. Valentine Daniel and Judy F. Pugh (eds), *South Asian Systems of Healing*. Leiden: Brill, pp. 46–59.
Robinson, Andrew. 2005. 'Towards an Intellectual Reformation: The Critique of Common Sense and the Forgotten Revolutionary Project of Gramscian Theory', *Critical Review of International Social and Political Philosophy* 8(4): 469–81.
Rogaski, Ruth. 2004. *Hygienic Modernity: Meanings of Health and Disease in Treaty-Port China*. Berkeley, CA: University of California Press.
Romanucci-Schwartz, Lola. 1969. 'The Hierarchy of Resort in Curative Practices: The Admirality Islands, Melanesia', *Journal of Health and Social Behavior* 10: 201–9. Reprinted in David Landy (ed.). 1977. *Culture, Disease and Healing*. New York: Macmillan, pp. 481–87.
Rodrigues, Carla F., Noémia Lopes and Anita Hardon. 2019. 'Beyond Health: Medicines, Food Supplements, Energetics and the Commodification of Self-Performance in Maputo', *Sociology of Health & Illness* 41(6): 1005–22.
Russell, Bertrand. 1922. *The Problem of China*. London: George Allen & Unwin.
Rutert, Britta. 2020. *Contested Properties: Peoples, Plants and Politics in Post-Apartheid South Africa*. Bielefeld: Transcript.
Sacks, Harvey, Emanuel A. Schegloff and Gail Jefferson. 1974. 'A Simplest Systematics for the Organization of Turn-Taking for Conversation', *Language* 50(4): 696–735.
Sagli, Gry. 2003. 'Acupuncture Reconceptualized: The Reception of Chinese Medical Concepts among Practitioners of Acupuncture in Norway', doctoral thesis. Oslo: University of Oslo.
———. 2008. 'Learning and Experiencing Chinese *qigong* in Norway', in Elisabeth Hsu (ed.), 'The Globalization of Chinese Medicine and Meditation Practices', special issue, *East Asian Science, Technology and Society: An International Journal* 2(4): 545–66.

## References

———. 2010. 'The Establishing of Chinese Medical Concepts in Norwegian Acupuncture Schools: The Cultural Translation of *jingluo* ("Circulation Tracts")', *Anthropology & Medicine* 17(3): 315–26.

———. 2017. 'Attentiveness to Nature in Learning *qigong* in Norway', *Asian Medicine* 12(1–2): 56–85.

Sangren, Steven P. 1987. *History and Magical Power in a Chinese Community*. Stanford, CA: Stanford University Press.

Saxer, Martin. 2013. *Manufacturing Tibetan Medicine: The Creation of an Industry and the Moral Economy of Tibetanness*. Oxford: Berghahn.

Scheid, Volker. 2002. *Chinese Medicine in Contemporary China: Plurality and Synthesis*. Durham, NC: Duke University Press.

———. 2007. *Currents of Tradition in Chinese Medicine 1626–2006*. Seattle, WA: Eastland Press.

Scheid, Volker, and Hugh MacPherson (eds). 2011. *Integrating East Asian Medicine into Contemporary Healthcare*. Edinburgh: Churchill Livingstone.

Scheper-Hughes, Nancy. 1992. *Death without Weeping: The Violence of Everyday Life in Brazil*. Berkeley, CA: University of California Press.

Schmoll, Pamela G. 1993. 'Black Stomachs, Beautiful Stones: Soul-Eating among Hausa in Niger', in Jean Comaroff and John Comaroff (eds), *Modernity and its Malcontents: Ritual and Power in Postcolonial Africa*. Chicago: University of Chicago Press, pp. 193–220.

Schrempf, Mona, and Lena Springer (eds). 2015. 'Efficacy and Safety in Tibetan and Chinese Medicine: Historical and Ethnographic Perspectives', special issue, *Asian Medicine* 10(1+2): 1–381.

Schütz, Alfred. 1971. *Collected Papers*, 3rd edn. The Hague: Nijhoff.

Schwabl, Herbert, and Jan M. A. van der Valk. 2019. 'Challenging the Biomedical Notion of "Active Substance": The Botanical Plasticity of Tibetan Medical Formulas', *Himalaya* 39(1): 208–18.

Scott, James C. 1999. *Seeing Like a State: How Certain Schemes to Improve the Human Condition Have Failed*. New Haven: Yale University Press.

Seaman, Gary. 1992. 'Winds, Waters, Seeds, and Souls: Folk Concepts of Physiology and Etiology in Chinese Gemancy', in Charles Leslie and Allan Young (eds), *Paths to Asian Medical Knowledge*. Berkeley, CA: University of California Press, pp. 74–97.

Seligman, Adam B., Robert P. Weller, Michael Puett and Bennett Simon. 2008. *Ritual and its Consequences: An Essay on the Limits of Sincerity*. Oxford: Oxford University Press.

Sennett, Richard. [2006] 2007. *The Craftsman*. London: Allen Lane.

Shahar, Meir, and Robert P. Weller. 1996. *Unruly Gods: Divinity and Society in China*. Honolulu, HI: University of Hawaii Press.

Sharp, Lesley A. 2006. *Strange Harvest: Organ Transplants, Denatured Bodies, and the Transformed Self*. Berkeley, CA: University of California Press.

Shimazono, Yosuke. 2003. 'Narrative Analysis in Medical Anthropology', MPhil dissertation. Oxford: University of Oxford.

———. 2014. 'Kidneys In-Between: An Anthropological Study of Live Kidney Transplantation in the Philippines', DPhil thesis. Oxford: University of Oxford.

Simmel, Georg. [1908] 1950a. 'The Secret and the Secret Society', in *The Sociology of Georg Simmel*, trans. and ed. Kurt H. Wolff. New York: The Free Press, pp. 307–76.

———. [1908] 1950b. 'The Stranger', in *The Sociology of Georg Simmel*, New York: The Free Press, pp. 402–8.

———. [1911] 1958. 'The Handle', trans. Rudolph H. Weingartner, *The Hudson Review* 11(3): 371–78.

Simmons, David. 2006. 'Of Markets and Medicines: The Changing Significance of Zimbabwean Muti in the Age of Intensified Globalization', in Tracy J. Luedke and Harry G. West (eds), *Borders and Healers: Brokering Therapeutic Resources in Southeast Africa*. Bloomington, IN: Indiana University Press, pp. 65–80.

Sivin, Nathan. 1987. *Traditional Medicine in Contemporary China: A Partial Translation of Revised Outline of Chinese Medicine (1972): With an Introductory Study on Change in Present-Day and Early Medicine*. Ann Arbor, MI: Center for Chinese Studies, University of Michigan.

———. 1991. 'Change and Continuity in Early Cosmology: The Great Commentary and the Book of Changes', in *Chugoku kodai kagaku shiron* [On the history of ancient Chinese science], issue no. 2. Kyoto: Institute for Research in Humanities, pp. 33–43.

———. 1995. 'Text and Experience in Classical Chinese Medicine', in Donald Bates (ed.), *Knowledge and the Scholarly Medical Traditions*. Cambridge: Cambridge University Press, pp. 177–204.

Smith, Arielle A. 2018. *Capturing Quicksilver: The Position, Power and Plasticity of Chinese Medicine in Singapore*. Oxford: Berghahn.

Snow, Philip. 1988. *The Star Raft: China's Encounter with Africa*. London: Weidenfeld and Nicolson.

Snyder, Peter Z. 1976. 'Neighborhood Gatekeepers in the Process of Urban Adaptation: Cross-Ethnic Commonalities', *Urban Anthropology* 5(1): 35–52.

Sobo, Elisa J. 1996. 'The Jamaican Body's Role in Emotional Experience and Sense Perception', *Culture, Medicine and Psychiatry* 20(3): 313–42.

Southall, Aidan. 1956. *Alur Society: A Study in Processes and Types of Domination*. Cambridge: W. Heffer.

Sperber, Dan, David Premack and Ann James Premack (eds). 1995. *Causal Cognition: A Multidisciplinary Debate*. Oxford: Oxford University Press.

Spronk, Rachel. 2009. 'Sex, Sexuality and Negotiating Africanness in Nairobi', *Africa* 79(4): 500–19.

———. 2012. *Ambiguous Pleasures: Sexuality and Middle Class Self-Perceptions in Nairobi*. Oxford: Berghahn.

Stafford, Charles. 2000. *Separation and Reunion in Modern China*. Cambridge: Cambridge University Press.

Star, Susan Leigh, and James R. Griesemer. 1989. 'Institutional Ecology, Translations and Boundary Objects: Amateurs and Professionals in Berkeley's Museum of Vertebrate Zoology, 1907–39', *Social Studies of Science* 19(3): 387–420.

Sterckx, Ruel. 2002. *The Animal and the Daemon in Early China*. Albany, NY: SUNY Press.

Stern, Daniel N., et al. 1998. 'The Process of Therapeutic Change Involving Implicit Knowledge: Some Implications of Developmental Observations for Adult Psychotherapy', *Infant Mental Health Journal* 19(3): 300–8.

Strahl, Hilde. 2003. 'Cultural Interpretations of an Emerging Health Problem: Blood Pressure in Dar es Salaam, Tanzania', *Anthropology & Medicine* 10(3): 309–24.

———. 2006. *Pressure of Life – Pressure of Blood: Local Illness Experiences Related to Hypertension in a Lower Middle Class Society of Dar es Salaam, Tanzania*. Herbolzheim: Centaurus Verlag.

Strathern, Marilyn. 1988. *The Gender of the Gift: Problems with Women and Problems with Society in Melanesia*. Berkeley, CA: University of California Press.

———. 1999. *Property, Substance and Effect: Anthropological Essays on Persons and Things*. London: Athlone Press.

Straus, Erwin Walter. [1935] 1963. *The Primary World of Senses: A Vindication of Sensory Experience*, trans. J. Needleman. New York: Free Press of Glencoe.

Street, Alice. 2012. 'Seen by the State: Bureaucracy, Visibility and Governmentality in a Papua New Guinean Hospital', *Australian Journal of Anthropology* 23(1): 1–21.

Stroeken, Koen. 2008. 'Sensory Shifts and "Synaesthetics" in Sukuma Healing', in Elisabeth Hsu (ed.), 'The Senses and the Social', special issue, *Ethnos* 73(4): 466–84.

Sullivan, Mark D. 1993. 'Placebo Controls and Epistemic Control in Orthodox Medicine', *Journal of Medicine and Philosophy* 18: 213–31.

Swantz, Lloyd. 1990. *The Medicine Man of the Zaramo of Dar es Salaam*. Uppsala: Scandinavian Institute of African Studies.

Tambiah, Stanley J. 1969. 'Animals are Good to Think and Good to Prohibit', *Ethnology* 8(4): 423–59.

Tan, Michael. 1994. 'The Meaning of Medicines: Examples from the Philippines', in Nina L. Etkin and Michael L. Tan (eds), *Medicines: Meanings and Contexts*. Quezon City: Health Action Information Network (HAIN), pp. 69–81.

Tao, Iven. 2008. 'A Critical Evaluation of Acupuncture Research: Physiologization of Chinese Medicine in Germany', in Elisabeth Hsu (ed.) 'The Globalization of Chinese Medicine and Meditation Practices', special issue no. 2, *East Asian Science, Technology and Society: An International Journal* 2(4): 507–24.

———. 2009. *Akupunktur zwischen Mythos und Moderne: Anregung, das Vorgehen klinischer Akupunkturstudien zu modernisieren*. Essen: KVC Verlag.

Taussig, Michael T. 1993. *Mimesis and Alterity: A Particular History of the Senses*. London: Routlege.

Taylor, Christopher. 1988. 'The Concept of Flow in Rwandan Popular Medicine', *Social Science & Medicine* 27(12): 1343–48.

———. 1992. *Milk, Honey, and Money: Changing Concepts in Rwandan Healing*. Washington, DC: Smithsonian Institution Press.

Taylor, Kim. 2001. 'A New, Scientific, and Unified Medicine: Civil War in China and the New Acumoxa, 1945–49', in Elisabeth Hsu (ed.), *Innovation in Chinese Medicine*. Cambridge: Cambridge University Press, pp. 343–69.

———. 2005. *Chinese Medicine in Early Communist China, 1945–63: A Medicine of Revolution*. London: Routledge.
Throop, C. Jason. 2010. *Suffering and Sentiment: Exploring the Vicissitudes of Experience and Pain in Yap*. Berkeley, CA: University of California Press.
Trawick, Margaret. 1987. 'The Ayurvedic Physician as a Scientist', *Social Science & Medicine* 24(12): 1031–50.
Tsing, Anna. 2012. 'Unruly Edges: Mushrooms as Companion Species', *Environmental Humanities* 1: 141–54.
Tu, Youyou 屠呦呦. 1977. '*Yizhong xinxing de beibantieneizhi: qinghaosu*—种新型的倍半萜内脂:青蒿素' [A New Sesquiterpene Lactone—Qinghaosu]. *Kexue Tongbao* 科学通报 [Science Bulletin]: 142.
———. 2011. 'The Discovery of Artemisinin (*qinghaosu* 青蒿素) and Gifts from Chinese Medicine', *Nature Medicine* 17: 1217–20.
Turner, Victor. 1968. *The Drums of Affliction: A Study of Religious Processes among the Ndembu of Zambia*. Oxford: Clarendon Press.
———. 1969. *The Ritual Process: Structure and Anti-Structure*. London: Routledge.
Turton, David. 2004. 'Lip-Plates and "the People Who Take Photographs": Uneasy Encounters between Mursi and Tourists in Southern Ethiopia', *Anthropology Today* 20(3): 3–8.
Tylor, Edward Burnett. 1871. *Primitive Culture: Researches into the Development of Mythology, Philosophy, Religion, Art and Custom*. London: John Murray.
Unschuld, Paul U. 1973. *Die Praxis des traditionellen chinesischen Heilsystems: Unter Einschluss der Pharmazie dargestellt und der heutigen Situation auf Taiwan*. Wiesbaden: Franz Steiner.
Valussi, Elena. 2014. 'Female Alchemy: Transformation of a Gendered Body', in Jia Jinhua, Kang Xiaofei and Yao Ping (eds), *Gendering Chinese Religions: Subject, Identity and Body*. Albany, NY: SUNY Press, pp. 225–252.
Van der Geest, Sjaak, and Susan Reynolds Whyte (eds). 1988. *The Context of Medicines in Developing Countries: Studies in Pharmaceutical Anthropology*. London: Kluwer Academic Publishers.
Van der Geest, Sjaak, Johan D. Speckmann and Pieter H. Streefland. 1990. 'Primary Health Care in a Multi-Level Perspective: Towards a Research Agenda', *Social Science & Medicine* 30(9): 1025–34.
Van der Geest, Jacques. 1992. 'Is Paying for Health Care Culturally Acceptable in Sub-Sahara Africa? Money and Tradition', *Social Science & Medicine* 34(6): 667–73.
Van der Valk, Jan M. A. 2017. 'Alternative Pharmaceuticals: The Technoscientific Becomings of Tibetan Medicines in-between India and Switzerland', PhD thesis. Canterbury: University of Kent.
Van Dijk, Rijk, Ria Reis and Maria Spierenburg. 1999. *The Quest for Fruition through Ngoma: The Political Aspects of Healing in Southern Africa*. Athens, OH: Ohio University Press.
Varela, Francisco G., Humberto R. Maturana and R. Uribe. 1974. 'Autopoiesis: The Organization of Living Systems, Its Characterization and a Model', *Biosystems* 5(4): 187–96.

# References

Vertovec, Steven. 2007. 'Super-Diversity and its Implications', *Ethnic and Racial Studies* 30(6): 1024–54.

Vilaça, Aparecida. 2005. 'Chronically Unstable Bodies: Reflections on Amazonian Corporalities', *The Journal of the Royal Anthropological Institute* 11(3): 445–64.

———. 2009. 'Bodies in Perspective: A Critique of the Embodiment Paradigm from the Point of View of Amazonian Ethnography', in Helen Lambert and Maryon McDonald (eds), *Social Bodies*. Oxford: Berghahn, pp. 129–47.

Viveiros de Castro, Eduardo. 1998. 'Cosmological Deixis and Amerindian Perspectivism', *Journal of the Royal Anthropological Institute* 4: 469–88.

Wahlberg, Ayo. 2006. 'Modernisation and Its Side Effects: An Inquiry into the Revival and Renaissance of Herbal Medicine in Vietnam and Britain', PhD thesis. London: London School of Economics and Political Science (LSE).

———. 2008a. 'Above and Beyond Superstition: Western Herbal Medicine and the Decriminalizing of Placebo', *History of the Human Sciences* 21(1): 77–101.

———. 2008b. 'Bio-Politics and the Promotion of Traditional Herbal Medicine in Vietnam', *Health* 10(2): 123–47.

———. 2012. 'Family Secrets and the Industrialisation of Herbal Medicine in Postcolonial Vietnam', in Laurence Monnais-Rousselot, Claudia Michele Thompson and Ayo Wahlberg (eds), *Southern Medicine for Southern People: Vietnamese Medicine in the Making*. Newcastle: Cambridge Scholars, pp. 153–78.

Waldram, James B. 2000. 'The Efficacy of Traditional Medicine: Current Theoretical and Methodological Issues', *Medical Anthropology Quarterly* 14(4): 603–25.

Waller, Richard D. 2003. 'Witchcraft and Colonial Law in Kenya', *Past & Present* 180: 241–75.

Wang, Yishan. 2017. 'A Critique of the Recent Medicalisation of Late-Life-Sexuality in Chinese Medicine in Reformist China', MPhil dissertation. Oxford: University of Oxford.

Warnier, Jean-Pierre. 2007. *The Pot-King: The Body and Technologies of Power*. Leiden: Brill.

———. 2009. 'Technology as Efficacious Action on Objects . . . and Subjects', *Journal of Material Culture* 14(4): 459–70.

Waxler, Nancy 1981. 'Learning to Be a Leper: A Case Study in the Social Construction of Illness', in Elliot George Mishler (ed.), *Social Contexts of Health, Illness, and Patient Care*. Cambridge: Cambridge University Press, pp. 169–94.

Weyl, Herrmann. 1952. *Symmetry*. Princeton, NJ: Princeton University Press.

White, Sydney. 1998. 'From "Barefoot Doctor" to "Village Doctor" in Tiger Springs Village: A Case Study of Rural Health Care Transformations in Socialist China', *Human Organization* 57(4): 1–9.

White, Nicholas J. 2008. '*Qinghaosu* (Artemisinin): The Price of Success', *Science* 320(5874): 330–34.

White, Nicholas J., Tran T. Hien and François H. Nosten. 2015. 'A Brief History of Qinghaosu', *Trends in Parasitology* 31(12): 607–10.

Whitehead, Alfred North. 1920. *The Concept of Nature: Tarner Lectures Delivered in Trinity College, November, 1919*. Cambridge: Cambridge University Press.

Whyte, Susan Reynolds. 1988. 'The Power of Medicines in East Africa', in Sjaak van der Geest and Susan Reynolds Whyte (eds), *The Context of Medicines in Developing Countries: Studies in Pharmaceutical Anthropology*. Dordrecht: Kluwer Academic Publishers, pp. 217–33.

———. 1997. *Questioning Misfortune: The Pragmatics of Uncertainty in Eastern Uganda*. Cambridge: Cambridge University Press.

Whyte, Susan Reynolds, Sjaak van der Geest and Anita Hardon. 2002. *Social Lives of Medicines*. Cambridge: Cambridge University Press.

Whyte, Susan Reynolds, and Godfrey Etyang Siu. 2015. 'Contingency: Interpersonal and Historical Dependencies in HIV Care', in Elizabeth Cooper and David Pratten (eds), *Ethnographies of Uncertainty in Africa*. London: Palgrave Macmillan, pp. 19–35.

Willcox, Merlin, et al. 2004. '*Artemisia annua* as a Traditional Herbal Antimalarial', in Merlin Willcox, Gerard Bodeker, Philippe Rasoanaivo and Jonathan Addae-Kyereme (eds), *Traditional Medicinal Plants and Malaria*. Boca Raton, FL: CRC Press, pp. 43–59.

Willcox, Merlin. 2016. 'Confidential Enquiry into Child Deaths in Two Contrasting Settings in Africa: An Exploratory Study', DPhil thesis. Oxford: University of Oxford.

Willerslev, Rane. 2004a. 'Not Animal not Not-Animal: Hunting, Imitation and Empathetic Knowledge among the Siberian Yukaghirs', *Journal of the Royal Anthropological Institute* 10(3): 629–52.

———. 2004b. 'Spirits as "Ready to Hand": A Phenomenological Analysis of Yukaghir Spiritual Knowledge and Dreaming', *Anthropological Theory* 4(4): 395–418.

Wilms, Sabine. 2002. 'The Female Body in Medieval China: A Translation and Interpretation of the "Women's Recipes" in Sun Simiao's *Beiji qianjin yaofang*, 備急千金要方, PhD thesis. Tucson, AZ: University of Arizona.

———. 2005. '"Ten Times More Difficult to Treat": Female Bodies in Medical Texts from Early Imperial China', *Nan Nü*. 2: 182–215.

Wimmer, Andreas, and Nina Glick Schiller. 2003. 'Methodological Nationalism, the Social Sciences, and the Study of Migration: An Essay in Historical Epistemology', *International Migration Review* 37(3): 576–610.

Winch, Peter, et al. 1996. 'Local Terminology for Febrile Illnesses in Bagamoyo District, Tanzania and Its Impact on the Design of a Community-Based Malaria Control Programme', *Social Science & Medicine* 42(7): 1057–67.

Witmore, Christopher L. 2007. 'Symmetrical Archaeology: Excerpts of a Manifesto', *World Archaeology* 39(4): 546–62.

Witt, Claudia M., Hugh MacPherson, Ted J. Kaptchuk and Ayo Wahlberg. 2011. 'Efficacy, Effectiveness and Efficiency', in Volker Scheid and Hugh MacPherson (eds), *Integrating East Asian Medicine into Contemporary Healthcare*. Edinburgh: Churchill Livingstone, pp. 123–38.

# References

Wolf, Angelika, and Viola Hörbst (eds). 2003. *Medizin und Globalisierung: Universelle Ansprüche -lokale Antworten*. Münster: Lit.

Woolgar, Steve, and Javier Lezaun. 2015. 'Missing the (Question) Mark? What is a Turn to Ontology?' *Social Studies of Science* 45(3): 462–67.

Wreford, Jo T. 2008. *Working with Spirit: Experiencing Lzangoma Healing in Contemporary South Africa*. Oxford: Berghahn.

Wright, Colin W. 2002. *Artemisia*. London: Taylor & Francis.

Wright, Colin W., Peter A. Linley, Reto Brun, Sergio Wittlin and Elisabeth Hsu. 2010. 'Ancient Chinese Methods are Remarkably Effective for the Preparation of Artemisinin-Rich Extracts of *Qing Hao* with Potent Antimalarial Activity', *Molecules* 15(2): 804–12.

Wu, Di. 2021. *Affective Encounters: Everyday Life among Chinese Migrants in Zambia*. London: Routledge.

Wu, Yi-Li. 2010. *Reproducing Women: Medicine, Metaphor, and Childbirth in Late Imperial China*. Berkeley, CA: University of California Press.

Wujastyk, Dagmar, and Frederick M. Smith. 2008. *Modern and Global Ayurveda: Pluralism and Paradigms*. Albany, NY: SUNY Press.

Yan, Hairong, Barry Sautman and Yao Lu. 2019. 'Chinese and "Self-Segregation" in Africa', *Asian Ethnicity* 20(1): 40–66.

Yates-Doerr, Emily. 2017. 'Where is the Local? Partial Biologies, Ethnographic Sitings', *HAU: Journal of Ethnographic Theory* 7(2): 377–401.

Young, Diana. 2001. 'The Colours of Things: Memory, Materiality and an Anthropology of the Senses in North West Australia', PhD thesis. London: University of London.

———. 2005. 'The Smell of Greenness: Cultural Synaesthesia in the Western Desert', in Regina F. Bendix and Donald Brenneis (eds), 'The Senses', special issue, *Etnofoor* 18(1): 61–77.

———. 2011. 'Mutable Things: Colours as Material Practice in the Northwest of South Australia', *Journal of the Royal Anthropological Institute* 17(2): 227–443.

——— (ed.). 2018. *Rematerializing Colour: From Concept to Substance*. Canon Pyon: Sean Kingston Publishing.

Young, Sera L. 2002. 'Critically Ecological Medical Anthropology: Selecting and Applying Theory to Anemia during Pregnancy on Pemba, Zanzibar', *Medische Anthropologie* 14: 321–52.

Zhan, Mei. 2001. 'Does it Take a Miracle? Negotiating Knowledges, Identities, and Communities of Traditional Chinese Medicine', *Cultural Anthropology* 16(4): 453–80.

———. 2009. *Other-Worldly: Making Chinese Medicine through Transnational Frames*. Durham, NC: Duke University Press.

Zhang, Everett. 2015. *The Impotence Epidemic: Men's Medicine and Sexual Desire in Contemporary China*. Durham, NC: Duke University Press.

Zhang, Yanhua. 2007. *Transforming Emotions with Chinese Medicine: An Ethnographic Account from Contemporary China*. Albany, NY: SUNY Press.

Zimmermann, Francis. [1982] 1987. *The Jungle and the Aroma of Meats: An Ecological Theme in Hindu Medicine*. Berkeley, CA: University of California Press.

## Premodern Texts

*Ben cao gang mu* 本草綱目 [Classified *Materia Medica*]. Ming, 1596. Li Shizhen 李時珍. 4 vols. Beijing: Renmin weisheng chubanshe, 1977–1981.

*Ben cao meng quan* 本草蒙筌 [Enlightenment of the *Materia Medica*]. Ming, 1565. Chen Jiamo 陳嘉模. Beijing: Renmin weisheng chubanshe, 1988.

*Fu ren da quan liang fang* 婦人大全良方 [Compendium of Efficacious Formulas for Women]. Song, 1237. Chen Ziming 陳自明. Beijing: Renmin weisheng chubanshe, 1985.

*Shi ji* 史記 [Records of the Historian]. Han, *c.* 86 BCE. Sima Qian.司馬遷. Beijing: Zhonghua shuju, 1959.

*Shan hai jing* 山海經 [Canon of the Mountains and Seas]. Warring States, Han dynasty. *c.* 1ˢᵗ century CE. Anon. References to *Shan hai jing jiao zhu* 山海經校注. Annotated by Yuan Ke 袁珂. Shanghai: Shanghai guji chubanshe, 1980.

*Zhou hou bei ji fang* 肘後備急方 [Emergency Recipes Kept in One's Sleeve]. Jin dynasty, *c.* 340 CE. Ge Hong 葛洪. References to *Wen yuan ge Si ku quan shu* 文淵閣 四庫全書 (The Wenyuan Pavilion's Collection of the Works from the Four Storehouses). Shangwu yinshuguan, Taibei, 1983.

## TCM Textbook s

*Fangjixue* 方剂学 [The study of TCM formulas], Xu Jiqun 许济群 & al. (eds) 1985. Shanghai: Shanghai kexue jishu chubanshe.

*Zhenjiuxue* 针灸学 [The study of acupuncture and moxibustion], Qiu Maoliang 邱茂良 & al. (eds) 1985. Shanghai: Shanghai kexue jishu chubanshe.

*Zhongyaoxue* 中药学 [The study of TCM drugs], Ling Yikui 凌一揆 & al. (eds) 1984. Shanghai: Shanghai kexue jishu chubanshe.

*Zhongyi neikexue* 中医内科学 [The study of TCM inner medicine], Zhang Boyu 张伯臾. & al. (eds) 1985. Shanghai: Shanghai kexue jishu chubanshe.

*Zhongyi zhenduanxue* 中医诊断学 [The study of TCM diagnosis], Deng Tietao 潭歇涛. & al. (eds) 1984. Shanghai: Shanghai kexue jishu chubanshe.

## Conferences, Unpublished Seminar Papers and Exhibitions

Bizard, Viola. 2014. 'Following the Season of Others: Rattan (Calamoideae arecaceae) Knowledge and Its Acquisition amongst Ngaju Dayak in Indonesian Borneo', *Botanical Ontologies Conference: A Cross-Disciplinary Forum on Human–Plant Relationships, 16–17 May 2014*. Oxford.

Krause, Kristine, Elisabeth Hsu and David Parkin (organisers): 'Revisiting Narrative in Medical Anthropology', held at the School of Anthropology and Museum Ethnography, University of Oxford, funded by the Max Planck Institut, Goettingen, and by Green Templeton College, Oxford; December 2012.

Kleinman, Arthur, Peter Kunstadter, E. Russell Alexander and James L. Gale (eds). 1975. 'Medicine in Chinese Cultures: Comparative Studies of Health Care in Chinese and Other Societies'. Papers and Discussions from a Conference held in Seattle, Washington, U.S.A., February 1974. Bethesda, MD:

US Dept. of Health, Education, and Welfare, Public Health Service, National Institute of Health, John E. Fogarty International Center for Advanced Health Sciences.

'Living and Dying', the Wellcome Trust Gallery, British Museum, London. See https://www.britishmuseum.org/collection/galleries/living-and-dying (accessed 10 January 2022).

Nyamnjoh, Francis B. 2021. 'Being and Becoming African as a Permanent Work in Progress: Inspiration from Chinua Achebe's Proverbs'. University of Oxford. Retrieved 10 January 2022 from https://podcasts.ox.ac.uk/people/francis-nyamnjoh.

Ott, Margus. n.d. *Ramifications of Embodiment: Embodied Cognition and Chinese Philosophy*. [A translation of Confucius's *Analects*]. Early draft.

Petit, Pierre, and Solange Chatelard. 2018. Chinese in Africa, Africans in China Research Network: 'China–Africa in Global Comparative Perspective', 5th International CA/AC Conference, 27–29 June 2018, University Libre de Bruxelles (ULB). Retrieved 10 January 2022 from https://africachinareporting.co.za/wp-content/uploads/2018/09/CAAC-Brussels-2018_Conference-Book.pdf.

Schipper, Kristofer. 2009. 'The Foods of Longevity: Food, Drugs and Longevity in a Comparative Perspective, with Special Reference to China', ArgO-EMR (Anthropology Research Group, at Oxford, on Eastern Medicines and Religions) seminar on 'Chinese Nurturing Life Practices', University of Oxford, 6 May 2009.

Sun, Xin, and Elisabeth Hsu. 2019. 'The First Emperor's Quest for the Herb of Immortality: Comparing Excavated with Received Textual Sources', talk presented at the 'Workshop on the Representations of the Qin Empire', Pembroke College, University of Oxford, June 2019.

Qiao, Wei. [2002] n.d. 'Traditional Chinese Medicine in Tanzania'. Unpublished manuscript.

# Grey Literature, Working Papers, Investigative Journalism and Work Written for Non-Academic Audiences

Castro, Joseph. 2013. 'Animal Sex: How Seahorses Do It', Live Science, August 27. Retrieved 10 January 2022 from https://www.livescience.com/39136-animal-sex-how-seahorses-do-it.html.

Dalrymple, Dana G. 2013. *Artemisia annua, Artemisinin, ACTs and Malaria Control in Africa: Tradition, Science and Public Policy*. Washington, DC: Politics and Prose Bookstore.

Galbi, Douglas. 2017. 'Donkeys, Penis Size, and Farting: Their Significance to Men', *Purple Motes*, April 9. Retrieved 10 January 2022 from https://www.purplemotes.net/2017/04/09/donkeys-penis-farting/.

Gess, Karol N. (in conjunction with Gaither International, Inc.). 1974. 'A Study of German Travel Habits and Patterns'. Washington, DC: US Department of Commerce.

Honigsbaum, Mark. 2001. *The Fever Trail: The Hunt for the Cure for Malaria*. London: Macmillan.

Hutchison, Alan. 1975. *China's African Revolution*. London: Hutchinson.

Köhle, Natalie. 2018. 'Feasting on Donkey Skin', in Jane Golley and Linda Jaivin (eds), *China Story Yearbook 2017: Prosperity*. Canberra: ANU Press.

Ribeiro, I. R., and P. Olliaro. 1998. 'Safety of Artemisinin and Its Derivatives: A Review of Published and Unpublished Clinical Trials', *Médicine tropicale: Revue du corps de santé colonial* 58 (3; Suppl): 50–53.

Silvester, Hans. 2009. *Natural Fashion: Tribal Decoration from Africa*. London: Thames and Hudson.

Wan, James. 2014. 'Get Rich or Die Trying: The Chinese Herbal Medicine "Death Sentence" in Uganda'. *Think Africa Press*. Accesed 22 March 2022. https://allafrica.com/stories/201406041416.html.

World Health Organization. 1996. 'Introduction', in *The Global Burden of Disease: A Comprehensive Assessment of Mortality and Disability from Diseases, Injuries, and Risk Factors in 1990 and Projected to 2020*. Harvard School of Public Health on behalf of the World Health Organisaiton and the World Bank, pp. 1–43.

———. 2005. 'Malaria Control Today: Current WHO Recommendations'. Retrieved 10 January 2022 from https://www.who.int/malaria/publications/mct_workingpaper.pdf. Retrieved in April 2022.

———. 2006. 'Guidelines for the Treatment of Malaria', first edition. Retrieved October 2021 from http://helid.digicollection.org/pdf/s13418e/s13418e.pdf. This document is no longer on the internet. Instead, see https://www.paho.org/hq/dmdocuments/2011/TreatmentGuidelines-2nd-ed-2010-eng.pdf. Retrieved in April 2022.

———. 2012. 'World Malaria Report 2012 FACT SHEET'. Retrieved 10 January 2021 from https://www.who.int/malaria/publications/world_malaria_report_2012/wmr2012_factsheet.pdf.

Zhang Jianfang. [2005] 2013. *A Detailed Chronological Record of Project 523 and the Discovery and Development of Qinghaosu (Artemisinin)*, trans. Keith and Muoi Arnold. Houston, TX: Strategic Book Publishing.

## Academic Publications by Elisabeth Hsu

Hsu, Elisabeth. 1992. 'The Reception of Western Medicine in China: Examples from Yunnan', in Patrick Petitjean, Catherine Jami and Anne Marie Moulin (eds), *Science and Empires: Historical Studies about Scientific Development and European Expansion*. Dordrecht: Kluwer, pp. 89–101.

———. 1994. 'Change in Chinese Medicine: *bian* and *hua*. An Anthropologist's Approach', in Viviane Alleton and Alexeï Volkov (eds), *Notions et perceptions du changement en Chine*. Paris: Collège de France, pp. 41–58.

———. 1996. 'The Polyglot Practitioner: Towards Acceptance of Different Approaches in Treatment Evaluation', in Søren Gosvig Oleson and Erling Høg (eds), *Communication in and about Alternative Therapies*. Odense: Odense University Press, pp. 37–53.

## References

———. 1999. *The Transmission of Chinese Medicine*. Cambridge: Cambridge University Press.

———. (ed.). 2001. *Innovation in Chinese Medicine*. Cambridge: Cambridge University Press.

———. 2002. '"The Medicine from China has Rapid Effects": Chinese Medicine Patients in Tanzania', in E. Hsu and E. Høg (eds), 'Countervailing Creativity: Patient Agency in the Globalisation of Asian Medicines', special issue, *Anthropology & Medicine* 9(3): 291–314 [partially elaborated on in Chapter 4].

———. 2005a. 'Time Inscribed in Space, and the Process of Diagnosis in African and Chinese Medical Practices', in Wendy James and David W. Mills (eds), *The Qualities of Time: Anthropological Approaches*. Oxford: Berg, pp. 155–70 [partially elaborated on in Chapter 1].

———. 2005b. 'Acute Pain Infliction as Therapy', in Regina F. Bendix and Don Brenneis (eds), 'The Senses', special issue, *Etnofoor* 18(1): 78–96.

———. 2005c. 'Tactility and the Body in Early Chinese Medicine', *Science in Context* 18(1): 7–34.

———. 2006a. 'The History of *qinghao* in the Chinese *Materia Medica*', *Transactions of the Royal Society of Tropical Medicine and Hygiene* 100(6): 505–8.

———. 2006b. 'Reflections on the "Discovery" of the Anti-malarial Qinghao', in J. Aronson (ed.), 'Future Developments in Clinical Pharmacology', *Special Issue, British Journal of Clinical Pharmacology* 61(6): 666–70.

———. 2007a. 'Zanzibar and its Chinese Communities', in Frank N. Pieke and Janet Salaff (eds), 'New Chinese Diasporas', special issue, *Population, Space and Place* 13: 113–24.

———. 2007b. 'The Biological in the Cultural: The Five Agents and the Body Ecologic in Chinese Medicine', in David Parkin and Stanley Ulijaszek (eds), *Holistic Anthropology: Emergences and Divergences*. Oxford: Berghahn, pp. 91–126.

———. 2007c. 'Learning to be an Acupuncturist, and not Becoming One', in Kent Maynard (ed.), *Medical Identities: Health, Well-Being and Personhood*. Oxford: Berghahn, pp. 101–16.

———. 2008a. 'Medical Pluralism', in Kris Heggenhougen and Stella R. Quah (eds), *International Encyclopedia of Public Health*, vol. 4. San Diego, CA: Academic Press, pp. 316–21.

———. 2008b. 'The History of Traditional Chinese Medicine in the People's Republic of China and its Globalization', in Elisabeth Hsu (ed.), 'The Globalization of Chinese Medicine and Meditation Practices', special issue no. 2, *East Asian Science and Technology Studies* 2: 465–84.

———. 2008c. 'Medicine as Business: Chinese Medicine in Tanzania', in Chris Alden, Daniel Large and Ricardo Soares de Oliveira (eds), *China Returns to Africa: A Rising Power and a Continent Embrace*. London: Hurst, pp. 221–35.

———. (ed.) 2008d. *The Senses and the Social. Special Issue. Ethnos* 73(4): 433–563.

———. 2009a. 'Chinese Propriety Medicines: An "Alternative Modernity?" The Case of the Anti-Malarial Substance Artemisinin in East Africa', *Medical Anthropology* 28(2): 111–40 [partially elaborated on in Chapter 7].

———. 2009b. 'Wonders of the Exotic: Chinese Formula Medicines on the East African Coast', in Kjersti Larsen (ed.), *Knowledge, Renewal and Religion: Repositioning and Changing Ideological and Material Circumstances among the Swahili on the East African Coast*. Uppsala: Nordiska Afrikainstitutet, pp. 280–99 [partially elaborated on in Chapter 8].

———. 2009d. 'Diverse Biologies and Experiential Continuities: Did the Ancient Chinese Know That *Qinghao* Had Anti-malarial Properties?', in F. Wallis (ed.), 'Medicine and the Soul of Science: Essays by and in Memory of Don Bates'. Special Issue. *Canadian Bulletin of Medical History* 26(1): 203–13.

———. 2010a. *Pulse Diagnosis in Early Chinese Medicine: The Telling Touch*. Cambridge: Cambridge University Press.

——— (in consultation with Frederic Obringer). 2010b. '*Qing hao (Herba Artemisiae annuae)* in the Chinese *Materia Medica*', in Elisabeth Hsu and Stephen Harris (eds), *Plants, Health and Healing: On the Interface of Ethnobotany and Medical Anthropology*. Oxford: Berghahn, pp. 83–130.

———. 2010c. 'Plants in Medical Practice and Common Sense: On the Interface of Ethnobotany and Medical Anthropology', in Elisabeth Hsu and Stephen Harris (eds), *Plants, Health and Healing: On the Interface of Ethnobotany and Medical Anthropology*. Oxford: Berghahn, pp. 1–48.

———. 2011. 'Treatment Evaluation: An Anthropologist's Approach', in Volker Scheid and Hugh MacPherson (eds), *Integrating East Asian Medicine into Contemporary Healthcare*. Edinburgh: Churchill Livingstone, pp. 157–72.

———. 2012a. 'Mobility and Connectedness: Chinese Medical Doctors in Kenya', in Hansjörg Dilger, Abdoulaye Kane and Stacey Ann Langwick (eds), *Medicine, Mobility and Power in Global Africa*. Bloomington, IN: Indiana University Press, pp. 295–315 [partially elaborated on in Chapter 5].

———. 2012b. '"Feeling Lighter": Why the Patient's Treatment Evaluation Matters to the Health Scientist', *Integrative Medicine Research* 1(1): 5–12.

———. 2012c. 'Medical Anthropology in Europe – Quo Vadis?', in Elisabeth Hsu and Caroline Potter (eds), 'Medical Anthropology in Europe: Shaping the Field', special issue, *Anthropology & Medicine* 19(1): 51–61.

———. 2013a. '"Holism" and the Medicalisation of Emotion: The Case of Anger in Chinese Medicine', in Peregrine Horden and Elisabeth Hsu (eds), *The Body in Balance: Humoral Medicines in Practice*. Oxford: Berghahn, pp. 197–217.

———. 2013b. 'What Next? Balance in Medical Practice and the Medico-Moral Nexus of Moderation', in Peregrine Horden and Elisabeth Hsu (eds), *The Body in Balance: Humoral Medicines in Practice*. Oxford: Berghahn, pp. 259–80.

———. 2014. 'How Techniques of Herbal Drug Preparation Affect the Therapeutic Outcome: Reflections on *Qinghao (Herba Artemisiae annuae)* in the History of the Chinese *Materia Medica*', in Tariq Aftab, Jorge F. S. Ferreira, M. Masroor, A. Khan, M. Naeem (eds), *Artemisia annua – Pharmacology and Biotechnology*. Heidelberg: Springer, pp. 1–8.

♣ *References*

———. 2015. 'From Social Lives to Playing Fields: "The Chinese Antimalarial" as Artemisinin Monotherapy, Artemisinin Combination Therapy and *Qinghao* Juice', in Laurent Pordié and Anita Hardon (eds), 'Stories and Itineraries on the Making of Asian Industrial Medicines', special issue, *Anthropology & Medicine* 22(1): 75–86 [partially elaborated on in Chapter 9].

———. 2016. 'Humour as a Mode of Cognition', in Lidia D. Sciama (ed.), *Humour, Comedy and Laughter: Obscenities, Paradoxes, Insights and the Renewal of Life*. Oxford: Berghahn, pp. 58–75.

———. 2017. 'Patients, Practitioners, and "Pots": Probing Chinese Medicine in East Africa', in Viola Hörbst, Pino Schirripa and René Gerrets (eds), 'Revisiting Medical Pluralism: An Old Concept Inspiring New Theoretical Horizons', special issue, *L'Uomo Società Tradizione e Sviluppo* 42(1): 27–47 [partially elaborated on in Chapter 3].

———. 2018a. 'The Iconography of Time: What the Visualization of Efficacious Movement (*shi*) Tells Us about the Composition of the *Yi jin jing* (Canon for Supple Sinews)', in Vivienne Lo and Penelope Barrett (eds), *Imagining Chinese Medicine*. Leiden: Brill, pp. 89–99.

———. 2018b. 'Diverse Biologies and Experiential Continuities: A Physiognomic Reading of the Many Faces of Malaria in the Chinese Materia Medica', in Aftab Tariq, M. Naeem, M. Masroor and A. Khan (eds), *Artemisia annua: Prospects, Applications and Therapeutic Uses*. Boca Raton, FL: CRC Press, pp. 1–15.

———. 2019. 'Durkheim's Effervescence and Its Maussian Afterlife in Medical Anthropology', *Durkheimian Studies* 23: 76–105.

———. 2021. 'The Healing Green, Cultural Synaesthesia and Triangular Comparativism', *Ethnos* 86(2): 295–308. DOI: 10.1080/00141844.2020.1768137.

———. 2022. 'Traditional Chinese Medicine: History, Ethnography, and Practice', in Dorothea Lüddeckens et al. (eds), *Routledge Handbook of Religion, Medicine, and Health*. London: Routledge.

Hsu, Elisabeth, and Erling Høg (eds). 2002. 'Countervailing Creativity: Patient Agency in the Globalisation of Asian Medicines', special issue, *Anthropology & Medicine* 9(3): 205–363.

Hsu, Elisabeth, and Caroline Potter (eds). 'Medical Anthropology in Europe: Shaping the Field', special issue, *Anthropology & Medicine* 19(1): 1–128. Reprinted as book in 2015 with London: Routledge.

Hsu, Elisabeth, and Chee Han Lim. 2016. 'Enskilment into the Environment: The *Yijin jing* Worlds of *jin* and *qi*'. MPIWG Preprint no. 486. Berlin: Max Planck Institut für Wissenschaftsgeschichte.

———. 2020. 'Enskilment into the Environment: The *Yijin jing* Worlds of *jin* and *qi*', in Julie Laplante, Ari Gandsman and Willow Scobie (eds), *Search after Method: Sensing, Moving, and Imagining in Anthropological Fieldwork*. Oxford: Berghahn, pp. 145–63.

Hsu, Elisabeth, Wu Zhongping, Yang Wenzhe, Zhou Xiaofei, Sun Xin and Peng Weihua. In preparation. *Handbook of Qinghao Recipes*.

# Index

Note: Page references with an *f* are figures; page references with a *t* are tables

abortions, 136, 137
*The Absent Body* (Leder), 110
ACT (Artemisinin Combination Therapy). *See* antimalarials
acupuncture, 11–12, 26, 60, 81, 115, 134, 135, 182, 360; *bi* obstructions, 157, 167; generating synchronicity, as diagnosis-*cum*-treatment, 64, 71–2; *guanyuan* acupuncture point, 131–32; miracle/miraculous and, 161–62, 175–77, 181–85, 228, 331, 355; needles and needling techniques, 131–32, 138, 144, 239; tacit knowledge, 72; rapid effects of, 345. *See also* Chinese medicine, TCM, TM/CAM
Adams, Vincanne, 2, 12, 38, 123, 313
'advanced' medicine, 3, 60, 69, 168–70, 171, 180, 265
affordance, concept of, 49, 51, 128–9, 257. *See also pots*, sensory affordances of
'African sexuality', stereotype of, 326, 338–9
'African time', stereotype of, 151
AIDS. *See* HIV/AIDS
Alter, Joseph S., 10, 13, 313
alterity. *See* self and the other
'alternative modernity', 37, 69, 137, 178, 265, 275, 333, 336; Chinese formula medicines (*zhongchengyao*) and, 154, 265–67, 282–94; PartySmart, 294–95. *See also* reformulation regimes; regulation multiple; Asian pharmaceuticals, reverse engineering, *zhongxiyi jiehe*
ambivalence, 112–3, 308, 358
ambiguities, 112, 152–6, 308; unambiguous, 68, 108
ancestors, and the power of place, 132–33, 304–05, 334–35; connecting to, through paternal lineage lands, 132, 305, 334–35; plant preparations, fresh, from those lands, 132, 334–35; *mzisi*, 274; *shirala*, 335. *See also* emplacement; empotment; healing
animate – inanimate, 140, 256, 258, 316, 332, 366; hunter killing prey, 315; *silva* germinating from *hyle*, 255–256, 336, 341; mater – matrix, 95, 332; *qi* as [animate] stuff, 250–51. *See also* matter/materialities
animal parts, ingestion of, 314, 315. *See* efficaciousness, folk medical meats; transspecies empowerment
animals: sexual and ritualised courting behaviours, 316–17. *See* efficaciousness
anti-Imperialist sentiment, 309
Anlo-Ewe, 86
anthropological analysis and interpretation: according to ANT (actor-network theory), 130–31, 244, 250; cognitive scientific, 56, 128, 253; cultural constructivist, 311, 317; ecological, 130, 249–250, 298, body ecological, 314, 317–319,

321, 336, 341, 359; epistemological, 140, 263, 276, 278, 312, 372; ethnoarchaeological, 344, 358–360; ethnobiological, 256–58, 278–80, 280–82, 282–94, 294–96, 299–301, 314–19, 333–37, 344, 358–360; 'ethnochemistry'–oriented, 154, 258, 275, 282–96; ethnomusicological, 67, 74, 78; gestalt psychological, 45–47, 50–51, 59, 141, 250–252, 263, 323, 326; linguistic pragmatic, 104–08, 111, 183, 185; Marxist, 140, 222, 254, 297, 317, not methodologically nationalistic, 367; ontological, 13, 48, 77, 140, 250–251, 263, 311, 312, 314, 303, 336, 372, with focus on doings, 3, 71, 128, 138, 142, 249, 255, 364; physiognomic, 50, 133, 149, 184, 269, 280–82, 299–301, 311, 320–26, 362, on phonemic perceptions, 100–16; pragmatist, 39, 125, 296, 304; relativist, 317; according to SPIDER (Skilled Practice Involves Developmentally Embodied Responsiveness), 250

antibiotics, 41, 98, 131, 133, 144, 155, 223, doxycycline, 352; penicillin, 131–132, 218; sulfonamides, 188, 267; microbial resistance to, 223, 344, 354–355, 365

antimalarials: analgesics as, 163, 352; *Artemisia annua* (*qing hao* in transcription system adopted for pre-twentieth century texts and *qinghao* in modern standard Chinese), 358–65; Artemisinin Combination Therapy (ACT), 343, 355–58, 364, 365–66, marketing of, 353, side effects of, 350, 354–55, with HIV/AIDs medication, 355; artemisinin (*qinghaosu*) monotherapy brands, 159–61, 167, 258, 343, 349–50, 350–54, recrudescence, 354–55, without side effects, 160, 166–67, 179, 344, 352; 'the Chinese antimalarial', 155, 159, 163–64, 167, 240, 259, as *dawa ya Kichina* (China's medicine), 155, 351; counterfeits of, 235; rapid effects of, 152, 154–56, 168, 171, 362; plant preparations, bitter, 282, as fresh juices, 344, 358–65, without side effects, 169, preventing resistance, 363; global health market and, 350–58; playing fields of, and their transfiguration, 344–45, 350–58; Western biomedical, 271, prophylactic, 352; Nivaquine (chloroquine), 271, 351; SP/Fansidar (sulfadoxine-pyremethamine), 271, 351. See also malaria

antihypertensive medication, 327. See also Apocynum compound tablets

anxiety, 102, 342. See also body parts, heart; hypertension

Apocynum compound tablets (*Fufang luobuma pian*), 286, 292–3. See also alternative modernity

Ardener, Edwin, 57, 299

*Artemisia annua* L. (*qing hao, qinghao*). See antimalarials; plants, fresh preparations

artemisinin. See antimalarials

arthritis, 161

articulations, 243–45

Arusha Declaration (Tanzania), 29

*Asian Medical Systems* (Leslie), 10

*Asian Medicine and Globalisation* (Alter), 11

Asian pharmaceuticals, 12–13; reformulation regimes of, 275–78; regulation multiple of, 275, reverse engineering, 276, 290, 293. See also alternative modernity; kaleidoscopic refractions

*asili, dawa za*, 334

aspirin, 155, 218

asthma, 161, 177, 271, 327

athlete's foot, 271

attention, education of (Ingold 2000), 71

## Index

attention, somatic modes of (Csordas 1993), 54, 66, 73–76
attentiveness, 125, 233, 251
attunement, mutual, 13, 47, 125, 128, 326, 371, bodily, 69, to 'situated biology', 283. *See also* self and other
Austin, John, 110
automorphic symmetry (Weyl 1952), 20, 188; automorphic symmetries, 18–19, 20, 34–35, 49, 131, 246, 258, 275; spatial textures and, 34–35
autonomous figuration (or spontaneous re-configuration), 372
autonomous pharmacy, distant from clinical practice, 277
autopoiesis, 19, 35, 245–49, 258

Barbira-Freedman, Françoise, 344
Bateson, Gregory, 250
belongingness, 139
Belt and Road Initiative (BRI), 8, 172, 373
Berlin Wall, fall of, 16
Bernard, Harvey Russell, 57, 145
*bi* obstructions, 157, 167
bifurcation of nature, 130
bingo, 236
bewitchment, 95, 150, 157–158, 182, 274, 309–10, 348–49. *See also* causation, illness; social distance
Blacking, John, 66, 74–77, 81
Blaikie, Calum, 12, 295–96, 320, 376
bloating, 161, 177
body. *See* the body in balance, body parts, the body in space, the body moving through space, body techniques
the body in balance, 3, 4, 169; blockages of flows, 4–5; body ecologic, concept of, 317 (*see also* anthropological analysis, ecological); body-enveloped-by-skin, 3–4, 53; openings and closings of, 4–5; social and sexual transgression (*chira*), 5, 39; technologies of temporality, 59–71, 71–72, 141, 326, 328
body parts, 99: digestive system, 272, 328, gall bladder, 103; heart, 102, 204, 342; kidneys, 72, 99, 169, 286–87, 316, kidney system, 81, 321; legs, 87, 93, 100, 135, 169, 175, 177, 181–83, 188, 341; liver, 72, 99, 259, 271, 287, 290, 324, 354–55, 397; lungs, 328; *mrite*, 321, 341; prickling on, 132; semiotics of, 96–100, 104; skin, 70, 120, 215, 327; spleen, 102, 290; testicles, 99, 104, 321, urogenital system, 175, 177. *See also* efficaciousness
the body in space, as aesthetic expression, 109; definition of the body, 370–71; emergence of the body, 54, 243; generalization and, 245; matter and, 255 (*see also* matter); perception and, 263; phenomenology of, 169, 370–71; sedimentation and, 243–44; the body moving through space, 45–46, 52, 60–72, 174, 241, 243, 258; the body creating space, 35, 38, 169; body and tools, mutual interdependencies of, 136, 142. *See also* events; sensory perception
body techniques, 7, 13, 38, 79, 131, 249–58, 370; actively squinting one's eyes, 47–52, 242, 249, 252; handling and sensing *pots*, 67, 124, 128, 135; rhythmicity of, 140–43, 243. *See also* body in space; *pots*; techniques of transformation
bone steaming, 287
Bourdieu, Pierre, 34, 46, 49, 59, 279, 345
*buyao* (supplementing medicines), 271, 286, 290

Çağlar, Ayse, 27, 196, 367, 368
CAM (complementary and alternative medicines). *See* TM/CAM
Cameroon, 133

Index

Canada, 198
cancer, 102, 227–28, 331
*caoyao* (folk medicines), 91, 285–89, 293, 314, 342, 351. *See also* efficaciousness; plants, fresh preparations of
capitalism, 298, 299; late-liberalism, 8, 25, 85, 123, 190, 220, 258, 297–99, post-independence cash crop, 297–99; post-socialism, 172; Protestant ethics and, 299. *See also* entrepreneurs, globalisation
Cartesian mind-body dualism, 33, 50, 52, 76, 102, 111, 130, 249, 251, 257, 259, 283–86, 294, 296; non-Cartesian theorising, 109, practical efficacy, 84, 129, 141; non-Cartesian 'new materialities', like *qi* or *rasa*, 252, 253, 279, 280; '*silva* is the germinative power', (Mauss), 255
causation, illness, 55, 56, contagion, 122, diet, 168. *See also* bewitchment
Chen Ziming, 137
China, 201, 202, 203, 295; socialist revolution of 1949, 14, Cultural Revolution (1966–76), 211, 297, victims of, 201, 208, Dengist reforms, 8, 22, 137, 201, 210, 211, doing business, 225, victims of, 230
China in Africa, Africa in China (CA/AC), 8–9, 10, 24, 369, Belt and Road Initiative (BRI), 8, 172, 373; foreign aid and, 9; ODA (official development assistance), to African states, 9; OOF (other official flows), 9. *See also* globalisation, capitalism
Chinese, cultural exchanges (*wenhua jiaoliu*), with African nation states, 26, 192, 233–34
Chinese, 'culture clash' between Africans and, 2, 3
Chinese Communist Party, 95, 208, 212. *See also* People's Republic of China (PRC)
Chinese cooking, 200, 218

Chinese formula medicines. *See zhongchengyao*
Chinese *materia medica*. *See zhongyao*
Chinese medical aid teams (*yiliaodui*), 153, 237, 351, 359; study of, 9, 187 (by Li Anshan)
Chinese medical formulas. *See zhongyi fangji*
Chinese medical practices, 2, 58, 62f; acupuncture in, 64; laboratory in, 63; as ritual space, 63, 112–13; spatial arrangements for divination, compared with, 63, 65–69, 95–108; storage rooms in, 64; patient movement through, 59, 60–65
Chinese medicine (*zhongyi*), 13–14. definition of, 1, 2, 13–14; *dawa ya Kichina* (China's medicine), 152–56, as used for treating malaria, 159–61; efficacy of, 12, 13, 166–70 (*see also* efficaciousness); hybridisation of, 15; integrated Chinese and Western medicine (*zhongxiyi jiehe*), 31, 212, 282–96; range of Chinese medical treatments sought, 131–39, 159–61, 161–64, 176–77, 180–84, 348–50. *See also* acupuncture, *zhongchengyao, zhongyao, zhongyi fangji, zhongxiyi jiehe*
Chinese medicine patients: acupuncture for, 176–77; education of, 211–12; farmers as, 180–83; health care choices, as perceived by, 164–66; rapid effects, as noted by, 154, 155; six-months follow up study on, 161–64; self-identified 'middle-class', 184, 239, 240, 294, 329; upwardly mobile, 156–59, 220–22. *See also* Chinese medical practices
Chinese medicine practitioners, 195; acupuncture, 202; as business people and entrepreneurs, 1, 63–64, 92–96, 100–1, 195–231; as Christians, 92, 222–27; education of, 197–201; government recognition of, 213; livelihood of,

416

208–11; paramedical professionals and auxiliary staff, 231–36; violence against, 235; *we*-relation with, 212–16. *See also* entrepreneurs, globalisation, mobility
*chong* (insect, dragon), 80, 324
Christianity, 92, 173, 174, 193, 218; disease encountered by missionaries, 349; narratives of converts, 222–27; non-governmental organizations (NGOs), 26, 31, 119, 359; a Christian *mganga*, 227–28. *See also* religious conversion
chronic conditions, 112, 162, 166, 187, 321, 283, chronic heart disease, 291, chronic tonsillitis, 161; chronic fevers, 163, chronic flu, 177, chronic typhoid, 179, skin asthma, 165. *See also* pain
cohabitation, symbiosis and, 246
colds, 271, 292
colour, the materiality of, 320–26, 325, 326
Commission for Science and Technology (COSTECH), 122
common sense/good sense, 38, 79, 102, 258, 317, 341, 358–9, 361–62. *See also* Gramsci
connectedness (*tong*), 201, 239; mobility and, 228–31; cutting and connecting, 4, 132, 316
contingency, as chance or opportunity, 229
contra Euclidean space, 33, 51, 57, 59, 95, 128, 242, 258, 345
contra Neo-Darwinism, 245, 247
contra solipsism, 73–76
conversions. *See* religious conversions
cooperative principle (Paul Grice), 104–8; flouting of, 112
copra, materiality of, 298, 300
co-presence, affective, 72, elated, 74, of heightened feelings, 75, 78, rhythmic, 85, 88, tactile, 71, 81, of spirits, 73. *See also* shared somatic states, synaesthesia, synchronicity

co-produced sensory/sensuous events, 299–301. *See also* events, self and other
coughs, 124, 169, 177, 183, 271
*Countervailing Creativity: Patient Agency in the Globalisation of Asian Medicines* (Hsu/Høg), 10
*Cours de linguistique générale* (de Saussure), 111
Craig, Sienna, 12, 376, 378
craft, 7, 131; craftmanship, 7, 141–43; Chinese *materia medica* as crafted artefacts, 281; the production of speech as a bodily craft, 111. *See also* body techniques, skills
Csordas, Thomas, 46, 50, 52, 54, 57, 67, 74–75, 77–78, 81, 128, 242, 257, 279, 313, 339
cultural difference, 142; clash due to, 2, 367; definition of, 249; embodiment of, 47, 48; heterogeneity and, 15; modern use of word, 6; perceptions of, 23; tolerance, 14. *See also* self and other, wholeness
customs. *See* port customs

da Gama, Vasco, 172
Davis, Christopher, 195, 239, 314, 335, 340, 373
*dawa ya Kichina* (China's medicine), 152–56, 165, 264, 296; 'the Chinese antimalarial' as, 155, 351; rapid effects of, 154–55, 168, 171. *See also* Chinese medicine
de Certeau, Michel, 38, 185, 373
decoctions, 301; material variability due to substitutions, 294–97; comparison with, tropical medicinal hardwood (*miti*), 273–74. *See also* *zhongyao*, *zhongyi fangji*.
'deep knowledge', 39, 79, 80, 317–18, 341
*dege dege*, 348. *See also* malaria
depression, 53, 240, 348–50
de Saussure, Ferdinand, 111
Despret, Vinciane, 244

diabetes, 63, 91, 158, 161–62, 175, 179, 271, 283, 287, 295, 330
diagnosis: in Chinese antiquity, of pulse and colour/complexion (*mai se*), 151; in East Africa, divination, 67–68, 74–75, 274; Siddha pulse, 81; to listen/smell (*wen*), 98; diagnoses of malaria, 159–61, 348–50, 359; Chinese pulse diagnosis, 70–71, 74, 267, 327; diagnosis *and* treatment, in two phases, 59–65, 69–71, 72; diagnosis *cum* treatment, 71–72, 73; diagnosis *is* treatment, 66; See also TCM, diagnostic methods (*sizhen*); pulse diagnosis
digestive problems, 154, 161, 167, 327, 342; heartburn, 91, 327; indigestion, 327. See also stomach ache
dizziness, 181, 287
Durkheim, Emile, 39, 254, 255

*East African doctors* (Iliffe), 20
ecology of materials, 249–50
economies in decline, 368
education and aspirations, 137, 168, 174, 179; for offspring, 211–12, 216, 230, 240; of paramedical professionals, 232; of Chinese medical practitioners, 156, 171, 197–201, 211–12; of Chinese medicine patients, 175, in comparison, 158
efficaciousness/efficacy: 219, 240, 258; 'the Chinese antimalarial', 359, 160; Chinese medical fresh *qing hao* juice, 362; Chinese formula medicines (*zhongchengyao*), 257, 263, 332; Chinese medicine, 12, 13; Chinese medicine practitioners and, 265; Chinese medicine patients and, 166–70; courting rituals of animals, and, 316–18; diagnostic touch and, 70, 74, 81, 326–7; financial expenses and, 161, 182, 220, 228, 298, 310, 324, 355; folk medical meats, 314–19 (*see also* transspecies empowerment); efficaciousness (efficacious action on matter) 257, 263; in comparison to efficacy, 311–12, 332; evidence-based medicine and, 311–12; handling and sensing *pots* and, 303–4; healing touch, 315, 327 (*see also* pulse diagnosis); incorporating, ingesting, injecting substances, and, 133, 304, 333–37; placebo and, 312–13. *See also* healing; play; techniques of transformation; trying out; TM/CAM, RCTs

ejiao (donkey hide), 314, 319
Elias, Norbert, 3, 18–19
embodiment paradigm, 47, 52–53, 74
emotional irritability, 53, 102
emplacement, 54, 133, 136; economic, 367–68
emplotment, 117, 128, 138, 141, 194, 372
empotment, 117, 128, 131, 134–39, 368, 372
entrepreneurs, 1, 22, 164, 211, 225; professional attire, 92–93; in Dar es Salaam, 309, in Kampala, 357, in Kenya, 190, 220; migrant entrepreneurs, 230, 367–68; laboratory technicians as, 175; medical practitioners as, 1, 92–96, 100–1, 207, 215; patients as, 149, 157, 184. *See also* globalisation, medical pluralism; mobility
epilepsy (*kifafa*), 271
events, 56, political, 209; sensory / sensuous events, co-produced, 241–43, 299–301; ritual as event, virtual dynamics of, 50, 55, 77, 80, 108; speech events as sensory events, 111, thought and speech, 110. *See also* sense perception; *pots*; self and other

fake malaria, 348
falciparum malaria, 348, 355

Fayers-Kerr, Kate, 3, 133, 239, 314, 335, 342
female fluids, 137; healers, 306; female organs, 99, 341; female professionals, 115, 138, 213, 231, 338–39
feminist research, 4, 20, 52–54. *See also* Haraway
fecundity/fertility, 99, 333–42; cutting and connecting, 4, 132, 316; genital cutting, 4; *lingzhi* mushroom, 330–31; longevity and, 11, 319–32, 337; potency-enhancing medicines, 310–29; slimming teas and, 329–32; 'things of our place', 333–42. *See also* ancestors, and the power of place; STD
fevers (*homa*), 159, 165, 287, 344, 349, 354. *See also* malaria
fieldwork methods (focused on the said): life history elicitation, 146, 191–94, 201–16, 225–26, 232; narrative analysis, 37, 73, 115, 125, 154, 190–95, 268–69; semi-structured interviews, 37, 145, 174, 183–84, 192–94
fieldwork methods (focused on doings): mapping, 47, 73; along vectors of time, 55–57; drawing maps, 58; mapping movement, 54–55; mapping spatial textures, 57–59; walking, 84–88
figure-ground images, 17, 47–51, 52, 61, 73, 242–43, 249–50, 308, 350, 352, 354. *See also* body techniques, actively squinting one's eyes; gestalt psychology; medical encounter, triadic; *pots*
fire/fireplace, the healer as steward of, 74
flu, 352, 359. *See also* chronic conditions
folk medicines (*caoyao*), 291, 314; folk-medical terms, 91. *See also zhongchengyao*, transspecies empowerment
Frazer, James, 255
freedom (*ziyou*), 207

Friedson, Steven, 78
fungal infections, 175

gambling, 235, 236. *See also* bingo
*ganzi* (numbness), 177, 181, 188
Gaudillière, Jean-Paul, 275–80, 301, 363
Ge Hong, 360–62
Geissler, P. Wenzel, 39, 59, 132, 195, 239, 335, 340, 341, 364
gender relations, 98, 174, 237, 240; distance between, 336; efforts to overcome it, with beauty, 329–32, virility, 322, 310–29. *See also* self and other, self-enhancement
Gerke, Barbara, 12, 376
germ theory, 55
*gesi* (gas, bloating), 91, 97, 99, 161, 177, 327, 342
gestalt psychology, 45–46, 47–51, 50, 51, 59, 141, 250–52, 263, 323. *See also* figure ground images, sensory perception
*Gesture and Speech* (Leroi-Gourhan), 86
Ghana, 349
Gibson, James, 51, 128
ginseng (*renshen*), 285, 289–90, 314, 319
Giriama people, 68, 296–98, 300–1
Glick Schiller, Nina, 27, 196, 207, 236, 367–36
globalisation, 1, 10–12; global health markets, 64, 124; global sexual leisure industry, 24, 340, 364; glocalisation, 170; migration studies and, 15; mobility patterns of connectedness, 201–5. *See also* entrepreneurs, migration, mobility
Good, Byron, 125, 154, 195, 238
Good, Mary-Jo DelVecchio, 125, 187, 190, 195
good sense. *See* common sense/good sense, Gramsci
government authorities, 218–20; Commission for Science and

Technology (COSTECH), 122;
Ministry of Commerce, 217;
Ministry of Health, (Tanzania;
Kenya), 171, 272, 310; 218, 219.
*See also* port customs
Gramsci, Antonio, 38, 79, 317, 341, 358, 362
Green, Maia, 239, 333–35, 340
Grice, Paul, 37, 104–13, 241, 373
Guantai, Anastasia, 215
*guanyuan* (acupuncture point), 131–32
Guilin Pharma, 353
Guo's slimming capsules (*Guoshi jianfei jiaonang*), 329–32

Haraway, Donna, 19–20, 35, 258, 318
Haudricourt, André, 252
headaches, 91, 102–3, 158, 177, 287, 352, 359
healing, 140, 239, 240, 329–32; etymology of the word, 3; focus of research on, 2; handling and sensing of *pots* and, 140 (*see also* empotment, PPP, *pots*); harming and, 297; reconnecting patients to ancestral lands, 132–33, 239, 333–42, ritual participation of the audience, 54; social distance and, 307 (*see also* social distance); self and other, vitality-enhancing implication of, 108; generating wholeness and, 3–4, 79, 113, 186–87, 370–71. *See also* efficaciousness; *homo ritualis*; techniques of transformation
health care: contingent, 229; palliative, 220, 272; pluralistic, 164–66; patients' seeking of, 125, 126–27, 129–31; profit-seeking providers, 31, 165, 229, 248, 363; public health, 2, 26, 240: campaigns, 144, 160. *See also* government authorities, medical pluralism
health policies, Tanzania, 29–32, 309
heat, all over, 181
haemorrhoids, 177, 181

hemiplegia, 161
herpes, 175
HIV/AIDS, 28, 62, 161, 163, 176, 190, 207, 214; antimalarials and, 352; Muhimbili clinic of, 89, 122, 123; treatments, 215, 224, 228, 264, Mocrea as treatment for, 179, 228, 273, 285, 289–90. *See also* COSTECH
Høg, Erling, 10, 187
*homo rationalis*, 79, 80, 96, 108, 240, 241, 263, 268
*homo ritualis*, 80, 96, 108–9, 116, 241, 263, 268–69
*How to Do Things with Words* (Austin), 110
hygiene, 39, 122, 135, 138, 200, 216
hypertension, 91, 102, 161, 175, 182, 283, 292, 327

Iliffe, John, 20–27, 29–30, 32, 41, 154, 172, 309
imagination, 81, 86, 227, 295–96, 299, 316; power of, 323, 320–26. *See also* healing, play
impotence, 81
infertility, 157, 166, 339
infusions, 282, 359, 363
Ingold, Tim, 18–19, 34, 84, 119, 130, 243, 249–52, 259
intercorporeal interdependencies, dynamic, 50, 75, 136. *See also* shared somatic states; attention; somatic modes of
interpreters, 233–34. *See also* paramedical professionals
Iraq, 351
Iraqw (northern Tanzania), 308

Jackson, Michael, 79
*jadi, dawa za*, 334
Janzen, John, 55, 124, 125
juice. *See* plant preparations, fresh, *qing hao*
Jullien, François, 38, 180, 186
Jung, Carl. G., 67

## Index

kaleidoscopic refractions, 17–20, 131, 293, 329, 367–68, 371–73
Kapferer, Bruce, 50, 54–55, 77–78, 80, 109, 125, 127
Kenya Medical Research Institute (KEMRI), 354
kidney depletion, 287
*kienyeji, dawa za,* 334
Kleinman, Arthur, professionalisation, 41; somatised affect, 53; psycho-boom, 115, illness narratives, 154; 195; health systems, 259
Kloos, Stephen, 278
Korean, i.e. North Korean, practitioners and medicines, 162, 166

laboratory technicians, 62–63, 97, 138, 151, 231–32. *See also* entrepreneurs, paramedical professionals
language-learning, 82–90; walking rhythms and, 84–88. *See also* fieldwork methods
Lambek, Michael, 320
Langwick, Stacy, 29, 30, 272, 274–75, 334
Latour, Bruno, 55, 127, 130, 144, 155, 244–45, 251, 257, 259, 265
Leder, Drew, 110
Lefebvre, Henri, 32–34, 46, 48–49, 79, 119, 243, 329, 345, 372
Leroi-Gourhan, André, 39, 86–88, 143, 252
Leslie, Charles, 10, 17
lethargy, 348–50
Lévi-Bruhl, Lucien, 255
Lévi-Strauss, Claude, 252, 320, 324
Lewis, Gilbert, 24, 55–56, 81, 95, 116, 310
licorice, 272–73, 289–90
life, Chinese philosophy of, 64
life expectancies (in Tanzania), 29
lifestyle, differences between Chinese and Africans, 233; lifestyle migration, 197, 208–11; livelihoods of Chinese medicine patients, 178–79; modern or traditional, 148, 178–80; Nairobi's climate, 216, 'fast life', 338
*lingzhi* mushroom, 330–31
Li Shizhen, 361–62
listlessness, 348–50, 359
liver depletion, 287
liver inflammations, 271
liver kidney blood depletion, 71, 72
Lock, Margaret, feminist research, 53; medical pluralism, 275; scars, 282; situated biologies, 283; transplant medicine, 316
Lowes, John Livingstone, 299
Luhmann, Niklas, 245

Maanda Uwa, 308
Ma Eun-Jeong, 278
magic, 150, 185; *ling,* 228; history and, 309–10, 314–19
Makerere University, 25
malaria, 62, 159–61, 163, 165, 167, 175, 177, 202, 240, 271; as burden of disease, 239, 348; *degedege,* 348; endemic malaria, symptoms of, 348–50, 359, fake malaria, 348; falciparum malaria, 348, 355; iatrogenic malaria, 169; local treatments for, 166. *See also* antimalarials
*malaya* (prostitute), 108
male *yang* potency, 271
Mandelbrot, Benoit, 19, 20, 246
Margulis, Lynn, 2, 19, 188, 245–49, 259
materiality/materials, 368: of brass, 322; of cash crops, 299; of colours, 325, 326; of copra, 298, 300; of *pots,* 345, of satin, 323; ecology of, 249–50; new materialities, 250–52; objective properties of, 282–94; *pots,* as handled and sense perceived, 243, 297 (*see also pots*); stuff, *qi,* 250; stuffy atmosphere, 45, 61, 67, 70, 73–75, 79, 90–91, 95, 105, 121;

421

Index

siting materialities, 51; materiality of sounds, 320–26; variability of a formula's composition, 320; variability due to substituted components, 294–97
matter, 252–56, 336, 368; definition of, 254. *See also* animate – inanimate, spatial textures
Mattingly, Cheryl, 128, 141, 194–95, 238, 394
Mauss, Marcel, 6, 7, 38–40, 111, 131, 141–43, 249, 252–57, 259, 278, 329, 332, 369, 370, 373; on economic pressure, 370
maxim of manner (Grice), 106–8, 109
medical encounter, triadic; beyond the patient-practitioner dyad, 124, 129–31; *tertium quid*, 127, 130, 144. *See also* PPP
medical pluralism, 124–26, 139, 238, 274–75; African (very diverse) patients, 3, 16, 60, 63, 95, 113–14, 117; Swahili-speaking practitioners, 4–5, 65–71; local herbs, 169, 304, 306–7, *ngetwa* and *ngoka*, 165; Arab physicians, 28; Arab patients, 157; Arab and South Asian practitioners, 307; Chinese medical services, range of, 240; a Christian pastor, 227–28; cultural brokers, 93–94; Indian patients, 175, pharmacists, 161, 353, practitioners, 90, 164, 179, 204, 271, medicine: Maha Sudarshan Chuma, 165; Muslim patients, 157, 173–75, Muslim practitioners, 347. *See also* TM/CAM
meditation, 234
menses, painful, 291, heavy bleeding, 104, 177, 179; treatment for, 319
mental health problems, 83. *See also* depression
miscarriage, 56
Merleau-Ponty, Maurice, 46, 48, 52, 54, 76–77, 86, 109–11, 116, 173, 241, 243–45, 258, 263, 279, 370, 371

meshwork, 119–24, 145, 194, 214, 242–43
migraines, 103
migration, 191, 217, 369; globalisation and, 15; superdiversity and, 14–17, 332, 358; lifestyle migration, 197, 208–11. *See also* mobility
Ministry of Health. *See* government authorities
minor surgery (*waikexue*), 135
miracles. *See* acupuncture; *dawa ya Kichina*, rapid effects, witchcraft (*uchawi*)
misunderstandings: Grice's cooperative principle, 104–8; overcoming social distance, 113–15; phenomenology of speaking, 108–15; phonemic (mis-)perception, 100–104; semiotics of the body, 96–100; thriving on, 90–108; trust and, 95–6, 112–13
*miti* (tropical medicinal hardwood), 273–74
mobility (*ling*), 1, 171; connectedness (*tong*) and, 228–31; motivations for, 206; patterns of mobility, star-like, 201–3, weblike, 203–5; upward mobility, 27, 156–59. *See also* migration, self and other
modern medicine, 20, anonymity of transaction, 69, consultation fees, 151, cost of treatments, 158; modern medicines, 22, 169, hygienic, 281, odourless, 281, packaged, 281, ready-made, 154, secret, 305. *See also* antimalarials; Western medicine; side effects
modern traditional clinics (MTCs), 60, 274; diagnosis in, 69, 70; patient movement through, 69–71
*Molecules*, 360
Morris, Katherine, 47–50, 128, 133
*mrite*. *See* body parts
Muhimbili hospital, 30, 85, 89, 122, 166, 214, 302
Mursi (or Mun), 133–34, 335
*mzisi* (ancestors, spirits), 274

422

*Nanbao* (treasure of men/manhood), 182, 310–20, 327–29, 337. *See also* efficaciousness/efficacy; *nguvu ya kiume* (strength of men)
National Institute for Medical Research (Tanzania), 119, 160, 354
Natural History Museum (Dar es Salaam), 84
*ngetwa* and *ngoka*, 165
*nguvu ya uchawi*, 158, 309–10; witchcraft (*uchawi*), 95, 152, 180, 257, 274, 297; bewitchment, 150, 274, 310, 348–49. *See also* causation, illness
*nguvu ya kiume* (strength of men), 158, 161, 183. *See* potency-boosters
Nichter, Mark, 127, 280
No-flu, 271, 292
Nyerere, Julius, 28, 30, 84, 152, 169, 207
Nyole people, 66, 67, 304, 305

obesity/overweight, 177, 271, 295, 330
obstructions, *bi*, 157, 167
odours, 281–82, 301, 304, *rasa*, 256, 279–80, 304; signatures of specific medical treatments, 281–82, social effects of, odoriferous substances, 280–82. *See also* scents/flavours/taste; sensory affordances
organ transplants, 316. *See also* animate – inanimate; efficaciousness, folk medical meats

pain, 157, 161, back pain, 161, 177; chest pain, 161, 177; chronic pain, 181; muscular pain, 157, 161; urethral pain, 177; in legs, 175, in womb, 175
*Palms, Wine and Witnesses* (Parkin), 297
palm wine, production of, 298–301
paramedical professionals and auxiliary staff, 231–36; education, 232; relationships with practitioners, 234. *See also* entrepreneurs
parasites, 354

Parkin, David, 5, 16, 27, 68, 73, 94, 296–98, 307
*Paths to Asian Medical Knowledge* (Leslie/Young), 10
PPP (patients, practitioners and *pots*), 47–51, 124–31, 131–39, 238, 253. *See also* empotment; figure-ground images; medical encounter, triadic
People's Republic of China (PRC), and Africa, 8–9; map of, 23; political history of, affecting individual life histories, 208–11, 212–16. *See also* Chinese medical aid teams (*yiliaodui*)
perception, 47f; body and, 46–47; existence of the other, 52; causal reasoning and, 55; sensory, as part of social relations, 241–42, 263. *See also* the body in space, figure-ground images, Merleau-Ponty
*The Perception of the Environment* (Ingold), 249
pharmaceuticals, industrially manufactured: Asian, Korean, Tibetan, Vietnamese, 12–13, 277–78, 322; [South] Asian reformulations, 275–78; Chinese formula medicines, 282–94 (*see zhongchengyao*); *dawa ya Kichina*, 152–56, Western biomedical, Chinese manufactured, 152; TM/CAM (traditional medicines/complementary and alternative medicines), 218; Western medical pharmaceuticals displayed as Traditional Chinese Medicines, 269–71. *See also* alternative modernity; medical pluralism; *zhongchengyao*
phenomenology: of perception (drawing on gestalt psychology), 47–51; of speaking, 108–15
*Phenomenology of Perception* (Merleau-Ponty), 46, 111, 263, 371
phonemic misperception, 100–4. *See also* anthropological analysis, physiognomic

pimples, 161, 175
placebo effect, 213, 257, 278, 312–13, 320
plants, fresh preparations of, coconut juice, 299–301, palm wine, 297–99, *qinghao* juice, 344, 358–65; wholeness (*uzima*) and, 3; select species for dried *zhongyao*, 284–86: *baishao* (*Paeonia lactiflora*), 285, *dahuang* (*Rheum officinale*), 286, *danggui* (*Angelica sinensis*), 285, *danpi* (*Paeonia suffruticosa*), 284, *fuling* (*Poria cocus*), 284, *gouqizi* (*Lycium barbarum, L. chinense*), 285, *guanmutong* (*Aristolochia manschuriensis*), 285, *muxiang* (*Saussurea lappa*), 285, *yejuhua* (*Chrysanthemum indicum*), 286. See also efficiousness, *pots*, sensory perception
play, 58, 125–26, bingo, 230, with clay, 134, foreplay, 316, wordplay, 315, 322–23, 325, 340
playful, banter, 335, interplay, 111, 320, recombination, 13, 69, 110, 275, 293–95, 296
playing fields, 27, 127, 258, 277, 344–45, 35–66
pleasures, of eating/food, 39, 188, 200, 217, 235, 334, of sex, 315, 339, 364; enjoyment of, autonomy, 204, 217, discovery, 185, each other's company, 1, 88, 93, 218; happiness and heartfelt joy, 36, 127, 214, 216. See also plants, fresh; scents/flavours/taste
port customs, 138; corruption, 267, 278; import-export bulk trade, 355–58, 364; quality control, 264–66; packaging and make-belief, 127, 149, 168, 256, 264–66, 272, 283–85, 309; outside 'pot' information versus inside contents, 263, 285, 314, 316, 319
Pordié, Laurent, 275–80, 294, 301, 363

potency-boosters, 320, 323, 324, 326; efficaciousness of, 310–37; through Chinese medical procedure, 326–29. See also *zhongchengyao*
*The Pot King* (Warnier), 128
pots, 50, 119–24; autopoiesis, 245–46; affecting disposition, 320–26; divinatory tool kit, 274; ecology of materials, 249–50; effectiveness of folk-medical meats, 314–19 (*see also* transspecies empowerment); efficaciousness of potency-boosters, 310–37; efficaciousness of the exotic other, 304–8; efficacy and, 303–4; empotment, 134–39 (*see* empotment); handling and sensing of, 61, 124, 128, 136–37, 141, 148, 266, 312, 326; materiality of, 345; materials, ecology of, 249–50; matter and, 252–56; new materialities and, 250–52; sedimentation and articulations, 243–45; sensory affordances of, 37, 128–29, 136, 155, 242, 251, 279–80, 296–301; sensory/sensuous events, co-produced, 299–301. *See also* perception, PPP, sensory perception
'pressure'. *See* antihypertensives, anxiety, hypertension
preventive health care, 29, 75, 133, 240, with condoms, 347; bathing and, 274, 335; plants, fresh preparation of, 300, 335, 358–63; prayer, 305; *shirala*, 335. *See also* healing
prevention of malaria, 344. *See also* antimalarials; malaria
primary health care, 26, 29, 31, 154, 220, 240, 268, 269; in socialist countries, 29
Prince, Ruth J., 39, 41 95, 132, 195, 299, 335, 340, 341, 364
*Prison Notebooks* (Gramsci), 317
problems of the heart, 271
procreation, medicines for, 336

*The Production of Space* (Lefebvre), 34
propensity of things (*shi*), 180, 184–87, 253, 268, 311, 345, 373
prostatitis, 100, 101
pulse diagnosis, 70, 72, 74, 81, 251, 267, 327

*qi*, 250, 287, 289, 319, 328
*qinghao* juice, 344, 358–65. *See also* plant preparations, fresh
*qinghaosu. See* antimalarials, ACTs, artemisinin
Qinshi Huangdi, 331

rhythm, 87; musical/technical rhythm, 87; physiological aesthetics, 86–87; rhythm of digestion, 87; rhythmic turn taking in conversation, 90, 111; walking rhythm, 84–88. *See also* spatial textures, techniques of transformation
Randomised Controlled Trials (RCTs). *See* TM/CAM
receptionists, 61, 64–65, 93, 107, 191, 231. *See also* paramedical professionals
reformulation regimes, 275–78, 363. *See also* alternative modernity; *zhongchengyao*
regulation multiple, 275, 309, 310. *See also* reformulation regimes; *zhongchengyao*
Rekdal, Ole Bjørn, 306–8
religion, 173; ancestral lands, 133, 333–42; occult practices, 297; prayer, 305; spells, Koranic, 304. *See also* healing, techniques of transformation
religious conversion to Buddhism, 234; Christianity, 218, 222–27; Islam, 347
rheumatism, 215, 271, 291
Rhodes, Lorna Amarasingham, 56, 126, 129
Russia, 201, 203, 223, 247
Rwanda, 232

sacrifice, 305. *See also* transformation
Sacks, Harvey, 105
sameness, 'culture' on the basis of, 17
*Sanhuangpian* (Tablets of the three yellows), 286
*Sanjinpian* (Three gold tablets), 284–85
*Sanjiu weitai* (Weitai 999 [Stomach health 999]), 285
Saxer, Martin, 278
Scent/flavour/taste (*wei*), 257, 278–80, 284–87, 304. *See also* materiality, new materilaties; *pots*; sensory perception; signatures
Schegloff, Emanuel, 105
Schlanger, Nathan, 6, 111, 141, 249
Schütz, Alfred, 37, 57, 75, 76, 104, 229, 373
sedimentation, 243–45. *See also Phenomenology of Perception*
self and other, 315, 369–70, co-presence of, 80; engaged with intersubjectively, 136, 146, 242; enhancement of, 77; self-perfection, joint effort of, 7, 143, 255, 329, 370. *See also* body techniques; synaesthesia; synchronicity
self-enhancement, 24, 196, 240, 315, 319, 330, 339, 363; selfhood, sexuality and, 338, 363; self-worth, 77, 339, *See also* self and other, sexual performance, transspecies empowerment
self-medication, 21–22, 139, 144, 363
self-similarity, 19–20, 243, 246, 258
sensory perception, 127, 129, 241, 242, 263; sensed/sensory affordances, 49, 128–29, 229, 296–301; sensed efficaciousness, 320–26; sensed medicine *pots*, 312–13 (*see also pots*); sensory/sensuous events, co-produced, 299–301; sensory illusions, 78, properties, 278–80, stimuli, 46. *See also* events, figure-ground images, *pots*

sexually transmitted disease (STD), 103, 136, 138, 187, 268; syphilis, 131–34
sexual performance, 319, 337–41; sexual pleasure, and the global leisure industry, 331–41. *See also* potency-boosters, self-enhancement
shared somatic states, 74. *See also* attention, somatic modes of; events
sickle cell anaemia, 177, 349
side effects: antihypertensive Apocynum compound tablets (*Fufang luobuma pian*) and, 286, 292–93; antimalarials, 160, 344, 350–58; Chinese medicine (*zhongyi*), 166
signature, of traditional medical formula, 256, 266, 278–80, 311
simultaneity, 68, 70, 106–15, 141. *See also* synchronicity
Six-flavour Rehmannia pill (*liuwei dihuangwan*), 284, 286–87
Six-spirits boluses (*liushenwan*), 284, 287–88
skills, 6–8, 38, 131; biomedical, 135, 137, 199, 220; Chinese medical, 72, 139; Ingold on, 249–50, 259; Jackson on, 79; skilled practice, 143, 187, 315, 352; skills and substances, 373; skills and tactics, 195. *See also* body techniques
skin, problems of (eczema and rashes), 161–62, 273–74
slimming teas, 329–32, 337, 340
Snow, Philip, 9
social distance, 303–4; efficaciousness of the exotic other, 304–8, 257; overcoming, 113–15; potency and, 333; between practitioners and patients, 59–65, 312, 314. *See also* gender relations
social lives of things, concept, 345
social morphology, 7
social relation of host and guest, 54, 156; ethnographer in, 86, 120, 300, 346–48; intimacy with strangers, 2–3, 39, 248–49, 340, 363. *See also* stranger
solipcism. *See* contra solipcism
space: bird's-eye view of space, 33; Euclidean, as empty container, 242; first-hand experience of, 238, 241–43; living beings as space, 35; meshwork, 119; sensory affordances, 49; spatial textures, 32–34, 45–46; tangible matter and, 252–56. *See also* automorphic symmetry, spatial textures
spatial textures, 32–34, 45, 59–72, 186; automorphic symmetries and, 34–35; movements through Chinese medical practices, 59, 60–65; local medical practices, 65–69; modern traditional clinics (MTCs), 60, 69–71, 274; Western medical practices, 62, 99
speech defects, 233
speech events. *See* events
Sri Lanka, 126
*Separation and Reunion* (Stafford), 228
stomach ache, 91, 158, 359; problems with, 165, 97–99, 158, 165, 289, 327, 342; stomach ulcers, 62, 162–63, 168, 175, 271, 239, 289, 352. *See also* digestive problems
strangers, 306, 308, 333, 336, intimacy with, 2–3. *See also* self and other, social relation of host and guest
Strathern, Marilyn, 18, 76
subjunctive mode, 125, 315. *See also* play
substances, 368, 373; anthropology of, 131–34; incorporation of and efficaciousness, 333–37. *See also* ancestors, and the power of place; materiality; matter
Sudan, 8
'sugar', 97. *See also* diabetes
swellings, 70, 132, 228
Swiss Tropical Institute (Basel, Switzerland), 362

symbiogenesis, 246–48; eukaryotic cell, 247–49, 333; prokaryotic holobionts, 248, 333
symbiosis, 246
sympathetic magic, 314–19
synaesthesia, 323, 340; rising smoke and scents, 73; smell of greenness, 326. *See also* synchronicity, techniques of transformation, technologies of temporality
synchronicity, 66f, 71–72; generating, 77–80, through touch, 73; simultaneity and, through incoherent speech, 109, 141; through substance injection, causing co-presence through pain, enabling empotment, 131–32. *See also* spatial textures, synaesthesia

taste. *See* scent/flavour/taste
TAZARA railway, 172, 180, 309
TCM (Traditional Chinese Medicine), 30, 65, 69, 89, 192; acupuncture, 72 (*see also* acupuncture); commodification of TCM, 170, 172, 266, 301, 330, 357; diagnostic methods, four (*sizhen*), 71, 280: to look (*kan*), to listen/smell (*wen*), to ask (*wen*), to take the pulse (*qie*), 70, 122, 267, 280, 326–27; education in, 171, 197; legislation of, 190; as a science, 168, 180, 168, 303, 358; women's medicine (*fuke*), 136. *See also* Chinese medicine; Western medicine
technical arts, 253
technical practice, 141–43
technical rhythms, 87
techniques of transformation, 140–43, 239, 303–4, 305; generating synchronicity, 71–72, 77–80, 81; spatial textures, 66f, 65–69, 71–72, 77–80; incorporating, injecting, ingesting substances, 131, 133, 359; tactics of the everyday, 155, 195, 206, 305. *See also* body techniques;

healing; technologies of temporality; transformation
*Techniques, Technologies and Civilization* (Mauss, edited by Schlanger), 6
technologies of temporality, 326–29. *See also* generating synaesthesia; synchronicity
technology as efficacious action on matter (Mauss, as interpreted by Warnier), 252–56
*tertium quid*, 127, 130
'things of our place', 333–37. *See* ancestors, and the power of place
*Thou*-orientation, 75–76, 104, 212–15, 230, 371, 372
Tibet, 107, 295, 322–23; pharmaceuticals, *sowa rigpa*, 12, 295
Tiens (Tianshui), 356–58
tinnitus, 287
TM/CAM (traditional medicines/ complementary and alternative medicines), 11, 27, 90, 173, 196–97, 276; efficacy of, based on Randomised Controlled Trial (RCT), 12, 28, 241, 312–13, 332, 365; legislation of, 219, 350, unregulated treatment, 272–73
toothache, 271
traditional medicine, 108, 140, 144, 169, 317, 336. *See also* body techniques; diagnosis; efficaciousness; healing; techniques of transformation; technologies of temporality; self and other, wholeness
Traditional Medicine Unit, 30
transformation: of conditions of life, 305; of medicines, 280; *pots* and, 140–43; spatial textures and, 60–71, 304. *See also* techniques of transformation
transgender allocation of caring roles, 318
transspecies empowerment, 314–19; bear bile, 302; cow bezoar, 302;

# Index

donkey hide (*ejiao*), 314, 319; elephant bezoar, 295; froth on deer antler, 325; kidney system of dogs, 314, 321, donkey, 319, goat, 321, horse, 321, deer, 321, water buffalo, 321, etc.; rhinoceros horn, 295; sea horse (whole animal); male moth antenna, 325; *mrite*, 321, 341. *See also* efficaciousness, folk medical meats; potency-boosters

transspecies fertilisation, 318

trickery, 91, 185, 315

trigger, 96, 108, 180, 186–87, 321, 350, 372. *See also* propensity of things

tropical medicinal hardwood (*miti*), 273–74

trust, 95–96, 148; *dawa ya Kichina* (China's medicine), 153; misunderstandings and, 112–13; overcoming social distance, 113–15

trying out, 3, 7, 39, 125, 174, 182, 294; pragmatic, 98, 125; probing attitudes, 7, 95–96, 126, 143, 238–39, 372. *See also* play

tumors, 228

Tu Youyou, 351, 360

typhoid, 63, 97–98, 157, 163, 175. *See also* chronic conditions

University of Nairobi, 215
urinary infection, 62, 179, 288

van der Valk, Jan, 278
Venegra, 323
Vertovec, Steven, 15–17
Viagra, 271, 323, 328
Vietnam, 13
Vilaça, Aperiçida, 47, 53

Wahlberg, Ayo, 278
Warnier, Jean-Paul, 128, 252, 253
*wei*. *See* scents/flavours/tastes
*wen* (to listen/to smell), 98. *See also* diagnosis, TCM, *zhongyao*

Western medicine, 14, 20; antimalarials, 351 (*see also* antimalarials); building boundaries between, 265; integrating Chinese and, 212 (*see also zhongchengyao, zhongxiyi jiehe*); Western medical practitioners working as TCM practitioners, 267–69; Western pharmaceuticals displayed as Chinese formula medicines, 269–71. *See also* alternative modernity, health care; TCM.

Weyl, Herrmann, 19–20, 35, 49, 188, 245

whole, definition of, 3; wholeness, 54, 72, 96, 127; efficaciousness and, 329–32; generating wholeness, 3–4, 79, 113, 186–87, 195, 242, 249, 329, 370–71; healing and the reconfiguration of, 78, 113, 242, 333–37; spatial production of, 5–8, *uzima* (wholeness, health), 3–4

Whyte, Susan Reynolds, 13, 39, 67–68, 125, 304–7

witchcraft. *See nguvu ya uchawi*

Witchcraft Act, 296

witchdoctors, 165. *See* TM/CAM

women: beauty, 329–32; blame and, 56; empotment and, 138; in Late Imperial China, 70; pills and, 282; roles of, 93. *See also* fecundity/fertility

women's medicine (*fuke*), 136–37

women's problems, 167, 271

words, materialities of, 320–26

World Bank, 9, 10, 30, 310, 350

World Health Organization (WHO), 29, 84, 160, 190, 310, 348, 350, 353–55, 364–66

Wright, Colin, 360

*xin* (matters of the heart), 151

Yan (legendary Emperor), 330
Yao Ji, 331

Yates-Doerr, Emily, 47, 51
*yiliaodui. See* Chinese medical teams
*yiliao renleixue* (medical anthropology), 192
*yin* and *yang* energies, 151, 319, 325, 328
Young, Diana, 323, 326

Zhan, Mei, 11, 123, 154, 161, 328
*zhongchengyao* (Chinese formula medicines), 22, 28, 64, 134, 153, 154, 263–65, 274–75, 282–94, 310–29; as alternative modernity, 265–67; *Danggui jingao pian* (*Angelica sinensis* plant extract), 285; *dawa ya Kichina* (China's medicine), 152–56; *Di'ao* (Mystery of earth), 286; *Fufang luobuma pian* (Apocynum compound tablets), 286; ethnochemistry of, 284–94; legitimacy of, 295, 308; *Leigongteng jingao pian* (*Tripterygium wilfordii* plant extract), 285; *Liuwei dihuangwan* (Six-flavour Rehmannia pill), 284; *Liushenwan* (Six-spirits boluses), 284; marketing of, 294; Mocrea, 285; *Niuhuang jiedu pian* (cow bezoar poison dissolving tablets), 286; packaging of, 364; as potency-boosters, 308, 336, 326–29; rationale of manufacture, 274–96; reformulation regimes, early stages, and, 275–78, 301; regulation multiple, 272–73; *Sanhuangpian* (Tablets of the three yellows), 286; *Sanjinpian* (Three gold tablets), 284–85; *Sanjiu weitai* (Weitai 999 [Stomach health 999]), 285; *zhongyao*, comparison with, 265–67, 280–82. *See also zhongyi fangji, zhongxiyi jiehe*
*zhongyao* (Chinese *materia medica*), 122, 135, 140, 153, 154, 219, 223, 257, 266, 359, 363; *buyao* (supplementing medicines), 272; ginseng as, 319; animate stuff, 280; man-made, 291; in powder form, 310; sensory affordances of *pots*, 128–29; substitutions of, 294–97; *wei* (scent/flavour/taste) of, 278–80; *zhongchengyao*, comparison with, 265–67, 280–82. *See also caoyao, zhongyao, zhongyi fangji*
*zhongxiyi jiehe* (integrated Chinese and Western medicine), 13–14. Chinese formula medicines (*zhongchengyao*), Western pharmaceuticals displayed as TCM, 269–71. *See* alternative modernity, Chinese medicine, TCM
*zhongyi. See* Chinese medicine, TCM
*zhongyi fangji* (Chinese medical formulas), 12, 72, 122, 134; age-old formula *dihuangwan* (Six-flavour Rehmannia pill), 284–86; basic treatment rationale, 167, 272; decoctions, 301; sensory experience as *pots* and, 311 (*see also pots*); signatures as taskonomies, 278–80. *See also* Chinese medicine, decoctions, technologies of temporality, *zhongchengyao, zhongyao*
Zimbabwe, 8, 234

www.ingramcontent.com/pod-product-compliance
Lightning Source LLC
Chambersburg PA
CBHW051523020426
42333CB00016B/1745